GENETICS OF FOCAL EPILEPSIES

Clinical Aspects and Molecular Biology

GENETICS OF FOCAL EPILEPSIES

Clinical Aspects and Molecular Biology

Editors

S.F. Berkovic
P. Genton
E. Hirsch
F. Picard

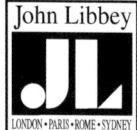

British Library Cataloguing in Publication Data

Current Problems in Epilepsy: 13

ISBN: 0 86196 569 8

ISSN: 0950-4591

Published by

John Libbey & Company Ltd, 13 Smiths Yard, Summerley Street,
London SW18 4HR, England
Telephone: (0) 181-947 2777 – Fax: (0) 181-947 2664
John Libbey & Company Pty Ltd, Level 10, 15–17 Young Street, Sydney, NSW 2000, Australia
John Libbey Eurotext Ltd, 6 rue Blanche, 92120 Montrouge, France
John Libbey/C.I.C. s.r.l., via Lazzaro Spallanzani 11, 00161 Rome, Italy

© 1999 John Libbey & Company Ltd. All rights reserved.
Unauthorized duplication contravenes applicable laws.

Printed in Rawang, Selangor, Malaysia by Kum-Vivar Printing Sdn Bhd

Table of contents

Part I
Introduction — 1

Chapter 1   The discovery of 'benign rolandic epilepsy'
Marc Beaussart, Pierre Loiseau and Joseph Roger — 3

Chapter 2   Genetics of partial epilepsies: new frontiers
Samuel F. Berkovic and Ingrid E. Scheffer — 7

Chapter 3   Clinical genetic and molecular genetic approaches to the familial partial epilepsies
Massimo Pandolfo — 15

Part II
The idiopathic age-related focal epilepsies — 33

Chapter 4   The genetics of benign childhood epilepsy with centro-temporal spikes
Orvar Eeg-Olofsson — 35

Chapter 5   Families with benign childhood epilepsy with centro-temporal spikes
Y.S. Choy, C.T. Tan and Asma Omar — 43

Chapter 6   The genetics of rolandic epilepsy and related conditions: multifactorial inheritance with a major gene effect
Bernd A. Neubauer, Ulrich Stephani and Hermann Doose — 57

Part III
Idiopathic focal epilepsies in infancy — 67

Chapter 7   Gene mapping for benign infantile familial convulsions
Michel Guipponi, Federico Vigevano, Bernard Echenne and Alain Malafosse — 69

Chapter 8   Benign partial epilepsies in infancy and early childhood: clinical description and genetic background
Kazuyoshi Watanabe — 73

Part IV
Autosomal dominant focal epilepsies — 79

Chapter 9 Autosomal dominant nocturnal frontal lobe epilepsy
Ingrid E Scheffer — 81

Chapter 10 Familial temporal lobe epilepsy
Samuel F. Berkovic — 85

Chapter 11 Genetics of autosomal dominant partial epilepsy with auditory features
Ruth Ottman, Christie Barker-Cummings, Joseph H. Lee and Susanna Ranta — 95

Chapter 12 Familial partial epilepsy with variable foci
Ingrid E. Scheffer — 103

Chapter 13 Autosomal dominant rolandic epilepsy with speech dyspraxia
Ingrid E. Scheffer — 109

Chapter 14 A clinical study of 21 European families with dominant partial epilepsy
F. Picard, G. Rudolf, R. Sebastianelli, F. Vigevano, S. Baulac, E. LeGuern, P. Thomas, M. Gavaret, P. Genton, R. Guerrini, C.A. Gericke, J.J. Poza, A. Lopez de Munain, I. An, M. Wolff, E. Hirsch, A. Brice and C. Marescaux — 115

Part V
Genetics of other focal epilepsies — 123

Chapter 15 Genetically determined forms of partial symptomatic epilepsies: clinical phenotype, neuropathology and neurogenetic basis of seizures
Renzo Guerrini, William B. Dobyns, Olivier Dulac, Alexis Arzimanoglou, Eva Andermann and Romeo Carrozzo — 125

Chapter 16 The genetics of febrile convulsions and temporal lobe epilepsy
Richard S. McLachlan and Dennis E. Bulman — 149

Chapter 17 Reading epilepsy: clinical and genetic background
Thomas Mayer and Peter Wolf — 159

Chapter 18 Pathophysiology and genetics of hot-water epilepsy
P. Satishchandra, Gautam R. Ulla, Anindya Sinha, S.K. Shankar — 169

Part VI
Molecular biology — 177

Chapter 19 Molecular biology in autosomal dominant nocturnal frontal lobe epilepsy
Ortrud K. Steinlein — 179

Chapter 20 Neuronal nicotinic acetylcholine receptor and epilepsy
B. Buisson, L. Curtis and D. Bertrand — 187

Chapter 21 Channelopathies: ion channels and paroxysmal disorders of the nervous system
Louis J. Ptáček — 203

Chapter 22	Homeobox genes in the developing brain	
	Edoardo Boncinelli, Antonio Faiella1, Silvia Brunelli, Renzo Guerrini	215

Part VII
Animal models   **227**

Chapter 23	Genetics of the EL mouse: a multifactorial epilepsy model	
	Thomas N. Seyfried, Michael J. Poderycki and Mariana Todorova	229
Chapter 24	Evidence for supernumerary GABAergic neurons and disinhibition in the hippocampus of seizure-sensitive gerbils	
	Gary M. Peterson and Charles E. Ribak	239
Chapter 25	Genetic predisposition to partial (focal) seizures and to generalized tonic/clonic seizures: interactions between seizure circuitry of the forebrain and brainstem	
	P.C. Jobe, P.K. Mishra, J.W. Dailey, K.H. Ko and M.E.A. Reith	251
Chapter 26	Transgenic animal models of epilepsy	
	Miklos Toth	261
Chapter 27	The epilepsy of the $GABA_A$ receptor β_3 subunit knockout mouse: comparison to the epilepsy of Angelman syndrome	
	Timothy M. DeLorey, Adrian Handforth, Gregg E. Homanics, Berge A. Minassian, Antonio Delgado-Escueta and Richard W. Olsen	267

Afterword   **277**

Author index   **279**

Subject index   **281**

PREFACE

The importance of genetic factors in the epilepsies has been recognized since the time of Hippocrates. In the modern era many studies have documented the major inherited component to the generalized epilepsies. In contrast, there has been an entrenched view that focal epilepsies are largely due to acquired cerebral lesions. It has recently emerged, however, that there are many forms of inherited focal epilepsy. Indeed, molecular genetic progress has actually been faster in the focal rather than the generalized epilepsies. From a neurobiological viewpoint, the idea that an inherited disorder can cause a focal disturbance of brain excitability is somewhat counter-intuitive. This puzzle poses an exciting and interesting challenge for neuroscience.

Major recent advances have included the identification of new inherited focal epilepsy syndromes, discovery of genetic linkages and basic molecular defects, and the marrying of concepts from animal models to man. Emerging concepts and data in this new field were crystallized at a meeting in Avignon, France, in September of 1996. The chapters in this volume are derived from that meeting and have been up dated to the present time. The compilation of knowledge in this volume should serve as an invaluable resource for the increasing number of clinicians, geneticists, molecular biologists, and basic neuroscientists attempting to solve the riddles of the inherited focal epilepsies.

The Editors

Part I
Introduction

Chapter 1

The discovery of 'benign rolandic epilepsy'

Marc Beaussart,[1] Pierre Loiseau[2] and Joseph Roger[3]

[1]10 avenue Kennedy, 59000 Lille, France; [2]Service de Neurologie, Hôpital Pellegrin, 33076 Bordeaux, France; [3]Centre Saint Paul, 13258 Marseille 09, France

In the 1980s, the Commission on Classification and Terminology of the International League Against Epilepsy proposed a classification of epileptic disorders (Commission, 1989), with two criteria for subdivision. The first is electroclinical, separating seizures of focal and seizures of generalized onset. The second is aetiological, with idiopathic epilepsies distinguished from symptomatic (or cryptogenic) epilepsies. Under the heading of localization-related, or partial, or focal epilepsies, are placed the idiopathic benign epilepsies of childhood. Among the latter, the most frequently occuring is benign rolandic epilepsy (BRE), officially designed 'benign childhood epilepsy with centro-temporal spikes' (BECTS). The fact that the characteristic abnormalities are sharp waves, and not spikes, is outside the subject of this paper. Even though outside our subject, we would like to underline the fact that 'benign' and 'idiopathic' are not synonymous, but semantically different terms: *idiopathic* refers to aetiology, while *benign* refers to outcome. All idiopathic syndromes are not benign. Some cryptogenic and even symptomatic epilepsies are easily controlled. So the syndrome is probably misnamed.

Idiopathic focal epilepsies of childhood represent approximately 25 per cent of epileptic seizures in children aged five to 14 years: they are more frequent than absence epilepsies (Cavazzuti, 1980). However, petit mal was recognized in the 19th century (Calmeil, 1824), and even earlier (Tissot, 1770), whereas the idiopathic focal epilepsies (IFE) remained totally ignored until the second half of the 20th century.

The early period

One has to admit that IFE went largely unrecognized by the clinicians, and that they were discovered by electroencephalographers. There may be several reasons for this. Under the influence of neurosurgeons, we were trained to consider that all focal seizures were due to a focal structural lesion. We were taught that partial epilepsies were either jacksonian or temporal, and there was no room for anything else. It is important to note that we tend to recognize, or accept, only what we are aware of. When we do not know, we do as if we knew and put the unfamiliar fact into a familiar category. Another reason is that neurologists did not trust EEG interpretations. The interictal EEG pattern of IFE of childhood is striking and cannot go unnoticed, whereas the associated clinical clinical features can.

In 1951, Yvette Gastaut gave a paper to the French EEG society on '*Un élément déroutant de la séméiologie électroencéphalographique, les pointes prérolandiques sans signification focale*' (a misleading element of the EEG semeiology – prerolandic spikes without focal significance) (Gastaut, 1952). Her opinion may be summarized as follows: it is confusing to find epileptiform abnormalities clearly focalized on a premotor area without any cortical lesion in this area. Her patients were children with various static conditions, but without epilepsy. Her presentation did not alert neurologists or electroencephalographers.

When considered from an electroencephalographic viewpoint alone, central (rolandic) epileptiform abnormalities have very heterogeneous clinical associations. In an early report on 200 cases (Smith & Kellaway, 1964), all the patients were children, but their ages varied from birth to adolescence, and only 40 per cent were in the 4–6 year age group. About 40 per cent experienced seizures; quite a few had neurological or mental impairment. However, a tendency toward disappearance of these foci was noted.

In 1952, the Gibbses demonstrated the existence of functional and transient EEG spike foci in the midtemporal area (Gibbs & Gibbs, 1964). The children were followed up, and their 1959 paper (Gibbs & Gibbs, 1959) is the first North American description of a benign focal epilepsy syndrome. However, they used the misleading term of temporal epilepsy. Furthermore, this paper came from an EEG laboratory, and gave no details on the clinical features. Lastly, it was not a pure series of benign childhood epilepsies, since the mandatory spontaneous remission was lacking in quite a few patients.

Two years earlier, in December 1957, Marc Beaussart presented at the French EEG Society the first European description of the EEG pattern (Nayrac & Beaussart, 1958). The analysis of the EEG characteristics was quite accurate: a slow spike, i.e. a sharp wave, followed or not by a slow wave; shifting of these changes from one hemisphere to the other; their possible disappearance. The pattern was seen exclusively in children, with various clinical conditions. As did Yvette Gastaut, the author considered the pattern as functional, without any associated rolandic lesion. Six months later, in a presentation at a meeting of the same society, Beaussart's number of cases was more than doubled. Most patients had seizures, but not all of them, and neither neurological deficits nor seizures were present in six children.

Once described, the EEG pattern was easily recognized. Interesting details were given in 1959 by authors from Lyon (Courjon & Cotte, 1959). They reported more variable localization than that of Nayrac and Beaussart. As became evident years later, the morphology of the sharp waves is more important than their precise localization. Enhancement by sleep, already noted by Beaussart, was confirmed. A retrospective study performed in the EEG laboratory of the main hospital in a large French city found some patients who had been followed up over several years, and ascertained the favourable outcome of the condition. However, at that stage, these functional changes observed in children and disappearing after puberty were not correlated with a particular type of epilepsy.

Pierre Loiseau was trained in clinical neurology, and started a private EEG practice in 1955. As he recorded many children with epilepsy, he accumulated over a short time a small series of cases with benign focal epilepsies and focal centro-temporal sharp waves. His first report was presented at the annual meeting of the French EEG society in December 1959 (Faure & Loiseau, 1960). The series included 15 otherwise healthy children, with onset of rare nocturnal seizures between the ages of four and 10. In keeping with Beaussart's findings, the EEG foci were of electrodes C5/C6, and not F7/F8. Their description was not flawless: in 13 children, the seizures were diagnosed as generalized. A favourable outcome was suggested, but the follow-up period was short. In subsequent papers, the existence of a particular form of childhood epilepsy with rolandic paroxysms was stressed. The syndrome appeared to have a real autonomy, and had to be removed from the heterogeneous group of functional rolandic spikes (Loiseau & Faure, 1961). Based on a series of 12 patients, more accurate symptomatology was delineated (Loiseau *et al.*, 1967). Partial seizures were found in 75 per cent of the children, and peculiar features were described. Oropharyngeal manifestations, speech impairment and hypersalivation were noted in at least one-third of the children. Forty patients had been seizure-free for at least 5 years, without medication and with a normal EEG.

Preaching in the desert?

For almost 20 years after the description of benign focal epilepsies in children, clinicians, and even some electroencephalographers, were not convinced. According to Gibbs & Gibbs (1970) : 'for reasons that are hard to explain, some of the most striking correlations and the most useful dinstinctions remain unrecognized by leading authorities. Even though there is a marked difference between the correlates of spike focus in the mid-temporal area and one in the anterio-temporal area, the distinction is more often disregarded than regarded'. As a subtitle, the authors added an old German saying: 'Bei Nacht sind alle Katzen grau' (at night, all cats are grey).

The concept of an 'idiopathic' focal epilepsy was clearly rejected at first, especially by adult neurologists. The old, 19th century tradition held that focal epilepsies belonged to neurology, and that generalized or 'genuine' epilepsies were for psychiatrists. Even those with a particular interest in childhood onset focal epilepsy failed to recognize the existence of an idiopathic form, and were only able to stress the better prognosis of epilepsies with rare seizures, with onset in school-age children and with focal rolandic changes .

However other authors were quick to recognized the existence of idiopathic and benign focal epilepsies in children. Cesare Lombroso published an outstanding paper with an accurate description of sylvian seizures and of their EEG correlates (Lombroso, 1967). He concluded: 'Their age incidence, the peripheral manifestations, the clinical and electrographic correlates, the mode of propagation, and their prognosis are sufficiently homogeneous to justify a special subgrouping'.

International recognition

Over the years, additional features of the syndrome were published, thanks to the identification of more and more cases in France (Beaussart, 1972). In 1973, 275 seizures observed in 190 patients were analysed (Loiseau & Beaussart, 1972). In Europe, Blom and Brorson (1966) and Lerman (1970) admitted the reality of a benign partial epilepsy of childhood with rolandic (or centro-temporal, which was the term used by Scandinavian authors) spikes or sharp waves. Very, very slowly, other groups, in other countries, 'discovered' the idiopathic focal epilepsies of childhood. Genetic studies of the clincial and of the EEG features of 'benign rolandic epilepsy' were performed even before the concept had gained international recognition: this volume, however, bears witness to the slowness of progress in this particular field. Towards the late 1970s, there was even a trend towards the delineation of several topographic and/or symptomatic forms (temporal/affective, frontal, occipital ...) of age-related, benign and idiopathic focal epilepsies, that will be discussed elsewhere in this volume.

As for our own discovery, we were helped by an identical EEG training and by our private practice. Both Pierre Loiseau and Marc Beaussart had attended Antoine Rémond's EEG laboratory at the Hôpital de la Salpêtrière, in Paris. Antoine Rémond did not use the international 10–20 electrode placing system. He placed low rolandic electrodes, corresponding to C5 and C6, and used very personal montages. Consequently, rolandic foci were clearly distinguished from temporal foci. Doctors in private practice have to listen to patients and to their parents. They establish a personal relationship with them. So it was that our new conviction, i.e. that not all partial epilepsies had a dismal outcome, was accompanied by deep personal feelings of relief.

Acknowledgements: The authors thank Jim Sneed, MD, and Pierre Genton, MD, for editorial assistance.

References

Beaussart, M. (1972): Benign epilepsy of children with rolandic (centrotemporal) paroxysmal foci: a clinical entity. Study of 221 cases. *Epilepsia* **13**, 795–811.

Blom, S. & Brorson, I.V. (1966): Central spikes or sharp waves (rolandic spikes) in childrens' EEG and their clinical significance. *Acta Paediatr. Scand.* **55,** 385–393.

Calmeil, L.F. (1824): De l'épilepsie étudiée sous le rapport de son siège et de son influence sur la production de l'aliénation mentale. *Thèse med.* Paris.

Cavazzuti, G.B. (1980): Epidemiology of different types of epilepsy in school children age of Modena, Italy. *Epilepsia* **13,** 57–62.

Commission on Classification and Terminology of the International League Against Epilepsy (1989): Proposal for revised classification of epilepsies and epileptic syndromes. *Epilepsia* **30,** 389–399.

Courjon, J. & Cotte, M.R. (1959): Les décharges pseudo-rythmiques localisées chez l'enfant et leur évolution à la puberté. *22ème Congrès de Pédiatrie de Langue Française,* pp. 247–250. Montpellier: Dehan.

Faure, J. & Loiseau, P. (1960): Une corrélation clinique particulière des pointe-ondes rolandiques sans signification focale. *Rev. Neurol. (Paris)* **102,** 399–406.

Gastaut, Y. (1952): Un élément déroutant de la séméiologie EEG: les pointes rolandiques sans signification focale. *Rev Neurol (Paris)* **87,** 488–490.

Gibbs, E L. & Gibbs, F.A. (1960): Good prognosis of mid-temporal epilepsy. *Epilepsia* **1,** 448–453.

Gibbs, F.A. & Gibbs, E.L. (1952): *Atlas of electroencephalography,* 2nd edition, vol.2. Reading, Mass.: Addison-Wesley Pub. Co.

Gibbs, F.A. & Gibbs, E.L. (1970): Clinical correlates and prognostic significance of various types of mid-temporal spike focus. *Clin. Electroenceph.* **1,** 45–64.

Lerman, P. (1970): Benign focal epilepsy in children. *Electroenceph. Clin. Neurophysiol.* **28,** 342 (abstract).

Loiseau, P. & Beaussart, M. (1972): The seizures of benign childhood epilepsy with rolandic paroxysmal discharges. *Epilepsia* **13,** 381–389.

Loiseau, P., Cohadon, F. & Mortureux, Y. (1967): A propos d'une forme singulière d'épilepsie de l'enfant. *Rev. Neurol. (Paris)* **116,** 244–248.

Loiseau, P. & Faure, J. (1961): Une forme particulière d'épilepsie de la seconde enfance. *J. Med. Bordeaux* **138,** 381–389.

Lombroso, C.T. (1967): Sylvian seizures and mid-temporal spike foci in children. *Arch. Neurol.* **17,** 52–59.

Nayrac, P. & Beaussart, M. (1958): Les pointes-ondes prérolandiques: expression EEG très particulière. Étude électro-clinique de 21 cas. *Rev. Neurol. (Paris)* **99,** 201–206.

Smith, J.M.B. & Kellaway, P. (1964). Central (rolandic) foci in children: an analysis of 200 cases. *Electroenceph. Clin. Neurophysiol.* **17,** 460 (abstract).

Tissot, S.A. (1770): *Traité de l'épilepsie, faisant le tome troisième du traité des nerfs et de leurs maladies.* Paris: Didot le jeune.

Chapter 2

Genetics of partial epilepsies: new frontiers

Samuel F. Berkovic and Ingrid E. Scheffer

Department of Medicine (Neurology), University of Melbourne, Austin & Repatriation Medical Centre, Studley Road, Heidelberg, Victoria 3084, Australia

For many years the presence of a family history of seizures in patients with partial epilepsies was regarded as an uncomfortable fact. Whilst the observation that generalized epilepsies are frequently inherited is easy to understand, the inheritance of a focal seizure disorder may appear at first to be counter intuitive. How genetic defects, that are presumably expressed widely and symmetrically in the brain, can cause partial epilepsies is unclear.

In this chapter an overview of some of the known and postulated mechanisms by which partial epilepsies may be inherited is presented. Second, reasons why a number of relatively common inherited partial epilepsies have only recently been recognized will be explored. Third, the problem of genetic heterogeneity as it applies to clinical and molecular genetic research in the partial epilepsies will be discussed. Finally, the issue of how epilepsy syndromes should be conceptualized for genetic research is addressed.

Mechanisms of familial partial epilepsies – previous views

The occurrence of a family history in a patient with partial epilepsy has traditionally had a number of explanations. First, it may occur by chance. At least one in 20 individuals will have a seizure at some time in their lives, and this general population frequency surely applies to the relatives of probands with partial epilepsy (Hauser *et al.*, 1993). Secondly, there has been a concept, going back to the time of Tissot of an 'epileptic diathesis'. Here there is a broad background predisposition to epilepsy that is inherited and the particular epileptic syndrome observed may depend on other factors including pre-natal, peri-natal and post-natal acquired insults, as well as effects of other modifying genes. This concept has been developed further in the neurobiological approach to epilepsy syndromes (Lennox & Lennox, 1960; Berkovic *et al.*, 1987; Berkovic *et al.*, 1994b). More specifically, in some probands with temporal lobe epilepsy and hippocampal sclerosis, Falconer recognized a family history of febrile seizures. The concept in these families was that the febrile seizure predisposition is inherited, but in certain individuals there are prolonged febrile seizures leading to secondary hippocampal damage and subsequently temporal lobe epilepsy (Falconer *et al.*, 1964; Falconer, 1971).

In a remarkable paper published nearly 30 years ago, Loiseau & Beaussart (1969) studied 53 patients with focal epilepsy and a family history of seizures. They recognized five subsets – benign rolandic epilepsy (15 cases), temporal lobe epilepsy with a family history of febrile seizures (13 cases), focal seizures due to hereditary brain diseases (10 cases), familial focal epilepsies (eight cases) and families with mixed partial and generalized epilepsies (seven cases). At that time they concluded that although there could be a familial element to partial seizures, this was an uncommon phenomenon and the focal character of epilepsy was usually not inherited. They reached the conclusion that hereditary partial epilepsy does not exist (Loiseau & Beaussart, 1969). It seems at that time the concept of inherited partial epilepsies was too revolutionary (Loiseau, personal communication) but their observations contain many of the elements upon which our current understanding of the familial partial epilepsies rests.

Familial partial epilepsies – current understanding of mechanisms

Current understanding of the possible mechanisms of inheritance of partial epilepsies are shown in Table 1. To date there are six partial epilepsies inherited in a simple mendelian fashion. Dominant inheritance of benign familial infantile convulsions was first clearly described in 1992 (Vigevano *et al.*, 1992) and the other five syndromes were first described in 1994 or later (Berkovic *et al.*, 1994a, 1996; Ottmann *et al.*, 1995; Scheffer *et al.*, 1994; 1995a, 1995b, 1995c). All are discussed in detail elsewhere in this volume. It is likely that other as yet unrecognized mendelian focal epilepsies exist and this remains a fruitful area for further clinical research.

Table 1. Mechanisms of inheritance of focal epilepsies

A.	**Simple (mendelian) inheritance**
	Benign familial infantile convulsions
	AD nocturnal frontal lobe epilepsy
	Familial partial epilepsy with variable foci
	Familial temporal lobe epilepsy
	Partial epilepsy with auditory features
	AD rolandic epilepsy with speech dyspraxia
B.	**Polygenic inheritance**
	Benign rolandic epilepsy
	Idiopathic occipital epilepsies
C.	**Acquired and genetic factors**
	Temporal lobe epilepsy with hippocampal sclerosis
D.	**Unsolved 'mixed' families**

Although benign rolandic epilepsy was once regarded as an autosomal dominant trait, at least with respect to the EEG marker, it now appears that it is inherited in a complex (polygenic or multifactorial) manner (Bray & Wiser, 1964; Heijbel *et al.*, 1975; Doose & Baier, 1989; Choy *et al.*, this volume). Similarly, the idiopathic occipital epilepsies, of which there are probably at least three subgroups, appear to show complex inheritance (Panayiotopoulos, 1989; Guerrini *et al.*, 1995; Ferrie *et al.*, 1997) There are hints that these partial epilepsies with complex inheritance may have some genetic relationship to the idiopathic generalized epilepsies, but this remains to be clarified.

The original observations of Falconer regarding a history of prolonged febrile seizures in probands with severe temporal lobe epilepsy and hippocampal sclerosis, and of febrile seizures in their relatives, have withstood the test of time (Falconer *et al.*, 1964; Falconer, 1971). There remains great debate regarding the mechanism of genesis of hippocampal sclerosis, but the occurrence of a family history of febrile seizures, or less commonly of generalized epilepsy, must be included in any explanation of the genesis of this important epileptogenic lesion. It is unusual, however, to observe more than one individual with temporal lobe epilepsy within an extended pedigree where many individuals have febrile seizures (Maher & McLachlan, 1995). It seems that there is a major acquired component, but genetic factors clearly also play a role, in this specific syndrome and in other symptomatic partial epilepsies (Andermann, 1982).

Finally, there are families where a mixture of epilepsy syndromes occurs. These families represent a challenge to explain. In some individuals there may be an obvious major acquired lesion causing partial epilepsy and a family history of generalized epilepsy, but this is relatively infrequently observed. More often, there is no obvious explanation and the concept of the neurobiological continuum of the epilepsies is perhaps the most sophisticated explanation we can make at the present time (Berkovic et al., 1987; Berkovic et al., 1994b). Once specific genes are identified in these families, the hypothesis of the neurobiological continuum can be specifically tested regarding the specific contribution of genetic factors in each individual.

Clinical lessons learnt

Why have the autosomal dominant partial epilepsies only been recognized in the last 5 years? There are a number of reasons for this. First, much of the literature on partial epilepsy deals with refractory cases, particularly those being considered for focal cortical resection. In such populations, a family history of epilepsy is uncommon, with the exception mentioned above of temporal lobe epilepsy sometimes occurring in families with a strong history of febrile seizures. In contrast, non-refractory partial epilepsies, which incorporates most patients with familial partial epilepsies, has not been as intensively studied.

A second set of reasons why this group of epilepsies has not been well recognized previously relates to the difficulties in clarifying the clinical history and the clinical genetics (see Table 2). The diagnosis of partial epilepsy may be missed in the proband. In autosomal dominant nocturnal frontal lobe epilepsy individuals may be thought to have non-epileptic disorders (Scheffer et al., 1995a). In individuals with familial partial epilepsies presenting with major convulsions, the symptoms of partial epilepsy may be overlooked. The family history may not have been adequately taken, perhaps due to a lack of expectation of positive findings. More importantly, the family history may not be known to the proband or the parents. Relatives may have been affected briefly many years ago and this may not be generally known within the family. Mildly affected relatives may not have been properly diagnosed, or they may have had such mild symptoms that they never sought medical attention. In some cases, other affected (particularly older) relatives may have hidden the diagnosis. Penetrance is often incomplete, thus masking the inherited nature. Finally, EEG studies in family members may be relatively unhelpful due to a lack of diagnostic changes or age-dependent penetrance.

Table 2. Barriers to diagnosing familial partial epilepsies

Diagnosis of focal epilepsy missed in proband

Family history not adequately taken

Family history not known to proband or parents
    Relatives hid diagnosis
    Relatives affected briefly many years ago
    Relatives mildly affected
    Relatives ignored mild symptoms

Incomplete penetrance of epilepsy

EEG studies in family members often unrewarding

These factors may thus mask recognition of a familial partial epilepsy. From a clinical point of view it is important to realize that clarification of a familial partial epilepsy is rarely achieved during a routine epilepsy consultation. The proband and attending relatives must be asked to probe back further into the family history and where necessary bring key older individuals back for a second interview.

For research purposes a more structured and rigorous protocol must be adhered to. An extensive family history must be taken in a systematized way. Usually, the older female relatives are the key to obtaining accurate and complete genealogical and medical information, particularly regarding events in early life of their children, grandchildren, nieces and nephews. The older relatives must be approached in a sensitive manner and appropriate information sought. In some families, formal genealogical research may be necessary. In our experience it is essential to take an epilepsy history directly from *all* available relatives. It is only by directly questioning that features of subtle and possibly ignored epilepsy will emerge and the true inherited nature will become clarified. A structured questionnaire is extremely helpful to avoid missing minor unrecognized symptoms (Reutens *et al.*, 1992). It is valuable to cross-check the histories from close relatives and to attempt to validate the histories from old medical records. This procedure can take many months. Construction of a large pedigree, however can be the clue to major progress in molecular genetics making the investment in this apparently tedious procedure more than worthwhile (Fig. 1).

Genetic heterogeneity

In order to find epilepsy genes clinical researchers must first identify 'pure' syndromes to allow the molecular geneticist to do linkage analysis, and subsequently identify specific genetic defects. If the clinician presents the molecular biologist with a heterogeneous sample, mapping of the relevant loci will be difficult, if not impossible. The ultimate confirmation of the genetic purity of a clinical sample is the demonstration of a specific genetic defects, but this leads to a circular problem of being unable to define a pure clinical sample to find a genetic defect because the genetic defect is not yet known (Berkovic, 1997).

The problem is even more difficult because of the emerging evidence of genetic heterogeneity even in clinically 'pure' samples. Locus heterogeneity, that is where mutations in different parts of the genome, affecting different genes, can cause the same clinical syndrome, is being increasingly recognized. In the epilepsies it was first described in benign familial neonatal convulsions where loci on 20q and 8q were identified (Leppert *et al.*, 1989; Lewis *et al.*, 1993) and subsequently two novel homologous potassium channels at those loci were found to be the responsible genes (Bievert *et al.*, 1998; Singh *et al.*, 1998; Charlier *et al.*, 1998). In autosomal dominant nocturnal frontal lobe epilepsy some families are linked to chromosome 20q and in others there is strong evidence that 20q is not involved. No clinical distinguishing features have been found to separate the molecular genetic subgroups (Steinlein *et al.*, 1995; Berkovic *et al.*, 1995; Hayman *et al.*, 1997; Oldani *et al.*, 1998). Moreover, allelic heterogeneity, where the same gene has different mutations in different families, is emerging as a cause of clinical variation in single gene disorders (Estivill, 1996). Finally, in some families with epilepsy, the same mutation appears to cause a variety of phenotypes, presumably due to the effect of modifying genes or perhaps environmental factors (Scheffer *et al.*, 1997).

Thus, there is evidence of a single genetic defect causing a variety of phenotypes and, on the other hand, different genetic defects causing the same phenotype. This obviously leads to considerable problems for the clinician in deciding what clinical material should be subject to molecular analysis. Choice of the clinical material will remain the most crucial step in the discovery of epilepsy genes and there are no easy answers to the problems outlined above. However, restricting analysis to single large families is a useful step in minimizing allelic and locus heterogeneity, but one must be careful to consider the possibility of additional pathogenic genes being introduced by spouses. Clinical and molecular genetic researchers need to have a flexible approach when analysing data on epilepsy phenotypes and perhaps consider analysing them with varying degrees of stringency regarding the specific diagnoses (Berkovic *et al.*, 1997).

Chapter 2 Genetics of partial epilepsies: new frontiers

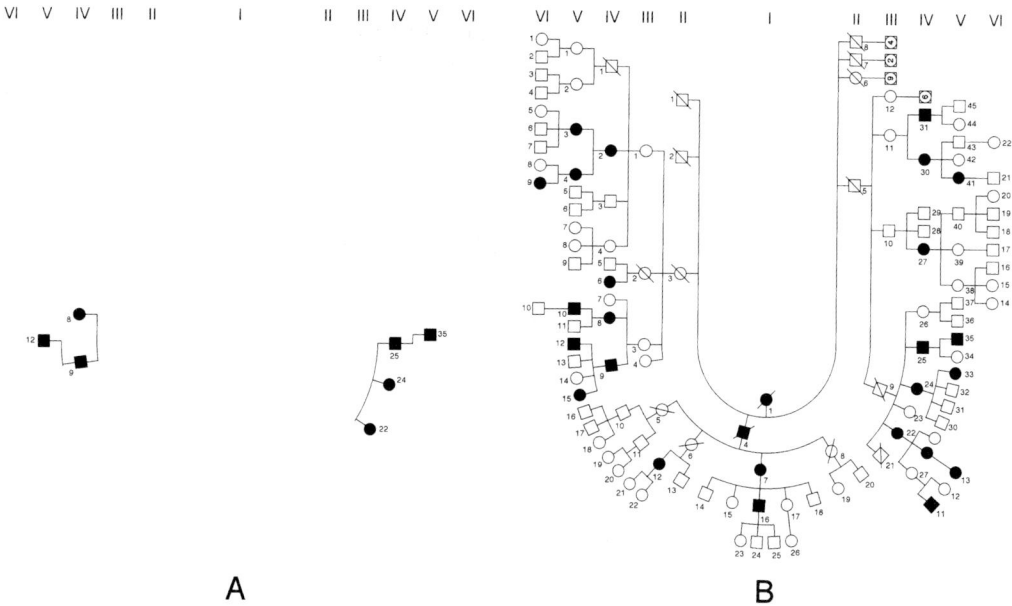

Fig. 1. Development of large family trees. On the left (A) are two small nuclear families with nocturnal frontal lobe epilepsy referred to us for study. Both families were from Adelaide, a city of one million people, and were not known to be related. Following 12 months of intensive research involving hundreds of phone calls, and two field trips to personally question and examine family members, the large pedigree (B) was created. This proved the two nuclear families were related and a total of 27 affected family members were identified. This clinical study led to the recognition of autosomal dominant nocturnal frontal lobe epilepsy and to subsequent discovery of its molecular basis.

Genetic epilepsy syndromes

The problem of genetic heterogeneity, and of the complexities in genotype-phenotype relationships are important when considering how we regard epilepsy syndromes. The ILAE classification of epilepsy syndromes is invaluable clinically for diagnosis of individuals, and has been central in development of research into specific disorders (Commission, 1989). However, it may be difficult to apply the classification to certain genetic epilepsies as outlined below.

For some inherited epilepsies the ILAE classification works well. For example, benign familial neonatal convulsions, where there is known locus heterogeneity, and Unverricht–Lundborg disease, where there is allelic heterogeneity, show essentially the same phenotype in affected relatives from the same or different families. Similarly, in the familial partial epilepsies, there is already evidence for both locus and allelic heterogeneity in autosomal dominant nocturnal frontal lobe epilepsy, but the phenotype is similar amongst different family members. In other inherited epilepsies, however, there is considerable phenotypic variation within families. This is the rule for epilepsies with polygenic inheritance such as idiopathic generalized epilepsies and benign rolandic epilepsy where if there are two affected individuals it is more likely that they will not have the same specific epilepsy syndrome. Variation in phenotype is also seen in some epilepsies where the molecular biology is known. For example in myoclonus epilepsy and ragged red fibre syndrome (MERRF) where there are mitochondrial mutations, most commonly affecting the tRNA for lysine a marked variation in phenotype can be seen (Berkovic et al., 1994b).

In other single gene epilepsies that have been recently described such as generalized epilepsy with

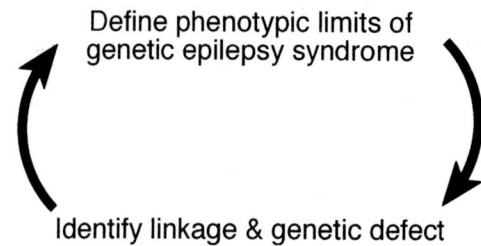

Fig. 2. Reciprocal relationship between clinical definition of a genetic epilepsy syndrome and molecular genetic analysis.

febrile seizures plus, and familial partial epilepsy with variable foci, a considerable variation in phenotypes is seen amongst family members and clarification of the genetic nature of these disorders can only be appreciated by examining large multiplex families.

We have therefore suggested the concept of *genetic epilepsy syndromes* where a number of individual epilepsy syndromes, as defined by the ILAE classification, may occur (Scheffer & Berkovic, 1997). Recognition of this phenomenon results in a particular challenge for clinical definition of these prior to molecular studies. As phenotypes may vary, it can be particularly difficult to determine the phenotypic limits of the genetic epilepsy syndrome. These families stretch to the limit our clinical skills in defining entities with biological meaning and highlight the major importance of a close interaction between clinicians and molecular geneticists in trying to unravel these fascinating disorders (Fig. 2).

It is likely that further study of the familial partial epilepsies will provide new surprises in the difficult problem of genotype–phenotype relationships in the epilepsies. Already, this group of newly recognized epilepsies has changed our concepts of the aetiology of the partial epilepsies.

References

Andermann, E. (1982): Multifactorial inheritance of generalized and focal epilepsy. In: *Genetic basis of the epilepsies*, Anderson, V.E., Hauser, W.A., Penry, J.K. & Sing, C.F. (eds), pp. 355–374. New York: Raven Press.

Berkovic, S.F., Andermann, F., Andermann, E. & Gloor, P. (1987): Concepts of absence epilepsies: Discrete syndromes or biological continuum? *Neurology* **37**, 993–1000.

Berkovic, S.F., Howell, R.A. & Hopper, J.L. (1994a): Familial temporal lobe epilepsy: a new syndrome with adolescent/adult onset and a benign course. In: *Epileptic seizures and syndromes*, Wolf, P. (ed.), pp. 257–263. London: John Libbey.

Berkovic, S.F., McIntosh, A.M., Howell, R.A., Mitchell, A., Sheffield, L.J. & Hopper, J.L. (1996): Familial temporal lobe epilepsy: a common disorder identified in twins. *Ann. Neurol.* **40**, 227–235.

Berkovic, S.F., Phillips, H.A., Scheffer, I.E. *et al.* (1995): Genetic heterogeneity in autosomal dominant nocturnal frontal lobe epilepsy. *Epilepsia* **36** (Suppl 4), 147.

Berkovic, S.F., Reutens, D.C., Andermann, E. & Andermann, F. (1994b): The epilepsies: specific syndromes or a neurobiological continuum?. In: *Epileptic seizures and syndromes*, Wolf, P. (ed.), pp. 25–37. London: John Libbey.

Berkovic, S.F. (1997): Genetics of epilepsy syndromes. In: *Epilepsy: a comprehensive textbook*, Engel, J. Jr & Pedley, T.A. (eds) pp. 217–224. Philadelphia: Lippincott-Raven.

Biervert, C., Schroeder, B.C., Kubisch, C., Berkovic, S.F., Propping, P., Jentsch, T.J. & Steinlein, O.K. (1998): A potassium channel mutation in neonatal human epilepsy. *Science* **279**, 403–406.

Bray, P.F. & Wiser, W.C. (1964): Evidence for a genetic etiology of temporal-central abnormalities in focal epilepsy. *N. Engl. J. Med.* **271**, 926–933.

Charlier, C., Singh, N.A., Ryan, S.G. et al. (1998): A pore mutation in a novel KQT-like potassium channel gene in an idiopathic epilepsy family. *Nat. Genet.* **18,** 53–55.

Commission on Classification and Terminology of the International League against Epilepsy (1989): Proposal for revised classification of epilepsies and epileptic syndromes. *Epilepsia* **30,** 389–399.

Doose, H. & Baier, W.K. (1989): Benign partial epilepsy and related conditions: multifactorial pathogenesis with hereditary impairment of brain maturation. *Eur. J. Pediatr.* **149,** 152–158.

Estivill, X. (1996): Complexity in monogenic disease (CF). *Nat. Genet.* **12,** 348–350.

Falconer, M.A., Serafetinides, E.A. & Corsellis, J.A. (1964): Etiology and pathogenesis of temporal lobe epilepsy. *Arch. Neurol.* **10,** 233–248.

Falconer, M.A. (1971): Genetic and related etiological factors in temporal lobe epilepsy: a review. *Epilepsia* **12,** 313–316.

Ferrie, C.D., Beaumanoir, A., Guerrini, R. et al. (1997): Early-onset benign occipital seizure susceptibility syndrome. *Epilepsia* **38,** 285–293.

Guerrini, R. et al. (1995): Idiopathic photosensitive occipital lobe epilepsy. *Epilepsia* **36,** 883–891.

Hauser, W.A., Annegers, J.F. & Kurland, L.T. (1993): Incidence of epilepsy and unprovoked seizures in Rochester, Minnesota: 1935–1984. *Epilepsia* **34,** 453–468.

Hayman, M., Scheffer, I.E., Chinvarun, Y., Berlangieri, S.U. & Berkovic, S.F. (1997): Autosomal dominant nocturnal frontal lobe epilepsy: demonstration of focal frontal onset and intrafamilial variation. *Neurology* **49,** 969–975.

Heijbel, J., Blom, S. & Rasmuson, M. (1975): Benign epilepsy of children with centro-temporal EEG foci: a genetic study. *Epilepsia* **16,** 285–293.

Lennox, W.G. & Lennox, M.A. (1960): *Epilepsy and related disorders*, pp. 548–574. Boston: Little Brown.

Leppert, M., Anderson, V.E., Quattlebaum, T.G., Stauffer, D., O'Connell, P., Nakamura, Y., Lalouel, J.M. & White, R. (1989): Benign familial neonatal convulsions linked to genetic markers on chromosome 20. *Nature* **337,** 647–648.

Lewis, T.B., Leach, R.J., Ward, K., O'Connell, P. & Ryan, S.G. (1993): Genetic heterogeneity in benign familial neonatal convulsions: identification of a new locus on chromosome 8q. *Am. J. Hum. Genet.* **53,** 670–576.

Loiseau, P. & Beaussart, M. (1969): Hereditary factors in partial epilepsy. *Epilepsia* **10,** 23–31.

Maher, J. & McLachlan, R.S. (1995): Febrile convulsions: is seizure duration the most important predictor of temporal lobe epilepsy? *Brain* **118,** 1521–1528.

Oldani, A., Zucconi, M., Asselta, R., Modugno, M., Bonati, M.T., Dalpra, L. et al. (1998): Autosomal dominant nocturnal frontal lobe epilepsy: a video-polysomnographic and genetic apraiasal of 40 patients and delineation of the epileptic syndrome. *Brain* **121,** 205–223.

Ottman, R., Risch, N., Hauser, W.A., Pedley, T.A., Lee, J.H., Barker-Cummings, C., Lustenberger, A., Nagle, K.J., Lee, K.S., Scheuer, M.L., Neystat, M., Susser, M. & Wilhelmsen, K.C. (1995): Localization of a gene for partial epilepsy to chromosome 10q. *Nat. Genet.* **10,** 56–60.

Panayiotopoulos, C.P. (1989): Benign childhood epilepsy with occipital paroxysms: a fifteen year prospective study. *Ann. Neurol.* **26,** 51–56.

Reutens, D.C., Howell, R.A., Gebert, K.E. & Berkovic, S.F. (1992): Validation of a questionnaire for clinical seizure diagnosis. *Epilepsia* **33,** 1065–1071.

Scheffer, I.E., Phillips, H.A., Mulley, J., Sutherland, G., Harvey, A.S., Hopkins, I.J. & Berkovic, S.F. (1995b): Autosomal dominant partial epilepsy with variable foci is not allelic with autosomal dominant nocturnal frontal lobe epilepsy. *Epilepsia* **36** (Suppl. 3), S28.

Scheffer, I.E. & Berkovic, S.F. (1997): Generalized epilepsy with febrile seizures plus: a genetic disorder with heterogeneous clinical phenotypes. *Brain* **120,** 479–490.

Scheffer, I.E., Bhatia, K.P., Lopes-Cendes, I., Fish, D.R., Marsden, C.D., Andermann, F., Andermann, E., Desbiens, R., Cendes, F., Manson, J.I. & Berkovic, S.F. (1994): Autosomal dominant frontal epilepsy misdiagnosed as sleep disorder. *Lancet* **343,** 515–517.

Scheffer, I.E., Bhatia, K.P., Lopes-Cendes, I., Fish, D.R., Marsden, C.D., Andermann, E., Andermann, F., Desbiens, R., Keene, D., Cendes, F., Manson, J.I., Constantinou, J., McIntosh, A. & Berkovic, S.F. (1995a): Autosomal dominant nocturnal frontal epilepsy: a distinctive clinical disorder. *Brain* **118,** 61–73.

Scheffer, I.E., Jones, L., Pozzebon, M., Howell, R.A., Saling, M.M. & Berkovic, S.F. (1995c): Autosomal dominant rolandic epilepsy and speech dyspraxia: a new syndrome with anticipation. *Ann. Neurol.* **38,** 633–642.

Singh, N.A., Charlier, C., Stauffer, D. *et al.* (1998): A novel potassium channel gene, KCNQ2, is mutated in an inherited epilepsy of newborns. *Nat. Genet.* **18,** 25–29.

Steinlein, O.K., Mulley, J.C., Propping, P., Wallace, R.H., Phillips, H.A., Sutherland, G.R., Scheffer, I.E. & Berkovic, S.F. (1995): A missense mutation in the neuronal nicotinic acetylcholine receptor a4 subunit is associated with autosomal dominant nocturnal frontal lobe epilepsy. *Nat. Genet.* **11,** 201–203.

Vigevano, F., Fusco, L., Capua, M. *et al.* (1992): Benign infantile familial convulsions. *Eur. J. Pediatr.* **151,** 608–612.

Chapter 3

Clinical genetic and molecular genetic approaches to the familial partial epilepsies

Massimo Pandolfo

*Centre Hospitalier de l'Université de Montréal; Departement de Médecine, Université de Montréal;
Department of Neurology and Neurosurgery, McGill University, Montréal, Québec, Canada*

All humans may have a seizure or develop epilepsy as a consequence of structural brain damage or due to altered metabolic states (DeLorenzo, 1991). Epilepsy arising in the presence of such an obviously acquired cause as trauma, infection or tumour, is called 'symptomatic'. Many individuals with epilepsy, however, have no gross structural brain lesions, no permanent neurological impairment, and show specific, often age-related, clinical and EEG features. These cases could in principle be due either to hidden acquired conditions or to a strong genetic predisposition to seizure activity, indeed so strong as to lead to recurring seizures without any evident precipitating cause. When such genetic predisposition is considered most likely, the condition is labeled as 'idiopathic epilepsy'. The International League Against Epilepsy (ILAE), in its International Classification of Epilepsies and Epileptic Syndromes (ICEES, ILAE Commission on Classification and Terminology, 1989) stressed that in idiopathic epilepsy *'there is no underlying cause other than a possible inherited predisposition'*, therefore excluding any symptomatic origin, detected or suspected. The term 'cryptogenic' is instead utilized when epilepsy is thought to be symptomatic, but no cause can be readily detected (ILAE Commission on Classification and Terminology, 1989).

The existence of idiopathic generalized epilepsy (IGE) has been widely accepted for decades. Accordingly, most genetic research in epilepsy has focused on investigating the genetic predisposition to generalized epilepsy, first through twin and family studies, more recently also through positional cloning. The concept of idiopathic partial epilepsy has instead encountered more difficulties, possibly because it is easier to imagine that a genetically determined enhancement in neural excitability may result in seizure activity involving the whole brain rather than just a part of it. Not long ago, with the possible exception of rolandic epilepsy of childhood (Nayrac & Beaussart, 1958), all partial epilepsy was considered symptomatic or cryptogenic. Even when familial aggregation was observed, it was attributed to shared environmental factors rather than to the effect of genes. In fact, there is no reason why a genetic abnormality should be more likely to result in generalized rather than partial epilepsy. Generalized epilepsy is the consequence of the hypersynchronized, paroxysmal firing of specific neural circuits as much as partial epilepsy. It is the nature of the primarily affected circuits that determines the resulting clinical and EEG features, partial or generalized. For example, a specific thalamo-cortical loop, not the 'whole brain', is thought to be involved in the pathogenesis of absences, a characteristic generalized seizure type occurring in several IGE syndromes. The anatomical specificity of a genetic syndrome may be explained by spatially restricted gene expression or by the special sensitivity of a specific circuitry to the abnormality of a more widely expressed gene (Ryan, 1995).

In the last few years an increasing number of idiopathic partial epilepsy syndromes has been described, a few of the underlying genes have been mapped, one has been identified. How recent is the development in this field is evidenced by the fact that the ICEES includes just a few of the currently recognized idiopathic partial epilepsy syndromes, many of which have been described only after 1989. In this chapter, the current clinical genetic and molecular genetic approaches to the idiopathic partial epilepsies will be summarized. By discussing some general and methodological issues, it is hoped that some useful indications will emerge about how these epilepsies should be approached clinically so that molecular geneticists may have the best chances of making progress. Some basic concepts in clinical and molecular genetics will be presented, along with the related methodological issues for molecular genetic studies.

Mendelian vs. polygenic inheritance

Diseases that are due to the effect of a single mutated gene are said to have mendelian inheritance. These diseases can be classified as autosomal or sex-linked, dominant or recessive, according to the specific pattern of transmission.

Polygenic diseases are instead caused by a combination of common functional polymorphisms in a set of interacting genes. Each susceptibility allele is not sufficient by itself to cause the disease, but it modifies the risk. The disease develops only when susceptibility alleles at several unlinked loci have been inherited. For this reason, relatives of affected individuals have a generally lower risk of developing the disease than in the case of single-gene disorders.

Multifactoriality

The aetiology of a disease is said to be multifactorial when it results from the combination of multiple acquired and genetic causes. The aetiology of most cases of epilepsy has been considered multifactorial (Andermann, 1981). This is a central concept, which should not be confused with that of polygenic inheritance. In its narrowest sense, the concept of multifactoriality is applied to those traits in which the combination of genetic and acquired risk factors is necessary to produce the phenotype, and none of these factors is *per se* sufficient. Multiple sclerosis may be an example. According to the prevalent views, in this disease several genetic polymorphisms contribute to a type of reactivity of the immune system that allows, after the appropriate environmental stimulus, the autoreactive aggression of the central nervous system myelin (Ffrench-Constant, 1994). Clearly, genetic and non-genetic factors are both necessary and neither is sufficient. In a wider sense, however, considering the multifactorial aetiology of a disease means taking into account how the interplay of many different factors can ultimately affect the phenotype. It is in fact difficult to find a disease that is not multifactorial, even among those with mendelian inheritance. Modifier genes and environmental factors such as diet, infection, lifestyle, trauma, can profoundly modify the phenotypes resulting from many gene mutations which are *per se* sufficient to cause disease. This broader meaning of multifactoriality provides a biological basis for much of the 'complexity' of mendelian traits that is discussed below.

Complexity of mendelian traits

Mendelian diseases may be somewhat genetically 'complex', because the correspondence between the phenotype and the underlying gene mutation is not always straightforward. In general, a given phenotype may be caused by different mutations, even in different genes. A given gene mutation may not necessarily result in a unique phenotype, and different mutations in the same gene may result in very different phenotypes. Some types of mutations in particular, as unstable repeat expansions, are associated with a high phenotypic variability. These points are illustrated below.

Genetic heterogeneity

The term genetic heterogeneity refers to the case in which the same disease phenotype may be caused by different mutations, either in the same gene (allelic heterogeneity) or in different genes (locus heterogeneity). Allelic heterogeneity does not generally interfere with the process of mapping a disease gene, but locus heterogeneity may be a major problem.

In the case of locus heterogeneity, how identical the phenotypes generated by mutations in different loci actually are may be sometimes a matter of discussion. In practice, this kind of heterogeneity will exist whenever the phenotypes determined by mutations at different loci are similar enough that they cannot be distinguished in the single patient despite a thorough clinical evaluation. Sometimes it is impossible to make a distinction even when examining multiple affected subjects from the same family. This is, for example, the case for tuberous sclerosis (TSC), which may be caused by mutations in the TSC1 gene on chromosome 9q or in the TSC2 gene on chromosome 16p (reviewed in Korf, 1997). Sometimes, statistical differences in the frequency of certain signs and symptoms may correspond to different mutations so, at least when several affected family members can be examined, it may be possible to consider one gene mutation more likely than others. For example, a number of signs and symptoms, as specific abnormalities of eye movements (Rivaud-Pechoux *et al.*, 1998), occur with different frequency in autosomal dominant hereditary ataxias caused by mutations at the SCA1, SCA2 or SCA3 loci, with slow saccades suggesting SCA2. If slow saccades and absent or reduced reflexes are consistently observed within a family, it is highly likely that the SCA2 gene mutation is responsible, but it would be unreliable to use these findings to make the clinical diagnosis of SCA2 in a single patient.

What is the biological basis of locus heterogeneity? In most cases, the different genes will encode proteins that are part of the same metabolic pathway or of the same oligomeric complex. The malfunction of the pathway or of the multiprotein complex will result in similar or identical consequences regardless of the primarily affected component. In the case of TSC, for instance, the TSC1 and TSC2 gene products, hamartin and tuberin, though dissimilar in terms of aminoacid sequence, have been recently demonstrated to interact with each other, forming a complex (van Slegtenhorst *et al.*, 1998). Alternatively, one gene may encode a regulatory protein that controls the expression of the other gene. Another possibility, observed in some dominant diseases, is that the mutations lead to a similar toxic gain of function regardless of the specific functions of their protein products. The diseases due to CAG trinucleotide expansions in the coding portions of the respective genes may be an example. An expanded polyglutamine tract in the encoded protein results from the CAG expansion in the gene, and it seems that polyglutamine proteins become toxic for neurons through the same mechanism, possibly the formation of intracellular, often intranuclear aggregates (Davies *et al.*, 1998). Hence, the overlap in the clinical phenotype among some of these diseases, such as the above mentioned cerebellar ataxias. In fact, the phenotypic differences among some of these diseases are currently more difficult to explain than the similarities.

Variable phenotypic effect of different mutations in the same gene

While in allelic heterogeneity different mutations affecting the same gene result in indistinguishable phenotypes, sometimes different mutations in the same gene may have widely different phenotypic consequences. The phenotypes may be so different that the discovery that they are due to allelic mutations comes as a surprise. The biological basis of this phenomenon must lie in the different effect on protein function of different mutations, principally in proteins with multiple functional and regulatory domains. Among the inherited neurological disorders, this variability has been observed in many cases (e.g. the different types of peripheral neuropathy caused by different mutations affecting the PMP22 gene on chromosome 17p, reviewed by Scherer, 1997), but particularly in the channelopathies, diseases caused by mutations in genes encoding components of ion channels. A striking example is provided by the brain-specific P/Q-type calcium channel a1 subunit gene on chromosome 19p13 (CACNA1A). Missense mutations in this gene cause familial hemiplegic migraine (FHM, Ophoff *et al.*, 1996), truncating mutations cause episodic ataxia type 2 (EA–2, Ophoff *et al.*, 1996), some missense mutations may cause FHM associated with ataxia (Terwindt *et al.*, 1998), and a small CAG expansion causes progressive ataxia (SCA6, Zhuchenko *et al.*, 1997), but its shortest pathological alleles may also cause episodic ataxia (Jodice *et al.*, 1997). Mutations in the homologous mouse gene (tottering) cause epilepsy in addition to cerebellar dysfunction (reviewed in Meisler *et al.*, 1997). Very importantly for the purposes of this chapter, all human idiopathic epilepsies whose genetic basis has so far been elucidated are channelopathies. It would not be surprising if different epileptic phenotypes will turn out to be caused by allelic mutations in the same ion channel gene.

Variable expressivity, pleiotropy and reduced penetrance

Some mutations may determine different phenotypes in terms of severity (variable expressivity) and of pattern of involvement (pleiotropy). In some individuals, mutations known to cause disease may even result in a normal phenotype (reduced penetrance). TSC offers a typical example of both variable expressivity and pleiotropy (Gomez, 1991). Striking differences in severity are commonly observed within families with TSC, with some individual showing just a few minor skin lesions while others are severely incapacitated by intractable epilepsy and mental retardation. As for pleiotropy, TSC may variably involve skin, brain, kidney, heart, lungs and endocrine glands, so that each of these target tissues is sometimes totally spared, sometimes very severely affected. The biological basis for these phenomena may be found in the effect of other genes (modifier genes), of environmental factors, and possibly of chance. This indicates how blurred may be the distinction between monogenic and multifactorial aetiology, so that even when it is clear that a single gene mutation is causing the disease, several other factors may intervene to profoundly modify the phenotype. We can again use TSC as an example. Though it is due to a gene mutation present in all cells, this dominant disease is characterized by multiple discrete hamartomatous lesions. The lesions are thought to result from an additional somatic mutation event that inactivates the normal copy of the gene in a single cell, whose behaviour then becomes abnormal (Korf, 1997). This so-called two-hit hypothesis therefore postulates that the mutation, dominant at the level of the whole individual, is recessive at the cellular level. A gene that affects DNA repair may then affect the development of the phenotype, as well as other genes that control cell growth and differentiation, environmental factors affecting somatic mutation rate, and, last but not least, chance.

Dynamic mutations

Dynamic mutations, such as hyperexpanded triplet repeat sequences, may determine widely variable phenotypes as a consequence of their instability during meiosis and during development. These mutations have now been found in dominant, recessive and X-linked diseases (reviewed in Ashizawa & Zoghbi, 1997). While it would be impossible to discuss this mutation mechanism exhaustively in this chapter, at least some basic points can be made. Diseases due to unstable repeats can be classified into two groups: type 1 diseases are caused by CAG expansions in the coding region of the respective genes, resulting in an expanded polyglutamine tract in the encoded protein; type 2 diseases are caused by expansions of other repeat sequences in non-coding portions of the respective genes, resulting in most cases in suppression of gene expression, i.e. in loss of function. Type 1 expansions are smaller, and in some cases the normal and pathological size ranges are separated just by 1–2 triplets, and the largest expansions may reach up to 100–150 triplets (4–5 times more than normal repeats). Type 2 expansions are larger, there is a wider separation between normal and pathological alleles, most expansions contain hundreds of triplets (one order magnitude more than normal repeats) and may reach lengths of more than a thousand triplets. Meiotic instability, i.e. a change in size of the expanded repeat upon parent-child transmission is commonly observed both in type 1 and type 2 diseases. As a consequence, the mutation is quantitatively different in each affected family member. Since for all these disease severity is proportional to the length of the expanded repeat, the intrafamilial heterogeneity in expansion sizes will be reflected in heterogeneity in disease severity. In some cases, the tendency is for expansion to increase in size in subsequent generations. With dominant inheritance, this results in an increasing level of severity and earlier onset of the disease, the phenomenon of anticipation. A parental bias is often present, with type 1 expansions usually increasing in size after paternal transmission, and type 2 expansions after maternal transmission. In the case of fragile X, instability and parental bias lead to a peculiar distortion of the usual mendelian sex-linked pattern of inheritance, called Sherman's paradox. Type 2 expansions also show extensive mitotic instability, i.e. instability during somatic cell divisions, that leads to heterogeneity of repeat sizes within the same individual. Therefore, in this type of disease not only individuals within the same family carry different mutations, but heterogeneity extends even to cells within the same individual, leading to additional variable expressivity and pleiotropy.

Strategies for genetic research

Despite the above described difficulties, mendelian disorders are ideal for gene mapping and positional cloning. Each issue has a way to be dealt with throughout the process leading from clinical studies and family collection to segregation analysis, gene mapping, gene cloning, mutation analysis and genotype-phenotype correlation analysis.

Polygenic traits are much more difficult to study by linkage analysis than mendelian traits. The most powerful methods to determine linkage rely on the definition of a mode of inheritance for the disease-causing allele, which is very uncertain in the case of a susceptibility allele. The alternative methods used for complex traits are less powerful and require very large samples, particularly to detect predisposing loci with a weak effect. In addition, even when linkage is established, the accurate definition of the candidate region is difficult, because recombination boundaries cannot be readily recognized.

How can we decide if a trait showing familial aggregation is in the first place due to the influence of genes, and, if that seems to be the case, if it is mendelian or polygenic? The traditional tool for this kind of investigation is the evaluation of how the risk of developing the disease (relative to the general population) varies according to: (1) the degree of relationship with an affected individual, i.e. the sharing of genes with this individual; (2) the sharing of a common environment with an affected individual. Twins are extremely useful for these studies. Monozygotic (MZ) twins share 100 per cent of their genes, while dizygotic (DZ) twins, like all sib pairs, share 50 per cent of their genes. In addition, all twins have shared the same uterine environment. The role of genetic factors in epilepsy, generalized and partial, has in fact been revealed by twin studies (Lennox, 1960; Gedda & Tatarelli, 1971; Berkovic et al., 1998). Sib- and other relative pairs can also be studied. The effect of shared genes and of shared environment can be assessed by evaluating how the relative risk of disease varies in MZ vs. DZ twins, sibs in general, and other relatives, and whether having been raised together or separately affects such relative risks. Analysis of adopted vs. biological sibs and of half-sibs raised in the same family is a good way of separating the effect of genes from that of the environment. It should be evident how such studies are much more sophisticated and demanding than just the report of 'a positive family history'. Once a genetic effect is demonstrated, the question of its mono-, oligo- or polygenic nature can be addressed by analysing how the relative risk varies in relatives of different degree. As shown by Risch (1990), polygenic inheritance, compared to monogenic inheritance, leads to a more rapid decrease of the relative risk as the distance from the affected individual increases. Pedigrees with many affected individuals are more likely to represent cases of mendelian inheritance, though this is not necessarily the case. Dominant inheritance, in particular, is associated with the presence of affected individuals through several generations. Pedigrees segregating a dominant trait are those in which the inherited nature of the trait is easiest to recognize and to study by linkage analysis. It is therefore fortunate that many familial partial epilepsies seem to conform to a mendelian, usually dominant model.

Identification of families, clinical and EEG studies

In the field of idiopathic partial epilepsy we are confronted with a variety of clinical presentations. To perform molecular studies, we have to assume that by clinical observation and segregation analysis we can identify genetically distinct subtypes of idiopathic partial epilepsy. This hypothesis guided the ILAE Commission when it distinguished the first three idiopathic partial epilepsy syndromes in the ICEES and was behind the subsequent description of 'new' idiopathic partial epilepsy syndromes (Scheffer *et al.*, 1994, 1995a, b; Berkovic *et al.*, 1996; Berkovic & Scheffer, 1997b; Andermann, 1997; Cendes *et al.*, 1998). Not only do these syndromes appear to be distinct genetic entities, but, very importantly, analysis of several of them has clearly shown that a single major locus (with mendelian-type inheritance) is operating in many of these cases (Berkovic & Scheffer, 1997a).

In some families not showing a clear mendelian segregation of epilepsy, it may be possible to dissect the trait into simpler components, each independently inherited and likely to have a less complex, possibly mendelian genetic aetiology. This operation seems to be possible particularly through the analysis of the associated EEG traits (Tsai *et al.*, 1989; Pedley, 1991). It has long been known that EEG abnormalities presented by epileptic subjects may also be found in individuals without seizures, and that relatives of epileptic individuals show such abnormalities more often than the general population. EEG abnormalities without clinical seizures may be the expression of a high liability to epilepsy, but not high enough to cause unprovoked seizures (Tsai *et al.*, 1989). In the case of IGE, the typically associated EEG trait, generalized spike-wave discharges, was proposed to be an autosomal dominant trait with age-dependent penetrance (Metrakos & Metrakos, 1972), long before molecular genetic studies became possible. Though the hypothesis of the Metrakoses is no longer accepted as originally stated, it had an important heuristic role for the subsequent clinical and molecular genetic research on IGE, and, in a modified form that takes into account genetic heterogeneity, it is probably still valid.

The accurate delineation of the phenotype is the essential first step in the investigation. It is important to define the phenotype as accurately as possible and to exclude symptomatic cases. A suggested protocol for evaluation may include the following:

1. Personal history, including examination of previous medical records.
2. General physical, neurological and neuropsychological examination.

The following diagnostic tests on inpatients:

1. Routine and sleep EEG.
2. 24-h video telemetry monitoring.
3. Magnetic resonance imaging (MRI), including volumetric MRI.

Functional MRI, and/or magnetic resonance spectrometry (MRS), and/or positron emission tomography (PET) for confirmation of epileptic foci may be performed on selected cases. Outpatients may be examined by routine and sleep EEG, daytime video telemetry monitoring (in selected cases), computerized tomography and/or MRI, including volumetric MRI.

Family history allows the identification of possible additional cases in relatives. It is important, however, to keep in mind that the routinely collected family history is not sufficient to discover large pedigrees. Only an intensive effort by specialized research personnel allows digging into the family history, contact relatives, collect medical records and do genealogical searches, all respecting ethical guidelines on informed consent and protection of privacy. When evidence of additional familial cases is obtained, consenting possibly affected family members have to be evaluated as the probands. Consenting asymptomatic family members have to undergo a neurological, neuropsychological, and EEG (routine and sleep) examination.

The clinical data need then to be critically and reliably evaluated. Well-characterized families, in which there is a consensus on the definition of the trait under study, on the affection status of each individuals, and on the most likely mode of inheritance are needed for molecular studies. Any of the above described tricks that nature may wish to play then can be effectively handled. More than one diagnostic scheme is perfectly acceptable and there are methods of dealing with this situation in linkage analysis. On the other hand, any *ad hoc* modification in the clinical status of some family members to forcefully fit the data with some appealing molecular hypothesis needs to be avoided. The lack of a sound analysis of the phenotype can lead to such a dubious practice even without any voluntary mishandling of the research. There is no magic recipe for the clinician, other than using her/his professional ability, good judgement, spirit of observation, and synthetic and analytical skills. Starting from the proband, the syndrome has to be accurately described and compared to known conditions. Then, all additional affected family members have to be compared with the proband and with one another. Is there any clear common feature that characterizes the family? In the rapidly evolving field of genetically determined partial epilepsy syndromes, it is still possible to find previously unrecognized syndromes. The possibility that, considering the high frequency of epilepsy, some family members may have epilepsy of a different kind must be always carefully considered. Subjects with obvious risk factors for epilepsy, such as a history of head trauma, should not be included among those considered affected for the molecular genetic studies, because the risk that their epilepsy has an unrelated cause is too high. On the other hand, as discussed above for genetic diseases in general under the rubrics of variable expressivity and pleiotropy, some genetic epilepsy syndromes may show variability from individual to individual in terms of severity and of type of seizures, even within the same family (e.g. consider the case of partial epilepsy with variable foci, in which variability is one of the characterizing features of the syndrome) (Berkovic & Scheffer, 1997b).

Analysis of the clinical data should indicate if a relevant portion of family members without epilepsy have EEG abnormalities, suggesting that an epilepsy-related EEG trait rather than an epilepsy syndrome directly results from the predisposing gene supposedly showing mendelian segregation in the pedigree. If this is the conclusion, the EEG trait should be defined as accurately as possible and differentiated from any other, non-specific EEG changes. A genetic EEG trait is usually rather homogeneous within a family, so its recognition should not be too problematic (for an example, see Zara *et al.*, 1998).

Criteria for selection for the linkage studies

In general, blood samples for DNA analysis should be obtained from all available consenting family members, including unaffected individuals and spouses, if knowledge of their genotypes adds information to the analysis. The choice of subjects for genotyping should be discussed between the clinician and the molecular geneticist to avoid missing important individuals or obtaining unecessary samples. Finding a pedigree with many affected individuals does not necessarily imply mendelian inheritance. The trait may be polygenic and multiple predisposing alleles may segregate in the family. It is probably an unnecessary effort to try to prove mendelian inheritance, or a specific type of inheritance, before performing linkage analysis. All pedigrees that by inspection seem to conform to a mendelian model should be considered. Simulation analysis (e.g. with the SLINK program by Weeks *et al.*, 1990) may be used to evaluate the power to detect linkage provided by each pedigree, assuming the mode(s) of inheritance suggested by inspection. Only the identification of linked markers will be the final evidence that the trait is mendelian and may also indicate the most likely type of inheritance.

It is recommended that smaller families with apparent mendelian inheritance are collected as well, because (1) they may be expanded in the future; (2) they may be used to test loci identified in larger families; and (3) families with a sufficiently homogeneous phenotype may be used together for primary linkage mapping, assuming that the causative locus is the same. In the last case, genetic heterogeneity will have to be considered when performing the analysis.

Collection of DNA samples and cell lines

A venous blood sample from each individual can be used for immediate extraction of DNA from peripheral blood lymphocytes (Lorenzetti et al., 1995). The rest of the sample may be used in selected cases to obtain EBV-transformed lymphoblastoid cell lines (Anderson & Gusella, 1988). Samples from difficult to reach, very old and seriously ill patients will be considered for establishment of cell lines. Informed consent must be obtained from each individual according to procedures approved by the local Institutional Review Board (IRB). Appropriate ethical guidelines must be followed at each step of such a research, being particularly careful to protect privacy and confidentiality. IRBs will usually indicate and enforce ethical standards, following guidelines established by national agencies.

Genotyping strategies

High heterozygosity DNA polymorphisms of the short tandem repeat (STR) type make the current standard for genetic markers. STRs have been developed by several laboratories and positioned in genetic and physical maps (Dib et al., 1996; Murray et al., 1994; Schuler et al., 1996). Specific marker sets for genome screens have been developed.

Gene mapping is best performed through a multi-step strategy. First, candidate regions may be tested, i.e. chromosomal regions where previous reports have indicated linkage with epilepsy syndromes, or harbouring genes known to cause epilepsy in animal models (Buchalter, 1993), or encoding proteins with a role in neuronal excitability. If no positive result is obtained, a whole genome screen is performed to identify potentially linked regions. A screening set of about 400 markers, spaced around 10 cM, provides a balance of good sensitivity with a relatively limited number of genotypings to perform. Confirmation of linkage and fine mapping is the final phase, when regions where linkage was suggested during the previous phases are re-examined with additional closely spaced markers and linkage is declared if the chosen significance level is reached. The cost-effectiveness of such a multi-step strategy has been established in several studies, as in Elston (1994).

Availability of a facility for automated, high-throughput genotype analysis is undoubtedly a plus, allowing a substantially accelerated gene mapping process. In such a facility, fluorescently-labeled PCR products generated in multiplex reactions can be analysed on an automatic sequencer.

The DNA chip technology may become the standard for genome screens in the near future. It is based on the automated analysis of a relatively large number (about 3,000) of biallelic polymorphisms scattered throughout the genome. Allele-specific oligonucleotides for all polymorphisms form an array on a silicon chip, which is hybridized with fluorescently-labeled PCR products corresponding to a short region surrounding each polymorphism. The hybridization pattern is read by a laser scanner and interpreted by a specialized software. This technology relies on products developed by Affymetrix Inc.

Linkage analysis for mendelian traits

The lod score method (parametric analysis) is the most appropriate for linkage analysis when a single major locus is analysed (Ott, 1985). For mendelian diseases, a lod score of 3 is usually sought to declare linkage, because it is thought to correspond to a 'posterior type 1 error probability' (or genome-wide significance) of about 0.05. In lod score analyses in humans with a dense map of markers, however, a lod score of 3.3 is probably necessary to obtain to a genome-wide significance level of 0.05 (Lander & Kruglyak, 1995).

Parametric analysis by definition needs the adoption of a model of inheritance for a disease locus contributing to the trait under study. Most families with apparently mendelian inheritance of partial epilepsy show dominant inheritance, although in some cases recessive inheritance appears likely. Given the high frequency of epilepsy, particularly when dealing with families with 'common' phenotypes, allowance must be given to the possibility that some affected individuals may not carry the risk genotype and conversely that some unaffected individuals may carry the risk genotype. This directly relates to the above described phenomena of genetic heterogeneity, variable expressivity and reduced penetrance. With an actual data set, several models may be attempted. However, this has been shown to lead to lod score inflation and increased false-positive rate (Weeks *et al.*, 1990). A sensible way to deal with this possibility is to correct the required significance level to declare linkage. If each model is considered an independent test, according to the Bonferroni correction the significance level should be multiplied by the number of models used for the analysis (k), which corresponds to increase the required lod score by $\log_{10} k$. This is perhaps an excessive caution, as the different models may not be really independent tests. Apart from this correction for multiple modeling, the use of a paramaterization of the disease locus that is 'unreal' does not appear to increase the false positive rate (Clerget-Darpoux *et al.*, 1986), but only reduces power and leads to overestimation of the recombination fraction. According to some authors (Greenberg, 1989; Greenberg & Berger, 1994) the model that becomes the most powerful in the analysis is the one closest to the actual mode of inheritance of the examined disease locus.

Genetic heterogeneity generates contrasting results in the mapping study. In addition to concentrating on large families, each of sufficient size to detect linkage when separately analysed, some statistical approaches can be utilized to evaluate linkage in the presence of heterogeneity, even if only smaller families are available. Obviously, for any test to reach statistical significance the number of families must be large enough, depending on the degree of heterogeneity (more families are needed as the number of loci increases). Genetic heterogeneity may be analysed using the A-test (Smith, 1963), which is easily performed and is implemented in the generally available HOMOG programme and its variants. HOMOG provides a likelihood ratio for linkage and linkage with heterogeneity vs. no linkage, which can be interpreted in terms of significance to the corresponding lod score, considering that an additional parameter (a, the fraction of families linked to a particular locus) is being estimated and therefore the critical level should be increased by $\log_{10} 2$. It also provides a maximum likelihood estimate of α and of θ (recombination fraction) for the linked families. The M-test is a different type of test that can be used when families that can be classified into distinct groups on the basis of some characteristics before performing the homogeneity analysis.

The goal of linkage analysis is to identify a minimum genetic region between flanking markers. These are identified as recombination boundaries. The problem is that often, because of the limited number of available meioses, the analysis of crossing-overs does not allow narrowing down of a candidate region to less than several centimorgans, i.e. several millions of base pairs of genomic DNA, which may harbour hundreds of genes. Even if direct recombination information is limited, when several families showing linkage to the same locus are found, a powerful method of pinpointing the location of the disease gene may be association (linkage disequilibrium) analysis, particularly if the families share a common ethnic background. Linkage disequilibrium is established when: (a) few ancestral mutations account for most of the disease-causing alleles in a population; and (b) the associated marker allele was present on one ancestral chromosome where a mutation arose at a very closely linked locus. If linkage disequilibrium is present, families segregating the same mutation inherited from a distant, common ancestor (founder), will share the same haplotype for the most closely linked markers. The shared haplotype will extend for a much narrower interval than the minimum genetic region established by direct recombination analysis, because it will include only markers that have not recombined through all the meioses connecting to the founder. The chances for fine mapping will therefore depend on how many of the investigated families share mutations at the same loci, and how many represent unique or very rare cases. Even if traits are mapped to relatively broad chromosomal regions, this will not necessarily prevent the successful identification of the corresponding genes within a reasonable time frame. The positional candidate approach, described below, offers the best chances in such cases.

Linkage analysis when polygenic inheritance is suspected

Polygenic inheritance is suspected for some forms of idiopathic partial epilepsy, particularly some common paediatric syndromes such as benign childhood epilepsy with centro-temporal spikes (BCECTS). One approach that can be attempted in these cases is the above mentioned possibility of trying to identify simpler components, such as an associated EEG trait, possibly showing mendelian inheritance. However, the final goal is to identify all components of the genetic susceptibility to the type of epilepsy under study. The above described lod score analysis can be utilized also when polygenic inheritance is suspected. Clearly, the model will be 'unrealistic', because the disease is in reality the consequence of several interacting genetic variants at different loci. However, the effect of these additional genetic loci can be considered as acting on the penetrance of the locus being examined and on the probability of showing an affected phenotype without carrying a mutation in this locus (i.e. of being a phenocopy). Decreased penetrance will reflect the necessity of having inherited additional genetic risk factors in order to express the phenotype, the phenocopy probability will reflect the possibility that a sufficient load of other genetic risk factors may suffice to produce phenotypic consequences. In this perspective, multifactoriality is also taken into account, because the same effect on penetrance and phenocopy frequency will be exerted by non-genetic risk factors that may intervene. The opinion of the author of this chapter is therefore that lod score analysis has a role and should be attempted even when polygenic inheritance seems likely. Clearly, its power will be lower than in the case of mendelian inheritance, but it can still be quite good. Other approaches can however be utilized to analyse linkage of polygenic traits. These methods do not require the assumption of a mode of inheritance for the disease, and are therefore called model-free or non-parametric. They are based on the statistical evaluation of the sharing of genomic regions (as identified by marker alleles) between pairs of affected relatives. The methods are aimed at identifying genomic regions that are more frequently shared by affected relatives than it would be expected on a random basis, and are therefore expected to contain genes that increase the risk of disease. Affected sib-pairs are mostly utilized. In the absence of linkage, the proportions of affected sib pairs sharing 0, 1 and 2 alleles at a marker locus are expected to be respectively 0.25, 0.5 and 0.25. If linkage is present the proportion of affected sib pairs sharing 0 alleles identical by descent will decrease. This decrease (δ) will be a function of the contribution of the locus to the phenotype (λ_S) and of the recombination fraction θ between the marker and the disease locus:

$$\delta = [0.25 - \theta(1-\theta)](\lambda_S -1)/\lambda_S \quad \text{(Risch, 1990b).}$$

A maximum likelihood approach for performing sib pair analysis that can utilize information from partially informative pairs and that can be extended to other relative pairs has been proposed by Risch (1990b, c) and modified by Holmans (1993). It derives a 'maximum lod score' (MLS) statistic. Lander & Kruglyak (1995), considering sib-pair analysis conducted using the Holmans method, calculated that an MLS of 3.6, corresponding to a point P value of 2.2×10^{-5}, corresponds to a genome-wide P of 0.05, and is therefore sufficient to declare linkage. The problem is that, in practical terms, a very large number of sib pairs is necessary to reach such an MLS if the effect of the contributing locus is minor, while, if the contribution is major, it can probably be detected also by parametric lod score analysis. Experience in other complex, polygenic diseases, such as insulin-dependent diabetes mellitus (IDDM) and multiple sclerosis seems to indicate that, by doing genome screens with about a hundred affected sib-pairs, it is relatively easy to identify major loci (such as HLA in IDDM), but then one is left with many minor MLS peaks, whose interpretation is bound to remain difficult (real or false positive?) unless much larger samples are analysed. The other problem is that, despite progresses in multipoint non-parametric mapping, it is very difficult with non-parametric methods to pinpoint a small candidate region on which to concentrate the subsequent cloning efforts, so the method is effective only if it indicates a chromosomal region where an *a priori* candidate gene is localized.

Cloning and analysis of candidate genes

Positional candidate genes

A positional candidate gene is a known gene localized to a linked chromosomal region and thought to be a candidate for the trait under study because of its function and/or pattern of expression. In the case of idiopathic partial epilepsy or of a focal EEG trait, a mutation in such a gene is expected to affect specific brain circuits (frontal, temporal, occipital) making them liable to episodes of hyperexcitation and hypersynchronization. Of course, multiple systems may be affected. Genes encoding ion channels are of particular interest, because they directly control neuronal excitability. It is remarkable that both human idiopathic epilepsy syndromes whose genetic basis is known (ADNFLE and BFNC) are channelopathies, even though one is focal and one is generalized. Also some mouse mutants with epilepsy have ion channel abnormalities. Other types of genes may be good candidates, e.g. those whose knock-out in the mouse induces recurring seizures. In addition to ion channels (Brusa et al., 1995; Patil et al., 1995; Fletcher et al., 1996; Burgess et al., 1997) these include neurotransmitters, receptors and transporters (Tecott et al., 1995; Erickson et al., 1996; Matsumoto et al., 1996; Tanaka et al., 1997), synaptic terminal proteins (Rosahl et al., 1995), and calcium-activated kinases (Butler et al., 1995). The definition of idiopathic epilepsy excludes any case with a structural brain lesion, suggesting that the involved genes should cause purely functional disturbances. However, the interdependence of structure and function in the nervous system and its plasticity make it difficult to exclude the possibility that subtle structural abnormalities may occur in idiopathic epilepsy. Advanced imaging techniques are revealing the presence of limited dysplastic lesions corresponding to the epileptic focus in many patients with partial epilepsies and no other neurological symptom, and some evidence of abnormally migrated neurons has been reported even in individuals with an IGE phenotype. Abnormalities of molecules involved in neuronal function may lead to changes in structure, as much as abnormalities of structurally important molecules may lead to abnormal neural function. Therefore, genes with a more 'structural' function, such as those encoding molecules that regulate neuronal migration or the establishment of circuits might as well, when mutated, cause subtle abnormalities that manifest only with epilepsy, or even only with an abnormal EEG, and should be included among the candidate genes for idiopathic types of epilepsy. Another category of candidates may include transcriptional regulators, which may affect the proper expression of sets of neural genes in terms of timing, level and spatial distribution.

Physical mapping of the region of interest and isolation of new genes

A search for new genes becomes necessary when linkage or linkage disequilibrium analysis point to a sufficiently narrow genomic region where no *a priori* candidate gene is mapped, or, if one such gene is present, its direct analysis has not yielded significant evidence of involvement in the disease. The availability of integrated physical/genetic maps for human chromosomes, containing contigs of yeast artificial chromosomes (YACs), bacterial artificial chromosomes (BACs), or P1 artificial chromosomes (PACs), anchored to the polymorphic markers used for linkage analysis has greatly accelerated identifications of clones covering the regions of interest (Chumakov et al., 1995). The availability of genomic clones in different vectors ensures a better coverage of the genomic region of interest, which may be more stable in one vector then in others. The huge effort to isolate and analyse genes from large contigs of genomic clones, is being greatly facilitated by the ever increasing availability of expressed sequence tags (ESTs). These are sequences from transcribed genes that are stored in a public database. Mapping of ESTs to the chromosomal regions where their respective genes are localized is now well under way, so a number of ESTs will be found in any genomic contig, indicating where transcribed genes are localized and providing some sequence information. Although it is reasonable to assume that epilepsy-related genes have to be transcribed in the brain, it is not unlikely that some genes may be expressed at sufficient levels only during a precise developmental time window.

Evaluation of candidate genes

When a candidate gene is identified, the demonstration of its involvement in the disease phenotype relies on the identification of mutations that are specifically associated with the disease phenotype. The predicted functional consequences of a sequence variation should differentiate a mutation with phenotypic effect (as expected for a gene determining a mendelian trait) from a simple polymorphism. Nevertheless, analysis of non-affected controls is necessary to exclude common polymorphisms. Eventually, the involvement of a candidate gene may be proven by gene addition or gene knockout experiments in animals, and these experiments may turn out to be extremely sensitive to the genetic background of the utilized strain.

Results of molecular genetic research in idiopathic epilepsy

So far, almost all successful molecular genetic research on epilepsy has focused on syndromes or EEG traits showing mendelian inheritance.

Among the IGE, autosomal dominant benign familial neonatal convulsions (BFNC), the IGE subtype with earliest onset, have been demonstrated to be genetically heterogeneous with a fraction of families showing linkage to chromosome 20q (Leppert *et al.*, 1989; Malafosse *et al.*, 1990) (locus EBN1), another fraction of families showing linkage to chromosome 8q (Lewis *et al.*, 1993) (locus EBN2), and some families not linked to either EBN1 or 2 (Lewis *et al.*, 1996). Very recently, both EBN1 and EBN2 have been shown to harbour potassium channel genes that are mutated in BFNC (Biervert *et al.*, 1998; Singh *et al.*, 1998; Charlier *et al.*, 1998). It is thought that defects in these K^+ channels interfere with repolarization and lead to enhanced neuronal excitability. The reasons for the ictal nature and age specificity of the ensuing phenotype are still unknown. From a methodological point of view, it is relevant to note that, after EBN1 was found to encode a K^+ channel gene, the EBN2 gene was promptly identified by looking for a related gene on chromosome 8q (Charlier *et al.*, 1998). Families segregating common subtypes of IGE have also been studied by linkage analysis with the hope of finding a major determining gene. Linkage between juvenile myoclonic epilepsy (JME), one of the most common types of IGE, and markers on the short arm of chromosome 6 (Greenberg *et al.*, 1988) has been a matter of dispute for several years, with studies confirming (Weissbecker *et al.*, 1991; Durner *et al.*, 1991) or rejecting (Whitehouse *et al.*, 1993; Elmslie *et al.*, 1996) the proposed localization. Analysis of a single large family with GSW associated with JME in some individuals allowed the confirmation of the presence of a locus on 6p (Liu *et al.*, 1995). The conflicting findings about the 6p locus are most likely due to genetic heterogeneity of JME, including the complex inheritance of most cases. A second JME locus has been recently proposed on chromosome 15q (Elmslie *et al.*, 1997). A preliminary, small-scale study of 11 families with various types of IGE analysed by non-parametric and parametric methods found suggestive evidence for a predisposing locus on chromosome 8q24, near or at EBN2 (Zara *et al.*, 1995). Very recent data (Delgado-Escueta, communicated at the Pan-American Epilepsy Meeting, Buenos Aires, 1997) seem to confirm the existence of an IGE locus on chromosome 8q24, indicating that this chromsomal region is linked to childhood absence epilepsy in a single family segregating this syndrome as an autosomal dominant trait. Recently, we have mapped a peculiar sharp slow-wave EEG trait segregating as an autosomal dominant trait in a single Italian family with IGE to chromosome 3p14 (Zara *et al.*, 1998).

Febrile convulsions (FC) are a genetically heterogeneous, most commonly multifactorial trait, which is found with increased frequency in individuals with IGE or with temporal lobe epilepsy (McLachlan, 1995; Abou-Khalil *et al.*, 1993), possibly for different reasons (common genetic background with IGE, predisposing factor for temporal lobe epilepsy). Again the analysis of extended families with mendelian segregation has allowed the identification of two chromosomal regions linked to FC, one on chromosome 8q13-q21 (Wallace *et al.*, 1996) and the other on chromosome 19p (Johnson *et al.*, 1998).

More directly relevant to the subject of this book, impressive results have recently been obtained for

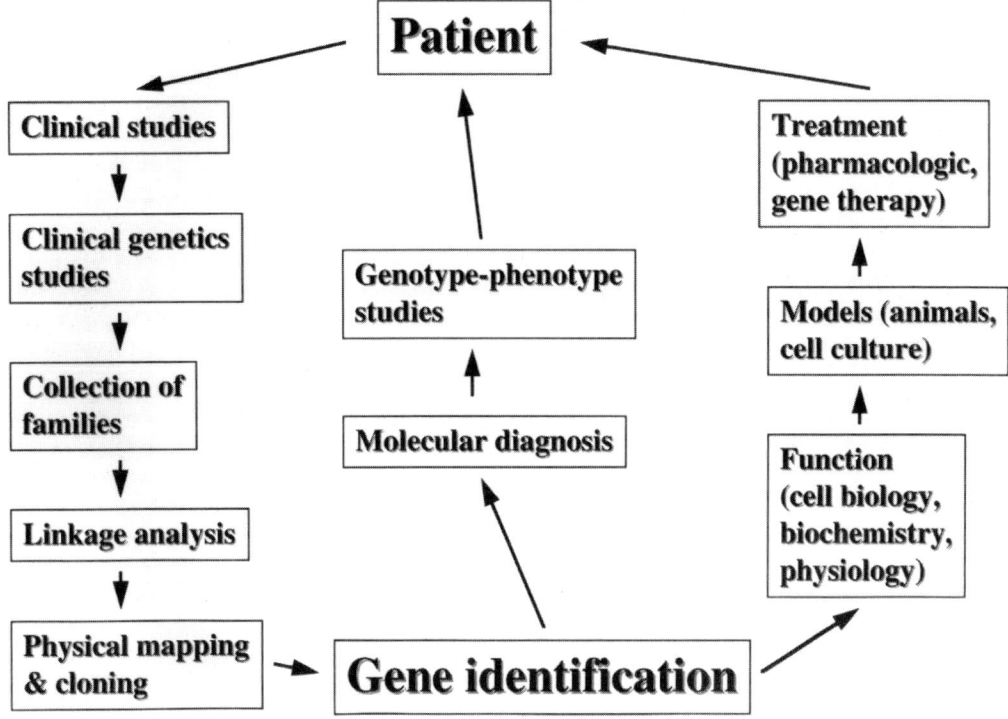

Fig. 1. Overview of the steps involved in molecular genetic research into human inherited diseases.

some mendelian idiopathic partial epilepsy syndromes. Just a brief overview of these results, extensively presented in other chapters, is given here. ADNFLE in an Australian family has been found to be due to a dominant mutation of a gene on chromosome 20q (Phillips et al., 1995). The gene encoding the alpha-4 subunit of the neuronal nicotinic acetylcholine receptor, known to map in that region, was analysed as a candidate and found to be mutated in this family (Steinlein et al., 1995), and subsequently in a Norwegian ADNFLE family (Steinlein et al., 1997). In both cases mutations affecting the lining of the ion channel portion of this receptor subunit were found but, surprisingly, the functional consequences of these mutations, analysed at the single-channel level, seem to be different. Ca^{2+} permeability, conductance, and gating of α4β2 receptors are affected in different and contrasting ways, but the resulting phenotypes are indistinguishable (Kuryatov et al., 1997; Steinlein et al., 1997). Many other families with ADNFLE studied so far do not show linkage to 20q. A rare mendelian form of TLE, partial epilepsy with auditory symptoms, has been mapped to chromosome 10q by analysis of a single large family (Ottman et al., 1995). Benign familial infantile convulsions, which have characteristics of focal epilepsy, have been mapped to chromosome 19 (Guipponi et al., 1997).

Conclusions

Increasing evidence indicates the importance of the genetic background in the aetiology of many cases of focal epilepsy. Several inherited partial epilepsy syndromes have recently been described and are being analysed using the methods of molecular genetics. The first important results have been reached, including the mapping of several genes causing inherited partial epilepsy and the identification of one of them, encoding the alpha-4 subunit of the neuronal nicotinic acetylcholine receptor, which is mutated in some families with autosomal dominant nocturnal frontal lobe epilepsy.

The continuing success of this research requires a close collaboration between clinicians and molecular geneticists. For this collaboration to be effective, each component must have a clear understanding of the research process, with all its problems and difficulties along with the appropriate approaches to deal with them.

Epilepsy is a major health problem because of its frequency, social impact, complex diagnosis, and sometimes difficult treatment. Identifying the genes underlying genetic epilepsy syndromes will have an enormous importance for the progress of our knowledge on normal and abnormal brain function, but in particular will allow new developments in diagnosis and treatment and ultimately have a great impact on patient care.

References

Abou-Khalil, B., Andermann, E., Andermann, F., Olivier, A. & Quesney, L.F. (1993): Temporal lobe epilepsy after prolonged febrile convulsions: excellent outcome after surgical treatment. *Epilepsia* **34,** 878–883.

Andermann, E. (1982): Multifactorial inheritance of generalized and focal epilepsy. In: *Genetic basis of the epilepsies*, Anderson, V.E., Hauser, W.A., Penry, J.K. & Sing, C.F. (eds), pp. 355–374. New York: Raven Press.

Andermann, E., Abou-Khalil, A., Berkovic, S., Javidan, M., Fish, D., Pandolfo, M. & Andermann, F. (1997): Deja-vu is the characteristic aura in benign familial temporal lobe epilepsy. *Epilepsia* **38** (Suppl. 8), 200.

Anderson, M.A. & Gusella, J.F. (1988): *In Vitro* **20,** 856–858.

Ashizawa, T. & Zoghbi, H.Y. (1997): Diseases with trinucleotide repeat expansios. *Curr. Neurol.* **17,** 79–136.

Berkovic, S.F., McIntosh, A., Howell, R.A., Mitchell, A., Sheffield, L.J. & Hopper, J.L. (1996): Familial temporal lobe epilepsy: a common disorder identified in twins. *Ann.. Neurology* **40,** 227–235.

Berkovic, S.F. & Scheffer, I.E. (1997a): Epilepsies with single gene inheritance. *Brain Dev.* **19,** 13–18.

Berkovic, S.F. & Scheffer, I.E. (1997b): Genetics of human partial epilepsy. *Current Opinions in Neurology* **10,** 110–114.

Berkovic, S.F., Howell, R.A., Hay, D.A. & Hopper, J.L. (1998): Epilepsies in twins: genetics of the major epilepsy syndromes. *Ann. Neurol.* **43,** 435–445.

Biervert, C., Schroeder, B.C., Kubisch, C., Berkovic, S.F., Propping, P., Jentsch, T.J. & Steinlein, O.K. (1998): A potassium channel mutation in neonatal human epilepsy. *Science* **279,** 403–406.

Brusa, R., Zimmermann, F., Koh, D.S., Feldmeyer, D., Gass, P., Seeburg, P.H. & Sprengel, R. (1995): Early-onset epilepsy and postnatal lethality associated with an editing-deficient GluR-B allele in mice. *Science* **270,** 1677–1680.

Buchalter, J.R. (1993): Animal models of inherited epilepsy. *Epilepsia* **34** (Suppl.), 31–41.

Burgess, D.L., Jones, J.M., Meisler, M.H. & Noebels, J.L. (1997): Mutation of the Ca^{2+} channel beta subunit gene Cchb4 is associated with ataxia and seizures in the lethargic (lh) mouse. *Cell* **88,** 385–392.

Butler, L.S., Silva, A.J., Abeliovich, A., Watanabe, Y., Tonegawa, S. & McNamara, J. (1995): Limbic epilepsy in transgenic mice carrying a Ca^{2+}/calmodulin-dependent kinase II alpha-subunit mutation. *Proceedings of the National Academy of Sciences U S A* **92,** 6852–6855.

Cendes, F., Lopes-Cendes, I., Andermann, E. & Andermann, F. (1998): Familial temporal lobe epilepsy: a clinically heterogeneous syndrome. *Neurology* **50,** 554–557.

Charlier, C., Singh, N.A., Ryan, S.G., Lewis, T.B., Reus, B.E., Leach, R.J. & Leppert, M. (1998): A pore mutation in a novel KQT-like potassium channel gene in an idiopathic epilepsy family. *Nat. Genet.* **18,** 53–55.

Chumakov, I.M., Rigault, P., Le Gall, I., Bellanné-Chantelot, C., Billault, A., Guillou, ?., Soularue, P., Guasconi G., Poullier, E., Gros, I., Belova, M., Sambucy, L., Susini, L., Gervy, P., Glibert, F., Beaufils, S., Bui, H., Massart, C., De Tand, F., Dukasz, F., Lecoulant, S., Ougen, P., Perrot, V., Saumier, M., Soravito, A., Bahouayila, R., Cohen-Akenine, A., Barilot, E., Bertrand, S., Codani, J.-J., Caterina, D., Georges, I., Lacroix, B., Lucotte, G., Sahbatou, M., Schmit, C., Sangouard, M., Tubacher, E., Dib, C., Fauré, S., Fizames, C., Gyapay, G., Millasseau, P., Nguyen, S., Muselet, D., Vignal, A., Morrissette, J., Menninger, J., Lieman, J., Desai, ?.?., Banks, A., Bray-Ward, P., Ward, D., Hudson, T., Gerety, S., Foote, S., Stein, L., Page, D.C., Lander, E.S., Weissenbach, J., Le Paslier, D. & Cohen, D. (1995): A YAC contig map of the human genome. *Nature* **377,** Supp., 175–183.

Clerget-Darpoux, F., Bonaiti-Pellié, C. & Hochez, J. (1986): Effects of misspecifying genetic parameters in lod score analysis. *Biometrics* **42**, 393–399.

Commission on Classification and Terminology of the International League Against Epilepsy (1989): Proposal for revised classification of epilepsies and epileptic syndromes. *Epilepsia* **30**, 389–399.

Davies, S.W., Beardsall, K., Turmaine, M., DiFiglia, M., Aronin, N. & Bates, G.P. (1998): Are neuronal intranuclear inclusions the common neuropathology of triplet-repeat disorders with polyglutamine-repeat expansions? *Lancet* **351**, 131–133.

DeLorenzo, R.J. (1991): The epilepsies. In: *Neurology in Clinical Practice*, pp. 1443–1478. Bradley, W.G., Daroff, R.B., Fenichel, G.M. & Marsden, C.D. (eds). Boston: Butterworth-Heinemann.

Dib, S., Fauré, C., Fizames, D., Samson, N., Drouot, A., Vignal, P., Millasseau, M., Hazan, J., Seboun, E., Lathrop, M., Gyapay, G., Morrissette, J. & Weissenbach, J. (1996): A comprehensive genetic map of the human genome based on 5,264 microsatellites. *Nature*, **380**, 152–154.

Durner, M., Sander, T. & Greenberg, D.A. (1991): Localisation of idiopathic generalized epilepsy on chromosome 6p in families of juvenile myoclonic epilepsy patients. *Neurology* **41**, 1651–1655.

Elmslie, F.V., Rees, M., Williamson, M.P., Kerr, M., Kjeldsen, M.J., Pang, K.A., Sundqvist, A., Friis, M.L., Chadwick, D., Richens, A., Covanis, A., Santos, M., Arzimanoglou, A., Panayiotopoulos, C.P., Curtis, D., Whitehouse, W.P. & Gardiner, R.M. (1997): Genetic mapping of a major susceptibility locus for juvenile myoclonic epilepsy on chromosome 15q. *Hum. Mol. Genet.* **6**, 1329–1334.

Elmslie, F.V., Williamson, M.P., Rees, M., Kerr, M., Kjeldsen, M.J., Pang, K.A., Sundqvist, A., Friis, M.L., Richens, A., Chadwick, D., Whitehouse, W.P. & Gardiner, R.M. (1996): Linkage analysis of juvenile myoclonic epilepsy and microsatellite loci spanning 61 cM of human chromosome 6p in 19 nuclear pedigrees provides no evidence for a susceptibility locus in this region. *Am. J. Hum. Genet.* **59**, 653–663.

Elston, R.C. (1994): P values, power, and pitfalls in the linkage analysis of psychiatric disorders. In: *Genetic approaches to mental disorders*, Gershon, E.S. & Cloninger, G.R. (eds), pp. 3–21. Washington (DC), London (England): American Psychiatric Press.

Erickson, J.C., Clegg, K.E. & Palmiter, R.D. (1996): Sensitivity to leptin and susceptibility to seizures of mice lacking neuropeptide Y. *Nature* **381**, 415–421.

Ffrench-Constant, C. (1994): Pathogenesis of multiple sclerosis. *Lancet* **343**, 271–275.

Fletcher, C.F., Lutz, C.M., O'Sullivan, T.N., Shaughnessy, Jr. J.D., Hawkes, R., Frankel, W.N., Copeland, N.G. & Jenkins, N.A. (1996): Absence epilepsy in tottering mutant mice is associated with calcium channel defects. *Cell* **87**, 607–617.

Gedda, L. & Tatarelli, L. (1971): Essential isochronic epilepsy in MZ twin pairs. *Acta Geneticae Medicae et Gemellologiae* **20**, 380–383.

Gomez, M.R. (1997): Phenotypes of the tuberous sclerosis complex with a revision of diagnostic criteria. *Ann. N.Y. Acad. Sci.* **615**, 1–7.

Greenberg, D.A. & Berger, B. (1994): Using lod-score differences to determine mode of inheritance: a simple, robust method even in the presence of heterogeneity and reduced penetrance. *Am. J. Hum. Genet.* **55**, 834–840.

Greenberg, D.A. (1989): Inferring mode of inheritance by comparison of lod scores. *Am. J. Med. Genet.* **34**, 480–486.

Greenberg, D.A., Delgado-Escueta, V.A. & Widelitz, H. (1988): Juvenile myoclonic epilepsy (JME) may be linked to the BF and HLA loci on human chromosome 6. *Am. J. Med. Genet.* **31**, 185–192.

Guipponi, M., Rivier, F., Vigevano, T., Beck, C., Crespel, A., Echema, B., Lucchini, P., Sebastianelli, R., Baldy-Mouliner, M. & Malafosse, A. (1997): Linkage mapping of beingn infantile familial convulsions (BIFC) to chromosome 19q. *Hum. Mol. Genet.* **6**, 473–478.

Holmans, P. (1993): Asymptotic properties of affected-sib-pair linkage analysis. *Am. J. Hum. Genet.* **52**, 362–374.

Jodice, C., Mantuano, E., Veneziano, L., Trettel, F., Sabbadini, G., Calandriello, L., Francia, A., Spadaro, M., Pierelli, F., Salvi, F., Ophoff, R.A., Frants, R.R. & Frontali, M. (1997): Episodic ataxia type 2 (EA2) and spinocerebellar ataxia type 6 (SCA6) due to CAG repeat expansion in the CACNA1A gene on chromosome 19p. *Hum. Mol. Genet.* **6**, 1973–1978.

Johnson, E.W., Dubovsky, J., Rich, S.S., O'Donovan, C.A., Orr, H.T., Anderson, V.E., Gil-Nagel, A., Ahmann, P., Dokken, C.G., Schneider, D.T. & Weber, J.L.(1998): Evidence for a novel gene for familial febrile convulsions, FEB2, linked to chromosome 19p in an extended family from the midwest. *Hum. Mol. Genet.* **7**, 63–68.

Korf, B.R. (1997): Neurocutaneous syndromes: neurofibromatosis 1, neurofibromatosis 2, and tuberous sclerosis. *Curr. Opin. Neurol.* **10**, 131–136.

Kuryatov, A., Gerzanich, V., Nelson, M., Olale, F. & Lindstrom, J. (1997): Mutation causing autosomal dominant nocturnal frontal lobe epilepsy alters Ca^{2+} permeability, conductance, and gating of human alpha4beta2 nicotinic acetylcholine receptors. *Neurosci.* **17**, 9035–9047.

Lander, E.S. & Krugliak, L. (1995): Genetic dissection of complex traits: guidelines for interpreting and reporting linkage results. *Nat. Genet.* **11**, 241–247.

Lennox, W.G. (1960): *Epilepsy and related disorders*, pp. 548–571. Boston: Little and Brown.

Leppert, M., Anderson, V.E. & Quattlebaum, T. (1989): Benign familial neonatal convulsions linked to genetic markers on chromosome 20. *Nature* **337**, 647–648.

Lewis, T.B., Shevell, M.I., Andermann, E., Ryan, S.C. & Leach, R.J. (1996): Evidence of a third locus for benign familial convulsions. *J. Child Neurol.* **11**, 211–214.

Lewis, T.B., Leach, R.J. & Ward, K. (1993): Genetic heterogeneity in benign familial neonatal convulsions: identification of a new locus on chromosome 8q. *Am. J. Hum. Genet.* **53**, 670–675.

Liu, A.W., Delgado-Escueta, A.V., Serratosa, J.M., Alonso, E., Medina, M.T., Gee, M.N. & Cordova, S. (1995): Juvenile myoclonic epilepsy locus in chromosome 6p21.1-p11: linkage to convulsions and electroencephalography trait. *Am. J. Hum. Genet.* **57**, 368–381.

Lorenzetti, D., Pareyson, D., Sghirlanzoni, A., Roa, B.B., Abbas, N.E., Scaioli, V., Pandolfo, M., Di Donato, S. & Lupski, J.R. (1995): A 1.5 Mb submicroscopic deletion in 17p11.2-p12 is frequently observed in Italian families with hereditary neuropathy with liability to pressure palsies. *Am. J. Hum. Genet.* **56**, 91–98.

Malafosse, A., Dulac, O. & Leboyer, M. (1990): Linkage studies of benign familial neonatal convulsions in six French families. *Epilepsia* **31**, 816.

Matsumoto, M., Nakagawa, T., Inoue, T., Nagata, E., Tanaka, K., Takano, H., Minowa, O, Kuno, J., Sakakibara, S., Yamada, M., Yoneshima, H., Miyawaki, A., Fukuuchi, Y., Furuichi, T., Okano, H., Mikoshiba, K. & Noda, T. (1996): Ataxia and epileptic seizures in mice lacking type 1 inositol 1,4,5-trisphosphate receptor. *Nature* **379**, 168–171.

McLachlan, M.J. (1995): Febrile convulsions. Is seizure duration the most important predictor of temporal lobe epilepsy? *Brain* **118**, 1521–1528.

Meisler, M.H., Sprunger, L.K., Plummer, N.W., Escayg, A. & Jones, J.M. (1997): Ion channel mutations in mouse models of inherited neurological disease. *Ann. Med.* **29**, 569–574.

Metrakos, J.D. & Metrakos, K. (1972): Genetic factors in the epilepsies. In: *The epidemiology of epilepsy*, Alter M. & Hauser, W.A. (eds), pp. 97–107. Bethesda, DHEW Publication NO. 73–390.

Murray, J.C., Bluetow, K.H., Weber, J.L., Ludwigsen S., Scherpbier-Heddema, T., Manion, F., Quillen, J., Sheffield, V.C., Sunden, S., Duyk, G.M., Weissenbach, J., Gyapay, G., Dib, C., Morissette, J., Lathrop, G.M., Vignal, A., White, R., Matsunami, N., Gerken, S., Melis, R., Albertsen, H., Plaetke, R., Odelberg, S., Ward, R., Dausset, J., Cohen, D. & Cann, H. (1994): A comprehensive human linkage map with centimorgan density. *Science* **265**, 2049–2054.

Nayrac, P. & Beaussart, M. (1958): Les pointe-ondes prérolandiques: expression EEG très particulière. *Rev. Neurol.* **99**, 201–206.

Ophoff, R.A., Terwindt, G.M., Vergouwe, M.N., van Eijk, R., Oefner, P.J., Hoffman, S.M., Lamerdin, J.E., Mohrenweiser, H.W., Bulman, D.E., Ferrari, M., Haan, J., Lindhout, D., van Ommen, G.J., Hofker, M.H., Ferrari, M.D. & Frants, R.R. (1996): Familial hemiplegic migraine and episodic ataxia type-2 are caused by mutations in the Ca^{2+} channel gene CACNL1A4. *Cell* **87**, 543–552.

Ott, J. (1985): *Analysis of human genetic linkage*. Baltimore: John Hopkins University Press.

Ottman, R., Risch, N., Hauser, W.A., Pedley, T.A., Lee, J.H., Barker-Cummings, C., Lustenberger, A., Nagle, K.J., Lee, K.S., Scheuer, M.L., Neystat, M., Susser, M. & Wilhelmsen, K.C. (1995): Localization of a gene for partial epilepsy to chromosome 10q. *Nat. Genet.* **10**, 56–60.

Patil, N., Cox, D.R., Bhat, D., Faham, M., Myers, R.M. & Peterson, A.S. (1995): A potassium channel mutation in weaver mice implicates membrane excitability in granule cell differentiation. *Nat. Genet.* **11**, 126–129.

Pedley, T.A. (1991): The use and role of EEG in the genetic analysis of epilepsy. In: *Genetic strategies in epilepsy research*, Anderson, V.E., Hauser, W.A., Leppik, I.E., Noebels, J.L. & Rich, S.S. (eds), pp. 31–44. Amsterdam: Elsevier.

Phillips, H.A., Scheffer, I.E., Berkovic, S.F., Hollway, G.E., Sutherland, G.R. & Mulley, J.C. (1995): Localization of a gene for autosomal dominant nocturnal frontal lobe epilepsy to chromosome 20q 13.2. *Nat. Genet.* **10**, 117–118.

Risch, N. (1990a): Linkage strategies for genetically complex traits. I. Multilocus models. *Am. J. Hum. Genet.* **46**, 222–228.

Risch, N. (1990b): Linkage strategies for genetically complex traits. II. The power of affected relative pairs. *Am. J. Hum. Genet.* **46**, 229–241.

Risch, N. (1990c): Linkage strategies for genetically complex traits. III. The effect of marker polymorphisms on analysis of affected relative pairs. *Am. J. Hum. Genet.* **46**, 242–253.

Rivaud-Pechoux, S., Durr, A., Gaymard, B., Cancel, G., Ploner, C.J., Agid, Y., Brice, A. & Pierrot-Deseilligny, C. (1998): Eye movement abnormalities correlate with genotype in autosomal dominant cerebellar ataxia type I. *Ann. Neurol.* **43**, 297–302.

Rosahl, T.W., Spillane, D., Missler, M., Herz, J., Selig, D.K., Wolff, J.R., Hammer, R.E., Malenka, R.C. & Sudhof, T.C. (1995): Essential functions of synapsins I and II in synaptic vesicle regulation. *Nature* **375**, 488–493.

Ryan, S. (1995): Partial epilesy: chinks in the armour. *Nat. Genet.* **10**, 4–5.

Scheffer, I.E., Bhatia, K.P., Lopes-Cendes, I., Fish, D.R., Marsden, C.D., Andermann, F., Andermann, E., Desbiens, R., Cendes, F., Manson, J.I., Constantinou, J.E.C., McIntosh, A. & Berkovic, S.F. (1994): Autosomal dominant frontal epilepsy misdiagnosed as sleep disorder. *Lancet* **343**, 515–517.

Scheffer, I.E., Jones, L., Pozzebon, M., Howell, R.A., Saling, M.M & Berkovic, S.F. (1995): Autosomal dominant rolandic epilepsy and speech dyspraxia: a new syndrome with anticipation. *Ann.. Neurol.* **38**, 633–42.

Scheffer, I.E., Bathia, K.P., Lopez-Cendes, I., Fish, D.R., Marsden, C.D., Andermann, E., Andermann, F., Debien, R., Keene, D., Cendes, F., Manson, J.A., Constantinou, J.E.C., McIntosh, A. & Berkovic, S.F. (1995): Autosomal dominant nocturnal frontal lobe epilepsy: a distinctive clinical disorder. *Brain* **118**, 61–73.

Scherer, S.S. (1997): Molecular genetics of demyelination: new wrinkles on an old membrane. *Neuron* **18**, 13–16.

Schuler, D., Boguski, M.S., Stewart, E.A., Stein, L.D., Gyapay, G., Rice, K., White, ?., Rodriguez-Tome', P., Aggarwal, A., Bajorek, E., Bentolila, S., Birren, ?., Butler, A., Castle, A.B., Chiannilkulchai, N., Chu, A., Clee, C., Cowles, S., Day, P.J.R., Dibling, T., Drouot, N., Dunham, I., Duprat, S., East, C., Edwards, C., Fan, J.-B., Fang, N., Fizames, C., Garrett, C., Green, L., Hadley, D., Harris, M., Harrison, P., Brady, S., Hicks, A., Holloway, E., Hui, L., Hussain, S., Louis-Dit-Sully, C., Ma, J., MacGilvery, A., Mader, C., Maratukulam, A., Matise, T.C., McKusick, K.B., Morissette, J., Mungall, A., Muselet, D., Nusbaum, H.C., Page, D.C., Peck, A., Perkins, S., Piercy, M., Qin, F., Quackenbush, J., Ranby, S., Reif, T., Rozen, S., Sanders, C., She, X., Silva, J., Slonim, D.K., Soderlund, C., Sun, W.-L., Tabar, P., Thangarajah, T., Vega-Czarny, D. Vollrath, S. Voyticky, T. Wilmer, X. Wu, M.D. Adams, C. Auffray, N.A.R. Walter, R. Brandon, N., Dehejia, A., Goodfellow, P.N., Houlgatte, R., Hudson, J.R. Jr., Ide, S.E., Iorio. K.R., Lee, W.Y., Seki, N., Nagase, T., Ishikawa, K., Nomura, N., Phillips, C., Polymeropoulos, M.H., Sandusky, M., Schmitt, K., Berry, R., Swanson, K., Torres, R., Venter, J.C., Sikela, J.M., Beckmann, J.S., Weissenbach, J., Myers, R.M., Cox, D.R., James, M.R., Bentley, D., Deloukas, P., Lander, E.S. & Hudson, T.J. (1996): A Gene Map of the Human Genome. *Science* **274**, 540–546.

Singh, N.A., Charlier, C., Stauffer, D., Dupont, B.R., Leach, R.J., Melis, R., Ronen, G.M., Bjerre, I., Quattlebaum, T., Murphy, J.V., McHarg, M.L., Gagnon, D., Rosales, T.O., Peiffer, A., Anderson, V.E. & Leppert, M. (1998): A novel potassium channel gene, KCNQ2, is mutated in an inherited epilepsy of newborns. *Nat. Genet.* **18**, 25–29.

Smith, C.A.B. (1963): Testing for heterogeneity of recombination fraction values in human genetics. *Ann. Hum. Genet.* **27**, 175–182.

Steinlein, O.K., Magnusson, A., Stoodt, J., Bertrand, S., Weiland, S., Berkovic, S.F., Nakken, K.O., Propping, P. & Bertrand, D. (1997): An insertion mutation of the CHRNA4 gene in a family with autosomal dominant nocturnal frontal lobe epilepsy. *Hum. Mol. Genet.* **6**, 943–947.

Steinlein, O.K., Mulley, J.C., Propping, P., Wallace, R.H., Phillips, H.A., Sutherland, G.R., Scheffer, I.E. & Berkovic, S.F. (1995): A missense mutation in the neuronal nicotinic acetylcholine receptor alpha 4 subunit is associated with autosomal dominant nocturnal frontal lobe epilepsy. *Nat. Genet.* **11**, 201–203.

Tanaka, K., Watase, K., Manabe, T., Yamada, K., Watanabe, M., Takahashi, K., Iwama, H., Nishikawa, T., Ichihara, N., Kikuchi, T., Okuyama, S., Kawashima, N., Hori, S., Takimoto, M. & Wada, K. (1997): Epilepsy and exacerbation of brain injury in mice lacking the glutamate transporter GLT-1. *Science* **276**, 1699–1702.

Tecott, L.H., Sun, L.M., Akana, S.F., Strack, A.M., Lowenstein, D.H., Dallman, M.F. & Julius, D. (1995): Eating disorder and epilepsy in mice lacking 5-HT2c serotonin receptors. *Nature* **374**, 542–546.

Terwindt, G.M., Ophoff, R.A., Haan, J., Vergouwe, M.N., van Eijk, R., Frants, R.R. & Ferrari, M.D. (1998): Variable clinical expression of mutations in the P/Q-type calcium channel gene in familial hemiplegic migraine. Dutch Migraine Genetics Research Group. *Neurology* **50**, 1105–1110.

Tsai, J.J. (1989): Generalized spike-and-wave paroxysms – subclinical signs of seizure liability in offsprings of patient with epilepsy. In: *Genetics of the epilepsies*, Beck-Mannagetta, G., Anderson, H. Doose, V.E. & Janz, D. (eds), pp. 127–136. Berlin-Heidelberg: Springer-Verlag.

van Slegtenhorst, M., Nellist, M., Nagelkerken, B., Cheadle, J., Snell, R., van den Ouweland, A., Reuser, A., Sampson, J., Halley, D. & van der Sluijs, P. (1998): Interaction between hamartin and tuberin, the TSC1 and TSC2 gene products. *Hum. Mol. Genet.* **7**, 1053–1057.

Wallace, R.H., Berkovic, S.F., Howell, R.A., Sutherland, G.R. & Mulley, J.C. (1996): Suggestion of a major gene for familial febrile convulsions mapping to 8q13–21. *J. Med. Genet.* **33**, 308–312.

Weeks, D.E., Ott, J. & Lathrop, G.M. (1990a): SLINK: a general simulation program for linkage analysis. *Am. J. Hum. Genet.* **47**, A204.

Weeks, D.E., Lehner, T., Squires-Wheeler, E., Kaufmann, C. & Ott, J. (1990b): Measuring the inflation of the lod scores due to its maximisation over model parameter values in human linkage analysis. *Genet. Epidemiol.* **7**, 237–243.

Weissbecker, K.A., Durner, M. & Janz, D. (1991): Confirmation of linkage between juvenile myoclonic epilepsy locus and the HLA region on chromosome 6p. *Am. J. Med. Genet.* **38**, 32–36.

Whitehouse, W.P., Rees, M., Curtis, D., Sundqvist, A., Parker, K., Chung, E., Baralle, D. & Gardiner, R.M. (1993): Linkage analysis of idiopathic generalized epilepsy (IE) and marker loci on chromosome 6p in families of patients with juvenile myoclonic epilepsy: no evidence for an epilepsy locus in the HLA region. *Am. J. Hum. Genet.* **53**, 652–662.

Zara, F., Bianchi, A., Castellotti, B., Di Donato, S., Avanzini, A., Patel, P.I. & Pandolfo, M. (1995): Mapping of genes predisposing to idiopathic generalized epilepsy. *Hum. Mol. Genet.* **4**, 1201–1207.

Zara, F., Labuda, M., Garofalo, P. G., Durisotti, C., Bianchi, A., Castellotti, B., Patel, P.I., Avanzini, G. & Pandolfo, M. (1998): Unusual EEG pattern linked to chromosome 3p in a family with idiopathic generalized epilepsy. *Neurology*, in press

Zhuchenko, O., Bailey, J., Bonnen, P., Ashizawa, T., Stockton, D.W., Amos, C., Dobyns, W.B., Subramony, S.H., Zoghbi, H.Y. & Lee, C.C. (1997): Autosomal dominant cerebellar ataxia (SCA6) associated with small polyglutamine expansions in the alpha 1A-voltage-dependent calcium channel. *Nat. Genet.* **15**, 62–69.

Part II
The idiopathic age-related focal epilepsies

Chapter 4

The genetics of benign childhood epilepsy with centro-temporal spikes

Orvar Eeg-Olofsson

Child Neurology Unit, University Children's Hospital, S–75 1 85 Uppsala, Sweden

Summary

The genetics of BCECTS is considered based on earlier genetic studies on epilepsy in general, and on earlier and recent genetic and incidence studies of the syndrome. It has been suggested that the EEG manifestation of centro-temporal epileptiform activity apparently is inherited as an autosomal dominant trait with age dependent penetrance. When, however, the full syndrome is considered there is definitely no evidence for a specific single gene inheritance. On the contrary, the inheritance probably is multifactorial as are most other epileptic syndromes.

One of the most well-known localization-related epileptic syndromes is benign childhood epilepsy with centro-temporal spikes (BCECTS). According to the International Classification of Epilepsies and Epileptic Syndromes (1989) it is 'a syndrome of brief, simple, partial, hemifacial motor seizures, frequently having associated somatosensory symptoms which have a tendency to evolve into GTCS. Both seizure types are often related to sleep. Onset occurs between the ages of 3 and 13 years (peak 9–10 years), and recovery occurs before the age of 15–16 years. Genetic predisposition is frequent, and there is male predominance. The EEG has blunt high-voltage centro-temporal spikes, often followed by slow waves that are activated by sleep and tend to spread or shift from side to side.' Experience has shown that the seizures can also be of the complex partial type.

The denomination of the syndrome has been variable with a number of other terms used as benign epilepsy of children with centro-temporal EEG foci or benign epilepsy of childhood with centro-temporal spikes (BECCT), benign epilepsy with centro-temporal spikes (BECTS), benign epilepsy of childhood with rolandic spikes (BECRS), benign childhood epilepsy with rolandic spikes (BCERS), benign focal epilepsy of childhood (BFEC), benign partial epilepsy with centro-temporal spikes (BECT), benign epilepsy with rolandic spikes (BERS), benign rolandic epilepsy (BRE), rolandic epilepsy, and sylvian seizures.

Early genetic studies in epilepsy

Long ago, Lennox, Gibbs & Gibbs (1940) reported that EEG changes in connection with epilepsy were inherited as a mendelian dominant trait. A decade later Lennox (1951) reported a higher prevalence of epilepsy in relatives of patients with 'essential' or 'genetic' epilepsy than in relatives of patients with 'symptomatic' or 'acquired' epilepsy, which again was higher than in controls. Lennox concluded 'that in every patient there is a unique combination of genetic and environmental factors interacting to produce the clinical phenotype'. Rimoin & Metrakos (1963) studied children with hemiparesis present from birth or early life, with or without convulsions, and their near relatives as well as controls. They found that relatives of patients with both hemiparesis and convulsions had a higher prevalence of convulsions and epileptiform EEG abnormalities than did relatives of children with hemiparesis without concomitant convulsions. Surprisingly, the last-mentioned group had a lower prevalence of both convulsions and epileptiform EEG abnormalities than did control relatives. Excellent studies of the genetic background of epilepsy were presented by Metrakos & Metrakos (1961). After a report on monozygotic and dizygotic twins, where they found a concordance for epilepsy in 60 and 10 per cent respectively, they reported results on genetic studies in 'centrencephalic' epilepsy. This corresponds to absence epilepsy in the current classification.

A summary of the results showed that siblings and offspring of patients with this form of epilepsy would have a 50 per cent risk of inheriting the gene for the spike-wave EEG trait, a 35 per cent risk of expressing the EEG trait during their lifetime, a 12 per cent risk of having one or more seizures, and an 8 per cent risk of developing absence epilepsy. Thus, the typical '3 Hz spike-wave' EEG pattern was suggested to be an autosomal dominant trait with age dependent penetrance. From these results it is also of importance to consider that several genetic and environmental factors probably must interact with this trait to produce the specific epilepsy.

Genetic studies in focal epilepsy were reported by Andermann (1982). In the families of 60 patients surgically treated for their focal epilepsy it was found that the risk figures for siblings and offspring having an epileptiform EEG was 20 per cent (with maximal expression between 5–14 years), one or more seizures 7 per cent, and 'chronic epilepsy' 4 per cent.

About BCECTS

When describing an epileptic syndrome it is of utmost importance to base the diagnosis and selection of patients upon both the characteristic EEG findings and the clinical seizure manifestations. Unfortunately, this has not always been taken into consideration, especially concerning BCECTS.

EEG

Gastaut (1952) was the first to descibe the EEG features. She noted that the typical prerolandic discharges could not be related to a focal lesion. Bancaud et al. (1958) followed this EEG pattern into puberty and confirmed its vanishing. Gibbs & Gibbs (1960) recognized the distinct mid-temporal spike focus and also mentioned that 'children with mid-temporal spike foci have a far better prognosis than those with anterior temporal lobe spikes'. Further desciptions of the EEG pattern have been presented by Lombroso (1967) and Blom et al. (1972). It must be emphasized that the typical EEG pattern seen in BCECTS in no way is specific for this syndrome. It can be seen in many various disorders (Lerman & Kivity, 1975). The pattern has also been described in 3 per cent of normal 2–13 year old children (Eeg-Olofsson et al., 1971).

Clinical symptoms

After the initial description of the clinical symptoms (Nayrac & Beaussart, 1958), many reports have been published on the topic. The most important reports are those of Lombroso (1967), Blom et al. (1972) and Loiseau & Beaussart (1973) as well as a review article by Lerman (1992). With few exceptions most patients with BCECTS recover before adolescence with disappearance of both clinical manifestations and EEG findings. Because of this apparently good prognosis Blom et al. (1972) proposed the term 'benign epilepsy of children with centro-temporal EEG foci'.

Genetic studies in BCECTS

BCECTS was considered an idiopathic (primary) epileptic syndrome and, thus, there may be a genetic origin. Bray & Wiser (1964, 1965a, b) evaluated the genetic mechanisms in patients with 'temporal-central focal' epilepsy and with epileptiform discharges in the mid-temporal or central regions. They came to the conclusion that the EEG abnormality was inherited as an autosomal dominant trait. However, when scrutinising their material just 19 of their 40 index cases had seizures, which were mainly generalized. The index cases were both children and adults. In the illustrated kindreds just one (kindred 35) fits both clinically and electrographically with BCECTS. The other kindreds consist of both children and adults, and the epileptiform EEG manifestations are mainly temporal. The peak incidence of the EEG abnormalities in relatives of index cases occurred between 6 and 10 years, which is in agreement with findings in BCECTS. It is also of interest that just 12 per cent of all individuals with the EEG trait ever had a seizure. The reports do not describe the total number of index cases and siblings with similarities to BCECTS.

Blom *et al.* (1972) retrospectively studied patients with centro-temporal EEG foci and 'seizures'. Only 40 individuals, who were 15 years old or more at the time of the follow-up, were studied in detail. It is of importance to notice that in the selection of probands only the EEG findings were used regardless of the nature of clinical seizures. Partial seizures only were seen in 12 cases, generalized tonic–clonic seizures only in 15 cases, partial seizures with secondarily generalization in 12 cases, and in one case no information was received. From the general description of seizure manifestations it is difficult to evaluate the number of individuals having the characteristic clinical pattern. A positive family history of seizures during childhood was reported in seven parents and siblings (18 per cent), and a general 'hereditary predisposition' in 40 per cent. The same research group also presented a pure genetic study in BCECTS (Heijbel *et al.*, 1975). Nineteen children with seizures and centro-temporal spikes or sharp waves (rolandic discharges) were selected as probands (in the same way as stated above). In addition 36 of their full parents, and 34 full siblings (32 for EEG) were included. Five siblings (16 per cent) had generalized seizures and rolandic discharges, and six (19 per cent) had rolandic discharges alone. Four parents reported the occurrence of seizures in childhood. One parent without a history of seizures showed rolandic discharges (!). The report concludes that an autosomal dominant gene with age-dependent penetrance is responsible for the EEG trait. This conclusion is similar to that of Bray & Wiser, even if the study groups apparently are not quite comparable.

Degen & Degen (1990) studied the EEGs of 69 siblings of 43 children with rolandic epilepsy and/or centro-temporal spikes. Out of the 43 probands 14 had partial and 22 generalized seizures, while seven did not have seizures but had typical EEG changes. Epileptic discharges were found in 26 (37.7 per cent) of the 69 siblings. Centro-temporal spike foci were found in three siblings, one showed an occipital focus, and the other 22 siblings showed generalized 2.5–4 Hz spike-wave complexes. None of the siblings had rolandic epilepsy while five siblings of three probands had seizures. As most epileptic activity was observed in the group 5–12 years (54.3 per cent) the authors supported the assumption of an autosomal dominant genetic factor for the EEG manifestations.

These three studies suggest that the EEG pattern of centro-temporal spikes or sharp waves apparently is inherited as an autosomal dominant trait with age-dependent penetrance. Thus, the frequently misquoted opinion of autosomal dominance in BCECTS concerns the EEG trait not including the genuine seizure type.

Doose (1989) tried to identify the clinical symptomatology of children with focal sharp waves of genetic nature. A total of 41 probands and their 44 siblings were found showing EEG changes with focal or multifocal sharp waves. Out of 41 probands, 36 had seizures of different types, and strict rolandic seizures occurred in three (8 per cent). The seizures developed between the 1st and 11th year of life in 36 probands (88 per cent). Central or centro-temporal EEG foci were found in nine probands (22 per cent), three of them, as mentioned above, showing the typical seizure manifestations of BCECTS. Out of the 44 siblings, 16 had seizures, six (38 per cent) of them strict rolandic seizures.

Nothing is mentioned concerning the occurrence of centro-temporal EEG manifestations in these siblings. In one kindred the proband had a syndrome with focal seizures, generalized tonic–clonic seizures, atypical absences, and atonic-myoclonic seizures, and the three siblings had rolandic seizures. In three siblings with rolandic seizures the probands respectively had febrile convulsions and rolandic seizures, rolandic seizures, and generalized tonic–clonic seizures. In the same material a history of febrile convulsions was found in 29 per cent of the probands and in 19 per cent of their siblings. The author concludes that the overlap of clinical and/or electrographic symptoms, and the variable clinical symptomatology of partial epilepsies, suggests that disorders that have been delineated as separate clinical entities are manifestations of a single multifaceted aetiopathogenetic complex.

Other clinical data and BCECTS

The relationship between BCECTS, febrile convulsions and migraine headache is of interest from the genetic point of view. Lerman & Kivity (1975) reported an incidence of febrile convulsions in 9 per cent, Doose (1989) in 33 per cent, Degen & Degen (1990) in 19 per cent, and Kajitani et al. (1992) in 18 per cent. In the last-mentioned material a positive family history of febrile convulsions within 3rd degree relatives was found in 48 per cent. These authors also reported that in seven families with a proband with BCECTS and siblings with febrile convulsions, all siblings exhibited rolandic discharges on EEG.

BCECTS, like other seizure disorders, has been associated with a higher than expected incidence of migraine headache. Bladin (1987) reported an association in 66 per cent and a family history of migraine in 70 per cent. However, Blom et al. (1972) noted an occurrence of migraineous headache in only 5 per cent.

The mentioned observations suggest a possible genetic link between BCECTS and febrile convulsions but also with migraine.

Discussion

The diagnosis of BCECTS must be established from both the typical clinical and EEG characteristics. This, however, has not always been practised. It is thus difficult to compare different studies and to delineate the syndrome. Incidence figures have also been drawn from different kinds of epilepsy populations. Lerman & Kivity (1975) in a follow-up study reported an incidence of typical BCECTS in 14.4 per cent. Deonna et al. (1986) found BCECTS to occur in 36 per cent of all neurologically normal children with partial seizures. Heijbel et al. (1975) reported that 11 out of 70 children (15.7 per cent) with their first seizure had seizures with rolandic discharges. However, in a follow-up report (Blom et al., 1978) on 43 children with epilepsy, 11 (25.6 per cent) had 'partial or generalized seizures with rolandic discharges'. This difference is not explained, but the results clearly show that EEG was not performed in three cases, and in three cases the EEG was normalized. In a community-based Swedish prospective incidence study of epileptic seizures in children (Sidenvall et al., 1993) BCECTS was the most common identified epilepsy syndrome, and noticed in 13.6 per cent. In another Swedish population-based study of childhood epilepsy (Braathen & Theorell, 1995), BCECTS defined as 'typical partial seizures and rolandic spikes on the EEG' was found in 11 per cent. When children with rolandic discharges and generalized tonic–clonic seizures were added, the figure increased to 22 per cent (Braathen et al., 1996).

The present review concerning the occurrence of BCECTS shows the difficulties in delineating the syndrome. This has also influenced the genetic considerations. Studies have also shown that it is very difficult to collect families with at least two individuals with BCECTS (Eeg-Olofsson, unpublished results). What apparently is true is the fact that the EEG pattern may be transmitted by an autosomal, dominant gene with age-dependent penetrance. As described above, the occurrence of BCECTS in first-degree relatives is much below the 25–50 per cent expected in single gene (mendelian) traits. The findings indicate that the tendency to have clinical seizures in children who have the typical EEG patterns is actually determined by other multiple aetiological factors such as different genetic and environmenal factors. In this context it is logical to mention the hypothesis on the pathogenesis of temporal lobe epilepsy by Ounsted *et al.* (1966). They suggested that if a child is genetically predisposed to febrile convulsions, 'the convulsions, when they occur, tend to be severe, and in the course of them Ammon's horn is damaged. Sclerosis follows and an epileptogenic lesion arises.' In the report by Andermann (1982) one of the most significant aetiological factors was postnatal infection, and in patients with this factor the highest genetic component (increased frequency of seizures and/or EEG abnormalities in relatives) was found.

The existence of a postnatal infectious mechanism is supported by the studies of Eeg-Olofsson *et al.* (1988) on immune dysfunction in patients with focal temporal lobe epilepsy and their families, as well as studies in Rasmussen encephalitis (Andermann *et al.*, 1991). A lack of the HLA haplotype A1,B8, a decreased mean level of serum IgA, and a low T4/T8 ratio was found. The following hypothesis has been suggested (Eeg-Olofsson *et al.*, 1995): the expression of haplotype A1,B8 is genetically determined. As this haplotype is the most common one in all populations, it is suggested that it must offer some biological advantage in protecting individuals from certain noxious agents, e.g. viruses. The HLA system in general is also of importance for the development and function of T and B Iymphocytes and, thus, also for the generation of immunoglobulins. If a defect of the HLA system exists, there will be no proper antigen(virus) peptide-HLA molecule complex available for the T cell receptor to recognize. The result will be a virus persistence with concomitant effects on the excitatory transmitter system leading to seizure manifestations.

A lack of the HLA haplotype A1,B8 was also found in BCECTS (Eeg-Olofsson *et al.*, 1982). Thus, it is fascinating to speculate that the benign and more malignant localized epilepsies represented by BCECTS and temporal lobe epilepsy respectively, may constitute the two poles in a biological continuum, where the expression of the HLA haplotype Al,B8 may be a main determinant.

The multifactorial pathogenesis in benign partial epilepsies and especially BCECTS was also discussed by Doose & Baier (1989). The occurrence of specific genetic EEG patterns such as 4–7 Hz rhythms, generalized spikes and waves, a photoparoxysmal response, and focal or multifocal sharp waves determine the level of cerebral excitability. The three first-mentioned have probably a polygenetic background, while the last-mentioned may have an autosomal dominant one. Another genetically determined factor of importance for BCECTS is the increased incidence of febrile convulsions. The age dependent symptoms of BCECTS and other benign partial epilepsies with disappearance at puberty justify the assumption of a 'hereditary impairment of brain maturation'. BCECTS is considered a part of a phenotypic spectrum 'with a single, albeit complex, pathogenesis'. The authors really have indicated a critical point in the issue of heredity in BCECTS. There is no indication for a specific single gene inheritance – it apparently is multifactorial. We really need to understand the clinical genetics of BCECTS, as a prelude to molecular studies.

Addendum (August 1998)

Recently a linkage of BCECTS to chromosome 15q14 has been found (Neubauer *et al.*, 1998).

References

Andermann, E. (1982): Multifactorial inheritance of generalized and focal epilepsy. In: *Genetic basis of the epilepsies*, Anderson,V.E. , Hauser, W.A., Penry, J K. & Sing, C.F. (eds). pp. 355–374. New York: Raven Press.

Andermann, E., Oguni, H., Guttmann, R.D., Osterland, K., Antel, J.P., Eeg-Olofsson, O. & Andermann, F. (1991): Genetic aspects of chronic encephalitis. In: *Chronic encephalitis and epilepsy: Rasmussen's syndrome*, F. Andermann (ed.), pp. 167–175. Boston: Butterworth/Heinemann.

Bancaud, J., Collomb, J. & Dell, M.B.(1958): Les pointes rolandiques: un symptôme EEG propre à l'enfant. *Rev. Neurol.* **99**, 206–209.

Beaussart, M. (1972): Benign epilepsy of children with rolandic (centro-temporal) paroxysmal foci. A clinical entity. Study of 221 cases. *Epilepsia* **13**, 795–811.

Bladin, P.F. (1987): The association of benign rolandic epilepsy with migraine. In: *Migraine and epilepsy*, Andermann, F. & Lugaresi, E. (eds), pp. 145–152. Boston: Butterworths.

Blom, S., Heijbel, J. & Bergfors, P.G. (1972): Benign epilepsy of children with centro-temporal EEG foci. Prevalence and follow-up study of 40 patients. *Epilepsia* **13**, 609–619.

Blom, S., Heijbel, J. & Bergfors, P.G. (1978): Incidence of epilepsy in children: a follow-up study three years after the first seizure. *Epilepsia* **19**, 343–350.

Braathen, G. & Theorell, K. (1995): A general hospital population of childhood epilepsy. *Acta Paediatr.* **84**, 1143–1146.

Braathen, G., Andersson, T., Gylje, H., Melander, H., Naglo, A.-S., Noren, L., Persson, A., Rane, A., Sjors, K., Theorell, K. & Wigertz, A. (1996): Comparison between one and three years of treatment in uncomplicated childhood epilepsy: a prospective study. I. Outcome in different seizure types. *Epilepsia* **37**, 822–832.

Bray, P.F. & Wiser, W.C. (1965b): The relation of focal to diffuse epileptiform EEG discharges in genetic epilepsy. *Arch. Neurol.* **13**, 223–237.

Bray, P.F. & Wiser, W.C. (1965a): Hereditary characteristics of familial temporal-central focal epilepsy. *Pediatrics* **36**, 207–211.

Bray, P.F. & Wiser, W.C., (1964): Evidence for a genetic etiology of temporal-central abnormalities in focal epilepsy. *N. Engl. J. Med.* **271**, 926–933.

Commission on Classification and Terminology of the International League Against Epilepsy (1989): Proposal for revised classification of epilesies and epileptic syndromes. *Epilepsia* **30**, 389–399.

Degen, R. & Degen, H.-E. (1990): Some genetic aspects of rolandic epilepsy: waking and sleep EEGs in siblings. *Epilepsia* **31**, 795–801.

Deonna, T., Ziegler, A. L., Despland, P.A. & van Malle, G. (1986): Partial epilepsy in neurologically normal children: clinical syndromes and prognosis. *Epilepsia* **27**, 241–247.

Doose, H. (1989): Symptomatology in children with focal sharp waves of genetic origin. *Eur. J. Pediatr.* **149**, 210–215.

Doose, H. & Baier, W.K. (1989): Benign partial epilespy and related conditions: multifactorial pathogenesis with hereditary impairment of brain maturation. *Eur. J. Pediatr.* **149**, 152–158.

Eeg-Olofsson, O., Petersen, I. & Sellden, U. (1971): The development of the electroencephalogram in normal children from the age of one through 15 years paroxysmal activity. *Neuropediatrics* **2**, 374–404.

Eeg-Olofsson, O., Säfwenberg, J. & Wigertz, A. (1982): HLA and epilepsy: an investigation of different types of epilepsy in children and their families. *Epilepsia* **23**, 27–34.

Eeg-Olofsson, O., Osterland, C. K., Guttmann, R. D., Andermann, F., Prchal, J.F., Andermann, E. & Janjua, N.A. (1988): Immunological studies in focal epilepsy. *Acta Neurol. Scand.* **78**, 358–368.

Eeg-Olofsson, O., Bergstrom, T., Osterland, C.K., Andermann, F & Olivier, A. (1995): Epilepsy etiology with special emphasis on immune dysfunction and neurovirology. *Brain Dev.* **17** (Suppl.), 58–60.

Gastaut, Y. (1952): Un élément déroutant de la séméiologie électroencéphalographique: les points prérolandiques sans signification focale. *Rev. Neurol.* **87**, 488–490.

Gibbs, E.L. & Gibbs, F.A. (1960): Good prognosis of midtemporal epilepsy. *Epilepsia* **1**, 448–453.

Heijbel, J., Blom, S. & Rasmuson, M. (1975): Benign epilepsy of childhood with centro-temporal EEG foci: a genetic study. *Epilepsia* **16**, 285–293.

Heijbel, J., Blom, S., Bergfors, P.G. (1975): Benign epilepsy of children with centro-temporal EEG foci. A study of incidence rate in out-patient care. *Epilepsia* **16**, 657–664.

Kajitani, T., Kimura, T., Sumita, M. & Kaneko, M. (1992): Relationship between benign epilepsy of children with centro-temporal EEG foci and febrile convulsions. *Brain Dev.* **14**, 230–234.

Lennox, W.G. (1951): Heredity of epilepsy as told by relatives and twins. *JAMA* **146**, 529–536.

Lennox, W.G., Gibbs, E.L. & Gibbs, F.A. (1940): Inheritance of cerebral dysrhythmia and epilepsy. *Arch. Neurol. Psvchiat.* **44**, 1155–1183.

Lerman, P. & Kivity, S. (1975): Benign focal epilepsy of childhood. *Arch. Neurol.* **32**, 261–264.

Lerman, P. (1992): Benign partial epilepsy with centro-temporal spikes. In: *Epileptic syndromes in infancy, childhood and adolescence*, Roger, J., Dravet, Ch., Dreifuss, F.E., Perret, A. & Wolf, P. (eds), 2nd edition, pp. 189–200. London: John Libbey.

Loiseau, P. & Beaussart, M. (1973): The seizures of benign childhood epilepsy with rolandic paroxysmal discharges. *Epilepsia* **14**, 381–389.

Lombroso, C.T. (1967): Sylvian seizures and mid-temporal spike foci in children. *Arch. Neurol.* **17**, 52–59.

Metrakos, K. & Metrakos, J.D. (1961): Genetics of convulsive disorders. II. Genetic and electroencephalographic studies in centrencephalic epilepsy. *Neurology* **11**, 474–483.

Nayrac, P. & Beaussart, M. (1958): Les pointes-ondes prérolandiques: expression EEG très particulière. Etude électroclinique de 21 cas. *Rev. Neurol.* **99**, 201–206.

Neubauer, B.A. *et al.* (1998): Centro-temporal spikes in families with rolandic epilepsy: Linkage to chromosome 15q14. *Neurology* (in press).

Ounsted, C., Lindsay, J. & Norman, M. (1966): Biological factors in temporal lobe epilepsy. In: *Clinics in Developmental Medicine 22*. London: The Spastic Society Medical Education and Information Unit in association with W. Heinemann Medical Books Ltd.

Rimoin, D.L. & Metrakos, J.D. (1966): The genetics of convulsive disorders in the families of hemiplegics. In: *Proc. 2nd Intern. Congr. Hum. Genes*, pp. 1655–1658. Rome: Instituto G. Mendel.

Sidenvall, R., Forsgren, L., K:son Blomquist, H. & Heijbel, J. (1993): A community-based prospective incidence study of epileptic seizures in children. *Acta Paediatr.* **82**, 60–65.

Chapter 5

Families with benign childhood epilepsy with centro-temporal spikes

Y.S. Choy[1], C.T. Tan[2] and Asma Omar[3]

[1]*Institute of Pediatrics, Kuala Lumpur Hospital, Malaysia;* [2]*Department of Medicine, University Hospital, Kuala Lumpur, Malaysia;* [3]*Department of Pediatrics, University Hospital, Kuala Lumpur, Malaysia*

Summary

Benign childhood epilepsy with centro-temporal spikes (BCECTS) or benign rolandic epilepsy (BRE) is a common childhood epilepsy with a typical clinical presentation and characteristic electroencephalographic (EEG) manifestations. The EEG trait for centro-temporal foci was thought to be controlled by a single dominant gene with low penetrance and was age dependent (Bray *et al.*, 1964, 1965; Heijbel *et al.*, 1975). Doose *et al.* (1990) hypothesized that the clinical manifestations of the seizure were probably multifactorial in origin with various predisposing factors influencing the expression of the clinical picture.

In a study carried out in University Hospital, Kuala Lumpur, 31 patients with BCECTS and their siblings were studied clinically and electroencephalographically. Only 21 families completed the study. Waking and sleeping EEGs were performed in 44 siblings of these 21 families. Family trees were constructed and analysed. Statistical calculations were made by chi-square test, Fisher Exact test, priori method and estimation of heritability.

Epileptiform activity was recorded in at least one sibling in 14 of 21 families (66.7 per cent) that completed the study. Eighteen of 44 siblings (41.8 per cent) demonstrated epileptic discharges in their EEGs. Five of 44 siblings (11.4 per cent) had classical EEG changes consistent with BECTS and two of them had seizures clinically. 9.3 per cent of siblings had generalized epileptiform discharges and 20.9 per cent of siblings had non-rolandic focal epileptiform discharges. These rates were significantly higher than the rates in the general population. Statistical tests and pedigree analysis suggested that the mode of inheritance was probably multifactorial in origin.

Additionally, BCECTS was found in both individuals in an identical twin pair, but only one twin in another sibship was affected. One family had BCECTS associated with autosomal dominant retinitis pigmentosa.

This study suggests that BCECTS is probably multifactorial in origin. It may be genetically linked to other types of focal epilepsy and even generalized epilepsy. Further molecular studies are necessary to determine the exact genetic factors involved.

Benign childhood epilepsy with centro-temporal spikes (BCECTS) or more commonly known as benign rolandic epilepsy (BRE) is one of the common forms of epilepsy encountered in childhood. It accounts for approximately 15 to 20 per cent of young epileptics under 15 years of age in the western world (Beaussart *et al.*, 1972; Lerman, 1992). There is a male preponderance, with a male to female ratio of 60 : 40. The exact incidence in Malaysia is unknown. However, it is found in 2 per cent of newly diagnosed epilepsy in all age groups and 6 per cent of children less than 15 years old in the University Hospital, Kuala Lumpur according to a recent study by Tan (1995).

The age of onset of seizure in BCECTS is between 3 to 13 years with a mean of 10 years (Lerman *et al.*, 1986). The seizures are usually mild with variable frequencies and they respond well to anticonvulsant therapy. Not all the children with rolandic spikes or centro-temporal spikes in the EEG have seizures. Eeg-Olofson *et al.* in 1971 reported rolandic discharges in 1.2 per cent of healthy children. The prognosis is excellent, as its name implies, even when it is associated with a brain lesion (Santanelli *et al.*, 1989). Complete recovery is the rule in most of the reports (De Romanis *et al.*, 1986; Loisseau *et al.*, 1988; Beaussart, 1981).

BCECTS is considered genetic in origin as there is frequently a family history of epilepsy varying from 17 per cent (Blom *et al.*, 1972) to 59 per cent of cases (Heijbel *et al.*, 1975). Bray & Wiser (1964) first pointed out genetic predisposition of rolandic spikes based on pedigree analysis. They postulated that the EEG trait of rolandic spikes was controlled by a single gene transmitted in an autosomal dominant fashion with low penetrance and strong age dependence. This was later supported by a genetic study by Heijbel & Blom (1975) based on EEG study on siblings and pedigree analysis. The hereditary characteristics were further confirmed by Degen *et al.* (1989). However, they concluded that the clinical manifestations of the seizure could be multifactorial in origin. In the same year Doose & Baier hypothesized that the EEG trait is autosomal dominant with variable age dependent penetrance but the syndrome of BCECTS is likely to be multifactorial in origin.

So far there are no detailed studies on BCECTS in Asian children particularly in terms of genetics. Hence, a study was carried out in 1993/1994 to determine the genetic influence on BECTS in a multiracial Asian population in Malaysia.

Materials & methods

Patients selected for this study were all diagnosed to have BCECTS based on both clinical and electroencephalographic criteria. They were followed-up in the paediatric neurology clinic from 1986 to 1994.

Inclusion criteria

Clinical criteria:

Nocturnal partial or generalized tonic–clonic seizures (GTCS) and/or daytime partial or secondary GTCS with normal developmental milestones and a normal neurological examination.

EEG criteria:

(a) normal background features.
(b) focal monomorphic, di- or tri- phasic sharp waves with blunted peaks (rolandic spikes) localized at T3, T4, C3 or C4 (Fig. 1).
(c) absence of focal slowing.

Exclusion criteria

Patients were excluded from the study if they had a past history of head injury, meningitis, birth asphyxia, kernicterus, metabolic encephalopathy, intrauterine infection or chromosomal abnormalities or any form of cerebral insult.

A total of 31 patients and 44 siblings from 21 families were included in the study. Patients were examined and history of seizures was checked. A detailed family history was obtained by personally interviewing both the parents. All of the study subjects were examined personally by one of the authors (Y.S. Choy) with special attention to neurological status, cognitive and mental functioning.

All the study subjects (patients and siblings) had a waking EEG immediately followed by a sleep EEG (induced by chloral hydrate 50 mg/kg or promazine hydrochloride 1 mg/kg). The waking EEG lasted an average of 40 min and sleep EEG an average of 1 h. Recording of the EEG was made in our neurophysiology lab using 21 channel instruments (San-ei). Electrodes were placed according to the international 10–20 system. Referential, longitudinal bipolar and transverse bipolar montages were employed. Nineteen surface disc electrodes with six other extra electrodes were applied with collodium. A time constant of 0.03 to 0.3 ms and high frequency filter of 120 Hz were used. Paper speed was 30 mm/s.

Data analysis

Family trees were constructed and pedigree analysis was carried out. To correct for the sampling errors (as no normal control population was included) and observation errors on the pedigrees, statistical tests of significance were carried out. The observed distribution of affected and non-affected children were tested against the expected from the autosomal dominant (AD) or autosomal recessive (AR) mode of inheritance as shown in Tables 1 and 2 (priori method of Stein *et al.*). The possibility of multifactorial inheritance was tested according to the theory of quasi-contiuous traits with threshold characteristics by Edwards (1969).

Table 1. Dominant mode of inheritance: 21 sibship; 64 children; q = 1/2

Size of sibship N	No. of sibship X	Expected proportion affected q'	No. affected Expected ($q'NX$)	No. affected Observed
1	2	1/2	1	2
2	5	2/3	6.7	5
3	7	4/7	12	9
4	5	8/15	10.7	7
5	1	16/31	2.6	1
6	1	32/63	3.1	2
		TOTAL	36.1	26

$X^2 = 7.39$; $D = 0.3$ ns.

Table 2. Recessive mode of inheritance: 20 sibship; 60 children; q = 1/4

Size of sibship N	No. of sibship X	Expected proportion affected q'	No. affected Expected ($q'NX$)	No. affected Observed
1	2	1	1	2
2	5	4/7	5.7	5
3	7	16/37	9.08	8
4	5	64/175	5.85	6
5	1	286/781	1.64	1
6	1	1024/3367	1.82	23
		TOTAL	26.09	23

$X^2 = 0.83$; $P = 0.9$.
nb. q = proportion affected according to genetic hypothesis; $q' = q/r(1-q)^n$.

Statistical inferences on various data were made based on chi-square test or Fisher exact test. Conventional *P* values of less than 0.05 were considered significant. To prove that the three EEG characteristics of the siblings were genetically related, estimation of heritability by Falconer's method was carried out.

Results

Family history

A summary of family history of the patients is given in Table 3. Twelve out of 31 patients (38.7 per cent) had a family history of epileptic seizures in their relatives. Four of the 31 patients (12.9 per cent) had more than one relative with the history of epileptic seizures. Five out of 31 patients (16.2 per cent) had a family history of epilepsy in their first degree relatives. Two mothers had a history of childhood epilepsy suggestive of BCECTS.

Table 3. Number of patients with a family history of epilepsy

Family history of epilepsy in:		Number of patients	Percentage
1st degree relative	Siblings	4	12.4
	Parents		6.4
	Mother	2	
	Father	2	
2nd degree relative	Grandparents	1	3.2
	Uncle/Aunts	5	16.1
3rd degree relative	Cousins	4	12.9

Table 4. EEG abnormalities in siblings by family history

Family history	No. of patients with EEG activation in siblings		Total
	Positive	Negative	
Positive	8 (88%)	1	9
Negative	7 (59%)	5	12
Total	15	6	21

Table 5. Epileptiform EEG changes in 44 siblings who have had EEGs

EEG changes	No. of siblings		Total	%
	Symptomatic	Asymptomatic		
Rolandic	2	3	5	11
Generalized	0	4	4	9
Focal, non-rolandic	3	6	9	21
Normal	1	25	26	59
Total	6	38	44	100%

Interestingly, the proband in family 8 has night blindness due to retinitis pigmentosa. Her mother and sister also have similar ocular problem. All of them have autosomal dominant form of retinitis pigmentosa.

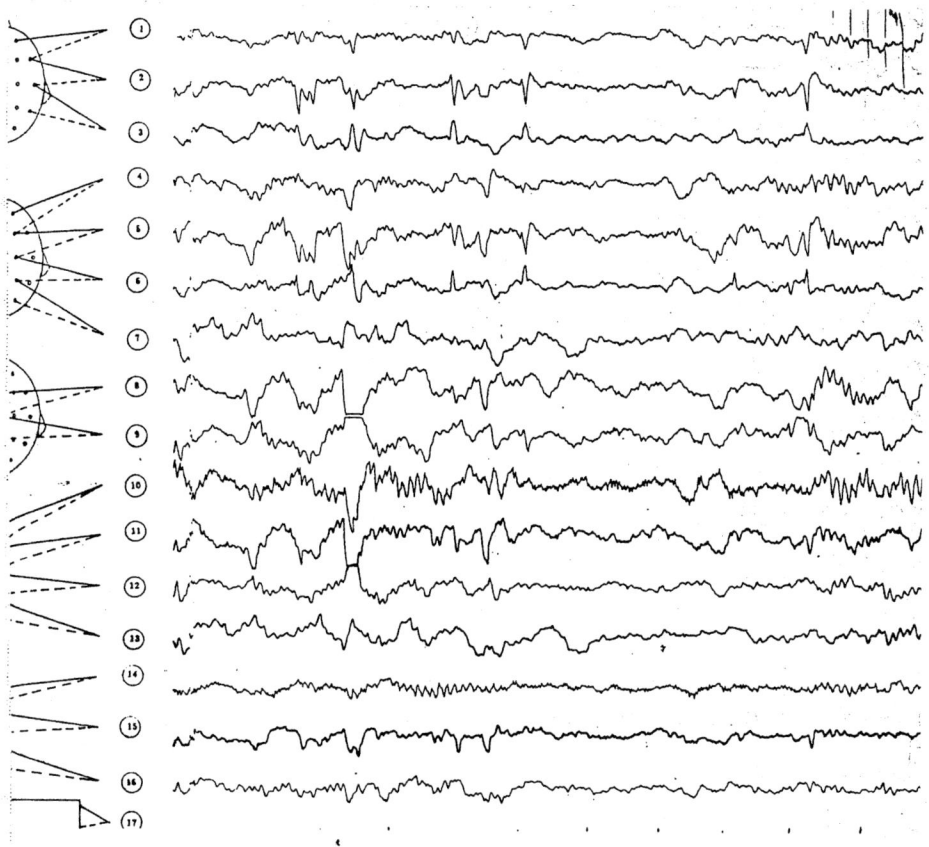

Fig. 1. Case 14, A, 11.5 year old Malay girl showing rolandic spikes on right side with dipole field, frontal positivity and temporal negativity, and Type 1 configuration.

EEG abnormalities in siblings

Forty-four siblings from 21 families completed the EEG study. A summary of the EEG findings in these siblings is given in Tables 4 and 5, and the findings are compared to the literature in Table 6. Examples of EEG changes are shown in Figs. 1–4. Overall, epileptiform activity was recorded electroencephalographically in at least one sibling in 14 of the 21 families (66.7 per cent). Eighteen of 44 siblings (40.9 per cent) showed definite epileptiform discharges in their EEG recordings, of which 13 were asymptomatic.

Five siblings (11 per cent) showed definite centro-temporal rolandic spikes. Four siblings (9 per cent) showed generalized epileptiform discharges and all four were clinically asymptomatic. Nine siblings (21 per cent) showed other focal epileptiform discharges (Table 5).

Epileptiform discharges were recorded only in waking in one sibling (2.2 per cent), only in sleep in eight siblings (18.1 per cent) and both sleep and waking in nine siblings (10.5 per cent). Hence, sleep is an important factor in the manifestation of this EEG trait.

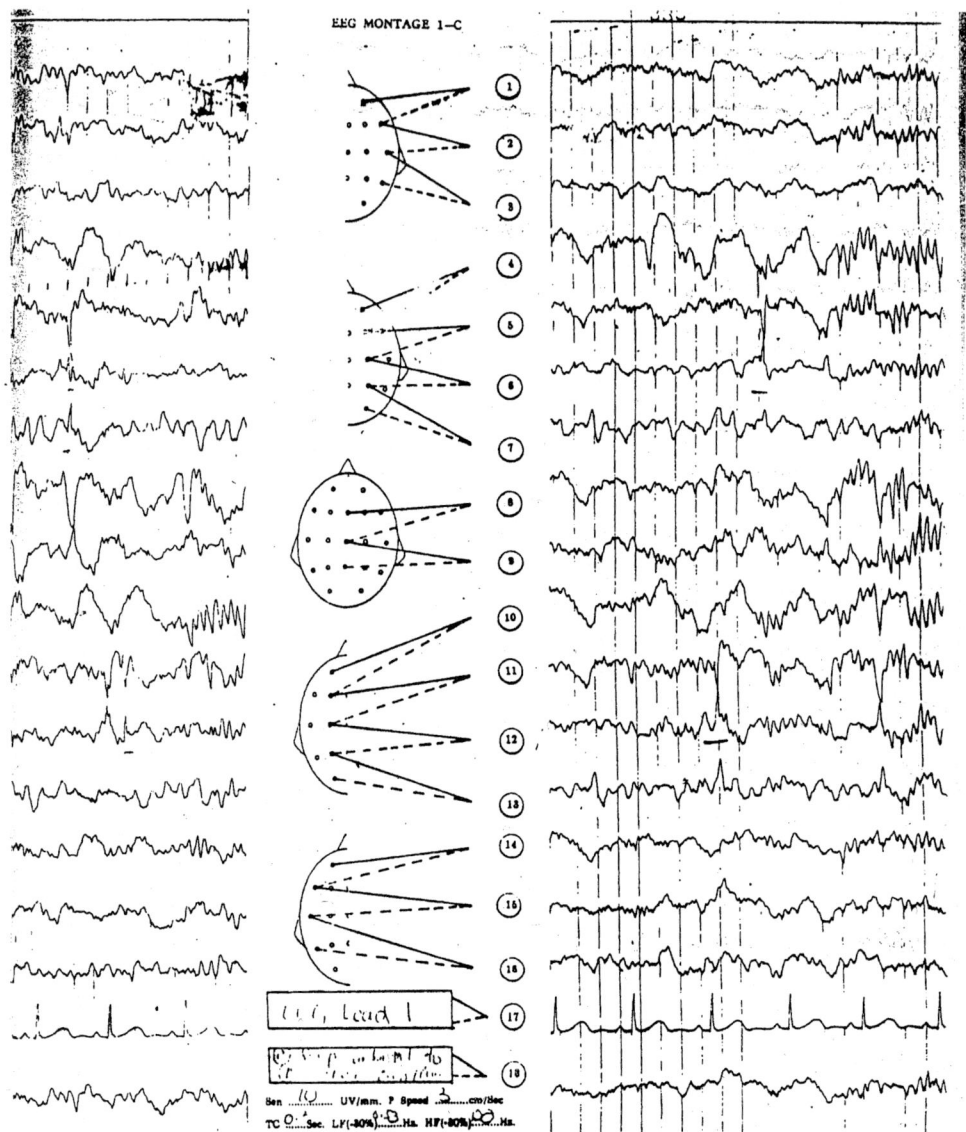

Fig. 2. K, 14 year old, asymptomatic sibling. EEG shows rolandic spikes which shift from side to side.

As shown in Table 7, the majority of the epileptic activity was observed in the age group between 3 to 14 years old (13 out of 18 = 72 per cent). Hence age is another important factor in EEG activation of BCECTS. When sex, race and socioeconomic states were considered, they were not significantly related to the EEG abnormalities of these siblings (Tables 8, 9 and 10)

The presence of a family history in this group of children seemed to correlate with a higher rate of EEG activation in their siblings; 88 per cent as compared to 59 per cent in those without family history of epilepsy (Table 4). A positive family history of epilepsy also apparently correlates with a higher rate of centro-temporal spikes in siblings (33 per cent) as compared to those without a family history of epilepsy (18 per cent).

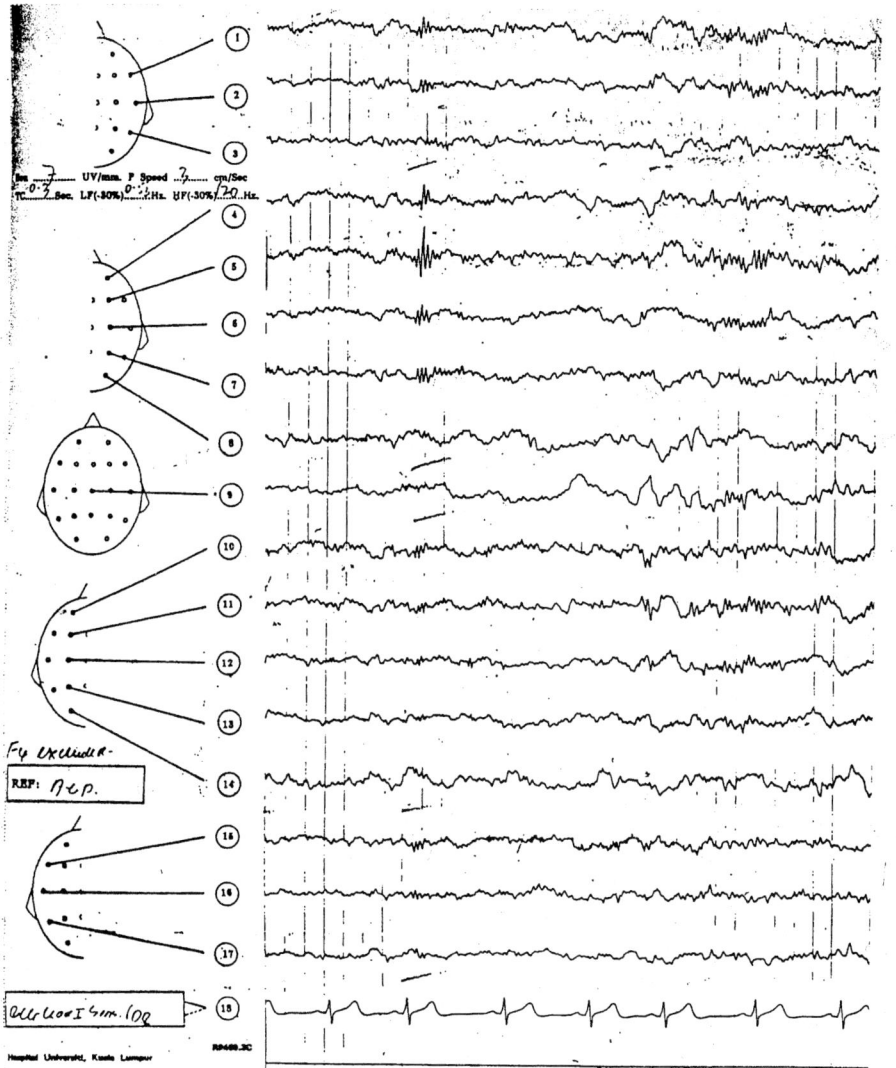

Fig. 3. NAN, 15 year old Indian boy, asymptomatic sibling shows polyspikes at right frontal region.

Pedigree analysis

The pedigrees of the 21 families completed the EEG studies were constructed (Fig. 5) and analysed. Different hypotheses concerning the mode of inheritance were tested on the families.

As shown in Fig. 5, the mother in family 1 had a past history of BCECTS and her daughter (proband) had BCECTS. Two other asymptomatic siblings had focal non-rolandic epileptiform discharges in their EEGs. Superficially, the inheritance appeared to be autosomal dominant (AD) since the phenotype appeared in every generation, the affected daughter had an affected mother. Even though, only one out of four siblings had centro-temporal spikes (25 per cent) the decrease in penetrance could be explained by strong age dependence or variability of gene expression resulting from influence of age. The apparently normal EEG in the youngest daughter (1.5 years old) could be the result of age dependency. Even though the incidence or recurrence rate of one in four was compatible, it was

49

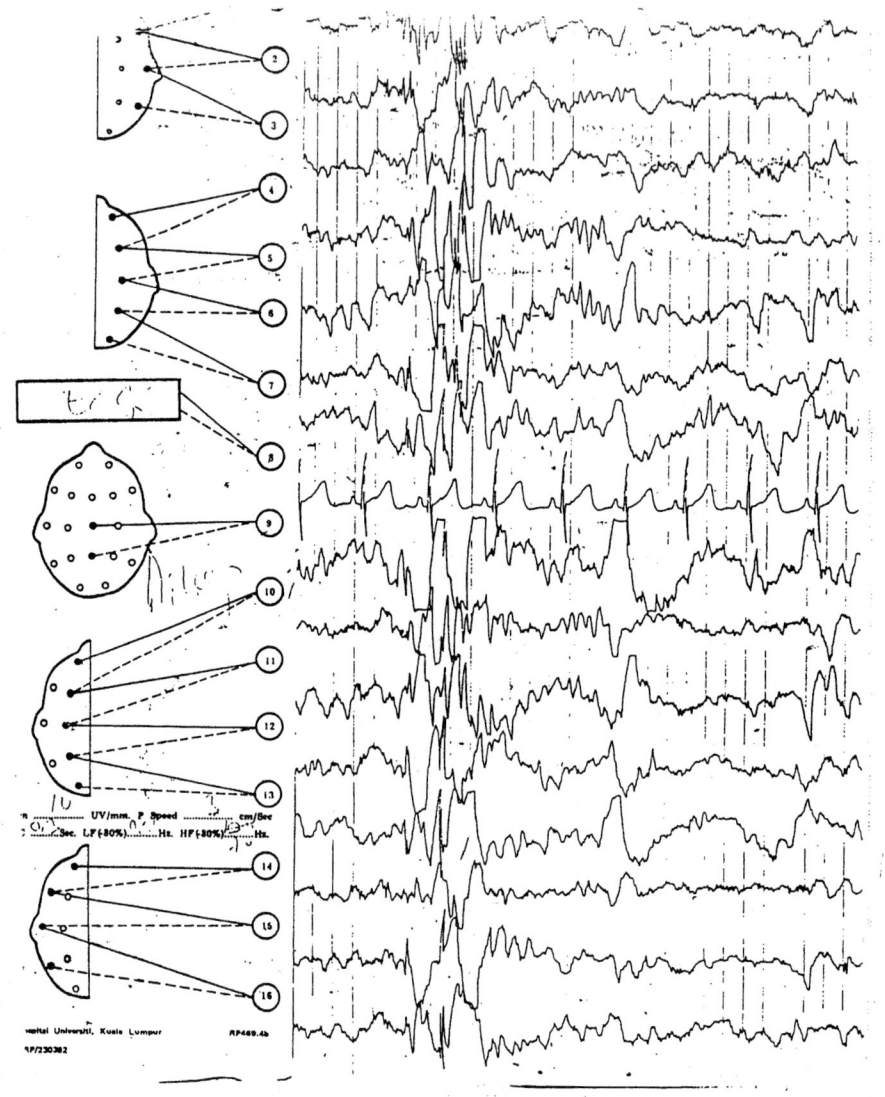

Fig. 4. LKN, 5 year old Chinese girl, asymptomatic sibling. EEG shows bursts of generalized spikes and waves.

unlikely to be autosomal recessive (AR) because the pattern of AR inheritance involves siblings of the proband and not parents or offsprings as in family 1 (i.e. horizontal pedigree pattern with importance of consanguinity). Neither is the inheritance X-linked recessive since there is transmission from mother to daughter. It is also not X-linked dominant as all the females would have been involved. Similar conclusions can be made from family 3 and family 8. Even though the parents of family 4 were normal and had no history of seizures, they could be heterozygotes/asymptomatic carriers of the EEG trait. Three out of four siblings (75 per cent) in this family had centro-temporal spikes and two of them were symptomatic. This frequency of occurrence was definitely compatible with AD mode of inheritance with variable penetrance. Similar conclusions can be made for family 15, 17 and 18.

Chapter 5 Families with benign childhood epilepsy with centro-temporal spikes

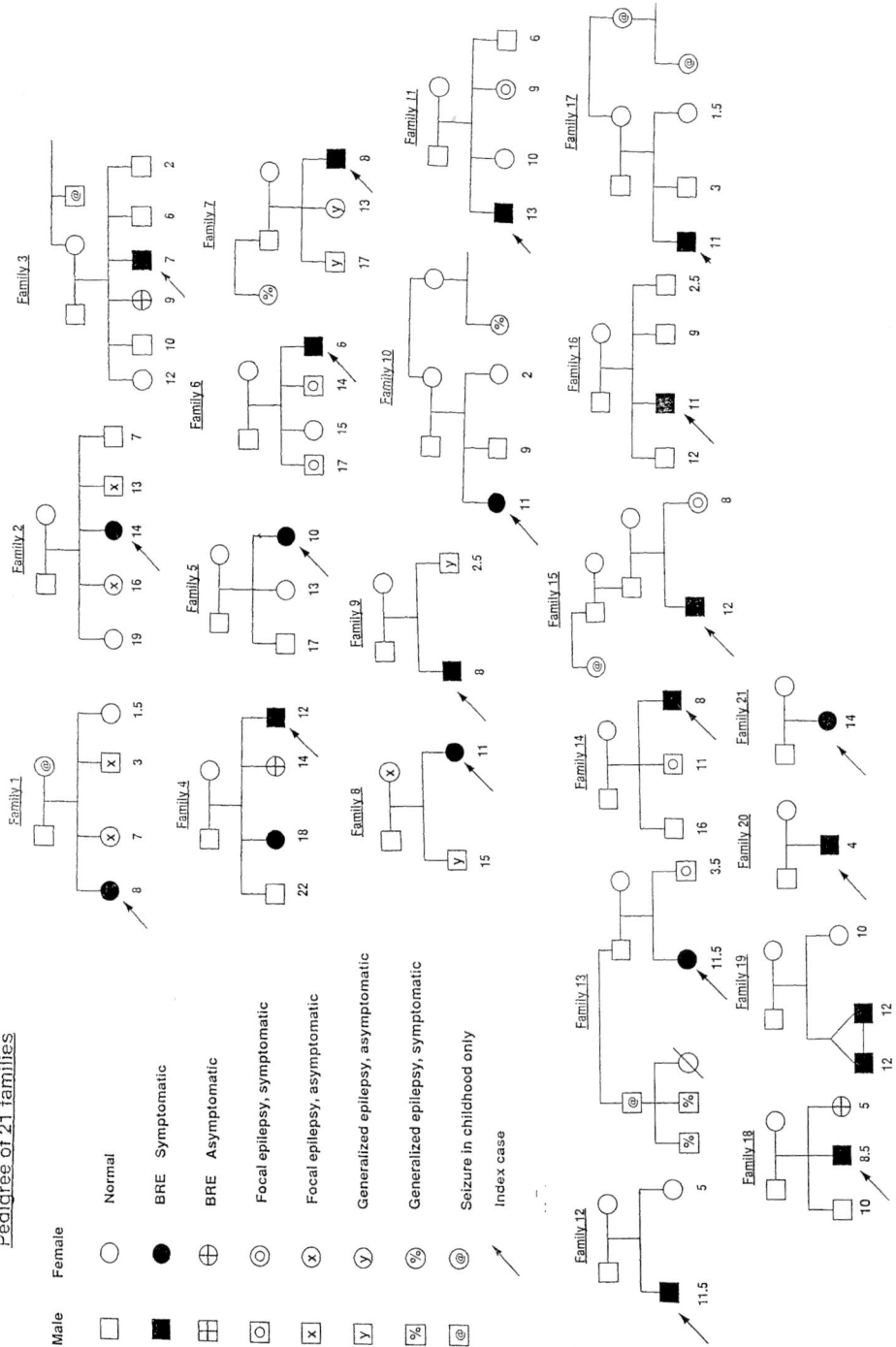

Fig. 5. Pedigree of 21 families.

GENETICS OF FOCAL EPILEPSIES

However, the pattern was not homogeneous for all the families. In 11 families (52 per cent, nos.y 2, 5, 6, 8, 9, 10, 11, 12, 13, 14 and 16) only one individual (the proband) had centro-temporal spikes. These family trees were non-diagnostic and the risks with other relatives were low. Hence, in these families, a sporadic case of a disorder could be the explanation. The affected individuals could be the result of a genetic or non-genetic process. These families could also represent AD with low penetrance or AR disorder. However, if variation in penetrance and expression reaches more than a certain level it becomes meaningless to consider the disorder following mendelian inheritance.

Among two pairs of identical twins, one pair was concordant, the pair was discordant. This is consoistent with multifactorial inheritance.

Table 6. EEG changes in siblings – comparison with two previous studies

EEG changes	Percentage of siblings		
	Present study	Heijbel, 1975	Degen, 1990
Rolandic spikes	11%	34%	6%
Generalized	9%		32%
Focal other than rolandic spikes	21%		
Total	41%	34%	38%

Table 7. EEG activation in siblings according to age

Age, years	Positive	Negative	Total
0–2	1	5	6
3–4	3	0	3
5–6	2	3	5
7–8	2	1	3
9–10	2	5	7
11–12	2	2	4
13–14	2	5	7
15–16	1	3	4
17–18	2	1	3
19–20	1	0	1
21–22	0	1	1
Total	18	26	44

Table 8. EEG activation in siblings by sex

EEG activation in siblings	Sex		Total
	Male	Female	
Positive	8	10	18
Negative	17	9	26
Total	25	19	44

$P = 0.17$

Table 9. EEG activation in siblings by race

EEG activation in siblings	Race			Total
	Malay	Chinese	Indian	
Positive	7	3	8	18
Negative	11	6	9	26
Total	18	9	17	44

Table 10. EEG activation in siblings by socio-economic status

Social class	EEG activation in siblings		Total
	Positive	Negative	
1	2	5	7
2	4	3	7
3	6	12	18
4	4	3	7
5	2	3	5
Total	18	26	44

Statistical analysis

Statistical analysis/test of significance was carried out to correct the sampling errors and observation errors on above pedigree analysis. The priori method was used. As shown in Tables 1 and 2, the difference between observed number of affected children and expected number were not statistically significant when the priori method was used to test the AD or AR mode of inheritance. Nevertheless, the pedigree analysis above has shown that AD or AR was unlikely to be the mode of inheritance.

The possibility of multifactorial inheritance was tested according to the theory of quasi-continuous traits with threshold characteristics; the risk among siblings should be at most square root of p, where p was the prevalence of the disease in the population. The prevalence of BCECTS in the population was estimated to be 0.001 according to the findings of CT Tan *et al*. Hence, 3.2 per cent of the siblings should be affected according to calculation. Only two out of 44 siblings (4.5 per cent) in these 21 families had BECTS. Hence, the observed prevalence was closed to estimated prevalence ($P < 0.05$) suggesting that the likely mode of inheritance is multifactorial.

If the prevalence of centro-temporal discharges was considered, the similarity was even greater between our siblings (11.4 per cent) and the expected value of 11 per cent calculated from the population prevalence of 1.2 per cent as described by Eeg-Olofsson *et al.* (1971). This was based on the assumption that the prevalence of centro-temporal spikes was similar between our population and his population. The difference in terms of the symptomatic BCECTS of ours 4.54 per cent versus 15 per cent of Heijbel could then be explained by other different precipitating factors or even different genetic factors.

Association with other epilepsies

One interesting finding in these pedigrees is the association of BCECTS with other forms of focal epilepsy and generalized epilepsy in 52 per cent of these families (i.e. family 1, 2, 6, 7, 8, 9, 10, 11, 13, 14, 15). They could either be asymptomatic with EEG changes or clinically affected with seizures.

The association has also been observed by other workers (Bray et al., 1965; Rodin et al., 1966; Ahmad Beydoun et al., 1992). To prove that the three EEG changes were actually phenotypically related, partitioning of chi-square test was carried out. In fact, P was much smaller than 0.05. Hence, we can conclude that there was significant phenotypic correlation between centro-temporal spikes and other focal spikes and generalized spikes and waves. Estimation of heritability by Falconer's method was carried out on all the three EEG traits to test if the phenotypic correlation was actually the result of genotypic correlation or genetically linked as shown in Fig. 6. Both centro-temporal spikes and other focal spikes had liability of inheritance of more than 110 per cent while it is about 70 to 80 per cent for generalized spikes and waves discharges. Hence, we can conclude that they are probably genetically linked.

Discussion

The findings described above were found on a fairly homogeneous group of patients and their families with BCECTS. Those patients with BECTS and neurological deficits were excluded from the study so as to achieve a more homogeneous population easier for statistical inference. EEGs were done on the siblings to detect asymptomatic carriers of the EEG trait for BECTS. Hence, it facilitated the pedigree analysis and the establishment of the mode of inheritance. EEG was not carried out on the parents as it was well recognized that the EEG trait normalizes after 20 years of age.

The data on family history suggests that genetics play an important role in BECTS as there is a high percentage of positive family history (38.7 per cent). This is comparable to the findings of Degen (39.5 per cent).

The finding of EEG activation in 41 per cent of siblings was also comparable to the previous studies done by Degen and by Heijbel as shown in Table 6. Those patients with a positive family history of epilepsy also had a higher rate of abnormal EEG in their siblings.

From the pedigree analysis, we can conclude that the mode of inheritance for both the EEG trait and clinical manifestation of BECTS is multifactorial. It is further evidenced by the strong association with sleep and age as shown above. Indeed, 64 per cent of the patients in this study had seizures only during sleep and 48 per cent of them had centro-temporal spikes only during sleep, comparable with the findings of Beaussart (1972) and Lerman & Kivity (1975). Therefore, sleep is important in both activation of centro-temporal spikes and seizures in BECTS.

Furthermore, some of our patients described various precipitating environmental factors relating to the onset of seizure. Three patients had emotional stress leading to seizure onset. One patient had onset of seizure with onset of menarche. One patient developed BECTS after head trauma. In fact, 4 per cent of Lerman patients had history of trauma.

The multifactorial mode of inheritance in BECTS is further evidenced by the statistical analysis carried out. Iit was found that centro-temporal spikes were significantly related to other non-rolandic focal discharges and generalized spikes and waves. This may suggest that there are genetically linked.

The association between BECTS and autosomal dominant retinitis pigmentosa may also suggest that they are genetically linked.

Conclusion

In conclusion, multifactorial inheritance is most likely for both the EEG trait as well as the clinical manifestation of BECTS. The presence of the EEG trait but absence of clinical seizure strengthens this hypothesis. Age, sleep and precipitating environmental factors such as stress appear to influence the pathogenesis of this epileptic syndrome. Other genes or regulatory genes may play an important role in the seizure threshold of this epilepsy. Association with generalized spikes and waves and other focal epileptiform discharges in the EEG suggest that they may be genetically linked. Furthermore, there is a significantly higher incidence of generalized epilepsy and focal epilepsy in these families. Further molecular studies need to be carried out to localize the gene for BECTS.

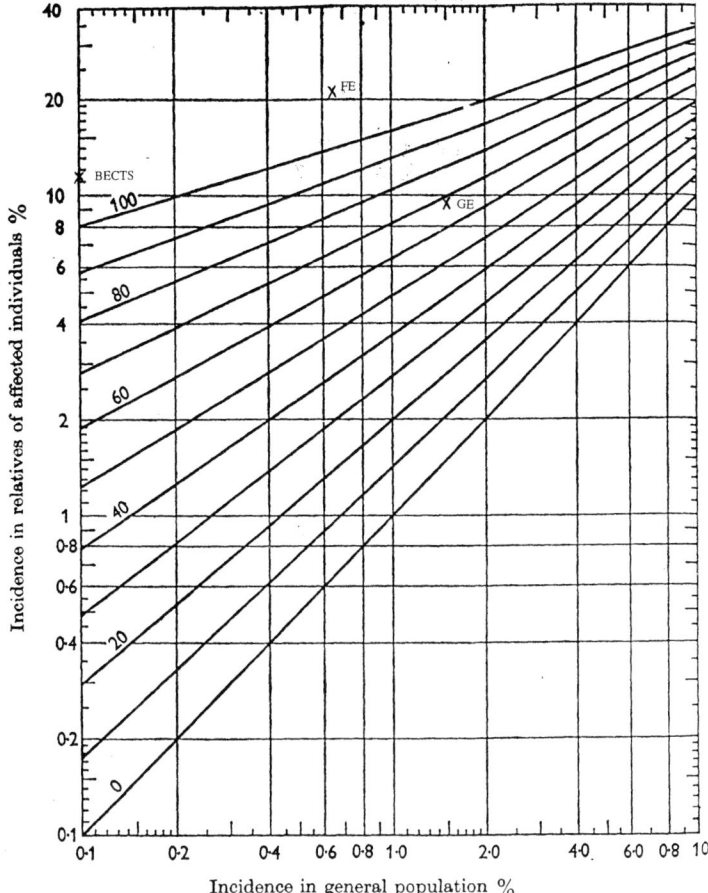

Fig. 6. The inheritance of liability to epilepsy as estimated from the incidence among relatives.

References

Ahmad Beydoun, E.A. (1992): Generalised spikes waves, multiple loci and clinical course in children with EEG features of BECTS. *Epilepsia* **33**, 1091–1096.

Beaussart, M. (1972): Benign epiepsy of children with rolandic centro-temporal paroxysm for a clinical entity : study of 211 cases. *Epilepsia* **13**, 795–811.

Beaussart, M. (1981): Crises épileptiques après guerison d'une épilepsie à paroxymes rolandiques. *Rev. EEG Neurophysiol.* **11**, 489–492.

Bray, F.P. & Wiser, W.C. (1964): Evidence for a genetic aetiology of temporal central abnormalities in focal epilepsy. *N. Eng. J. Med.* **271**, 926–933.

Bray, F.P. & Wiser, W.C. (1965): Hereditary characteristics of familial temporal central focal epilepsy. *Pediatrics* **30**, 207–211.

Degen R. & Degen H.E. (1990): Some genetic aspects of rolandic epilepsy: Waking and sleep EEGS in siblings. *Epilepsia* **31** (6), 795–801.

De Romanis, F., Deliani, M. & Ruggieri, S. (1986): Rolandic paroxysmal epilepsy: a long term study in 150 children. *Ital. J. Neuro. Sci.* **7,** 77–80.

Doose, H. & Baier, W. (1989): Genetic aspects of childhood epilepsy. *Cleveland J. Med.* **56,** Suppl. Part 1, 105–110.

Edwards, J.H. (1969): Familial predisposition in man. *Brit. Med. Bull.* **25,** 58–64.

Eeg-Olofsson, O., Peterson, I. & Sellden, V. (1971): The development of EEG in normal children from the age of 1 to 15 years. *Neuropédiatrie* **4,** 376–404.

Eeg-Olofsson, O., Tedroff, K., Mohlin, A.K., Gustavson, K.H. & Wadelins, C. (1993): Molecular genetic studies in families with benign epilepsy of childhood with rolandic spikes. *Epilepsia* **34** (Suppl. 2), 149–150.

Falconer, D.S. (1965): Inheritance of liability to certain diseases estimated from the incidence among relatives. *Ann. Hum. Genet., London* 29–51.

Heijbel, Blom, S. & Bergfors, P.G. (1972): Benign epilepsy of children with centro-temporal EEG foci, prevalence and follow up study of 40 patients. *Epilepsia* **13,** 609–619.

Heijbel, Blom S. & Rasmussen, M. (1975): Benign epilepsy of childhood with centro-temporal EEG foci: a genetic study. *Epilepsia* **16,** 285–293.

Lerman, P. & Kivity, S. (1975): Benign focal epilepsy of childhood. a follow up of 100 recovered patients. *Arch. Neurol.* **32,** 261–164.

Lerman, P. & Kivity, S. (1986): The benign focal epilepsies of childhood. In: *Recent advances in epilepsy. Vol III,* Pedley. T.A. & Meldrum, B.S. (eds), pp. 136–137. Edinburgh: Churchill Livingstone.

Lerman, P. *et al.* (1992): Benign partial epilepsy with centrotemporal spikes. In : *Epileptic syndromes in infancy, children and adolescence*. London: John Libbey.

Loisseau, P., Duche, B., Cardora, S., Dartiques, J.F. & Cohadon, S. (1988): Prognosis of benign childhood epilepsy with centro-temporal spikes: a follow up study of 168 patients. *Epilepsia* **29** (3), 229–235.

Rodin, E. & Gonzales, S. (1966): Hereditary components in epileptic patients. *JAMA* **198,** 131–135.

Stein, C. (1960): *Principal of human genetics*, p. 753. San Francisco: Freeman.

Tan, C.T. *et al.* (1995): A study of newly diagnosed epilepsy in Malaysia. *Epilepsia* **36,** S15.

Chapter 6

The genetics of rolandic epilepsy and related conditions: multifactorial inheritance with a major gene effect

Bernd A. Neubauer, Ulrich Stephani and Hermann Doose

Department of Neuropediatrics, Christian-Albrechts-Universität, Kiel; and North German Epilepsy Centre, Raisdorf, Germany

Summary

Focal spikes and sharp waves (FSW) with predominantly centro-temporal localization are the electroencephalographic hallmarks of rolandic epilepsy (RE), i.e. benign childhood epilepsy with centro-temporal spikes (BCECT). This EEG trait has been reported to follow a monogenic autosomal dominant mode of inheritance. Investigations of multiplex families with several siblings affected by this trait indicate that the clinical spectrum associated with this neurobiological marker is broader than pure RE. The majority of FSW carriers does not suffer from epilepsy or seizures. Amongst those individuals with documented seizures, generalized genetic EEG patterns are additionally found at a high percentage. Together with family data these findings strongly favour a multifactorial mode of inheritance for the trait associated epilepsies, e.g. RE. Genetic analysis at the molecular level of common disorders with a complex mode of inheritance are difficult and frequently unrewarding. Following the FSW trait therefore raises hopes of finding a possibly monogenic entry into the polygenic pathogenesis of this childhood epilepsy.

Rolandic epilepsy or BCECT accounts for 15–20 per cent of childhood epilepsies and thereby represents the most common epilepsy syndrome in this age group (Lüders *et al.*, 1987). Even though the first description of a rolandic seizure dates back to the 16th century (van Huffelen, 1989) the disorder basically went unrecognized until the historic descriptions of Y. Gastaut (1952) and Gibbs *et al.* (1954) in the early 1950s. In its pure form RE is characterized by a benign and self-limiting course. In most cases seizures are nocturnal and infrequent and by this only rarely impose a threat to the child's health. If treatment is required, the epilepsy responds well to anticonvulsive drugs. Therefore classic RE does not represent a major challenge to the practicing epileptologist (concisely reviewed by Dravet, 1994; Lerman, 1992; Lüders *et al.*, 1987)

However, recently an increasing body of evidence has accumulated showing that the disease definition given by the ILAE (Commission, 1989) merely covers part of a large spectrum. Adopting these diagnostic criteria, authors state that atypical features in RE are frequent and may rather be the rule than the exception (e.g. Wirrell *et al.*, 1995). This was first enunciated by Loiseau *et al.* (1967) when he argued that RE 'does not exist' in clinical practice, referring to its pure, typical form. One has to be aware that to the extent definitions of syndromes are based on the clinical symptomatology of selected typical cases they are based on circular reasoning and therefore cannot possibly delineate the whole spectrum of any disorder. While the current ILAE classification has proven extremely useful in clinical practice, and allows description of results that can be reproduced by the scientific community, from a neurobiological point of view it cannot be applied in general. For example normal intelligence and normal neurological findings are considered a prerequisite for diagnosis of RE. However it is hard to conceive that RE protects against other types of neurological disorders. One would rather expect to find it equally distributed in all groups of the population (Doose et al., 1996).

But how can this dilemma be overcome? How can we allow for the whole spectrum of a disease without introducing diagnostic uncertainties? Of course this problem can never be solved completely, and all efforts to do so will be arduous and require large cohorts of patients and many years of follow up. Another, however unsatisfactory solution might be to subdivide a given disorder into a (over time increasing) number of different but closely related syndromes. In RE, the story is somewhat less complicated for in fact we do have a 'laboratory test' for this disorder in the form of the characteristic FSW in the EEG, frequently but not exclusively with centro-temporal localization (Lüders et al., 1987; for review). This EEG trait, the electroencephalographic hallmark of RE, has been found to be genetically determined and can serve as a neurobiological marker for the increased risk of developing RE (Bray & Wiser, 1964, 1965; Heijbel et al., 1975). The trait is rare in the general population (Eeg-Olofsson et al., 1971) but is invariably found in individuals with RE. Therefore it is obvious that the genetics of RE cannot be separated from the genetics of the associated EEG trait. This opens a new perspective. Families can be sampled with several members displaying FSW in the EEG thereby selecting for genetically determined focal sharp waves and greatly reducing the numbers of phenocopies. This approach allows delineation of the symptomatology inherent to a neurobiological marker now quite precisely defined by the features of the EEG.

As could be expected the observed symptomatology is broader and not always as benign as known from pure RE (Doose, 1989; Doose & Baier, 1989). Therefore we rather refer to these epilepsies as 'idiopathic partial epilepsies of childhood with focal spikes and sharp waves' i.e. RE and related disorders, with RE as their best known and most common representative. In the following review we confine ourselves to the terminology used by the individual author.

Spikes and sharp waves characteristic of rolandic epilepsy (and related disorders)

In this field terminology always was a problem that we cannot ameliorate. However for any genetic study discussion and definition of what will serve as inclusion criteria is crucial. The EEG features characteristic for RE has received a plethora of designations in the literature: prerolandic sharp waves, midtemporal sharp waves, rolandic sharp waves, central sharp waves, temporal-central sharp waves, centro-temporal sharp waves, sylvian sharp waves, prerolandic sharp waves without focal significance etc. (Lüders et al., 1987; for review), centro-temporal spikes as incorporated in the current classification of the ILAE (Commission, 1989). All of these terms refer to location and are therefore only partially correct. One of the first reports on spikes and sharp waves in RE that were not solely confined to the centro-temporal region came from Beaussart (1972) and was readily confirmed by many other authors. Today it is generally accepted, that not the location but rather the typical morphology of the spikes and sharp wave is the essential characteristic (Lüders et al., 1987). Therefore it might be advantageous to use the term 'focal spikes and sharp waves' (FSW) as introduced by Eeg-Olofsson et al. (1971), thereby not falsely restricting them to the centro-temporal region.

FSW are negative discharges of high amplitude lasting from 50–100 ms generally preceded by a high-frequency, low amplitude positive wave that is followed by three further positive or negative sharp waves. The last positive wave is frequently superposed by faster waves and therefore difficult to recognize at low amplitude. Generalization of FSW is accompanied by increasing amplitude, with emphasis of the third and fifth component. Occipital and frontal FSW show a pronounced slow wave.

In the waking state they frequently appear in clusters and pseudorhythmic sequence. Sleep almost invariably induces marked activation.

This EEG trait, just like the epilepsy, is age dependant. Parieto-occipital foci usually occur before the fourth birthday, while midtemporal foci peak around the 8th year of life (reviewed by Doose et al., 1996; Lüders et al., 1987). Almost invariable the epilepsy and the EEG findings resolve after puberty. Phenocopies of course do exist and have been demonstrated in cases with proven neoplasma, trauma, several migration and gyration anomalies (reviewed by Dravet, 1994). Younger children tend to show a more occipital location of the FSW and during maturation they tend to 'migrate' to centro-temporal and sometimes even more frontal regions (Loiseau et al., 1992). Even in a single EEG recording a 'shifting' of the focus, sometimes even from one hemisphere to the other, can be observed (Kellaway, 1981). This only reflects the well known fact that there is no underlying lesion but rather a functional abnormality causing this EEG phenomenon.

Prevalence of rolandic epilepsy and the EEG trait

Heijbel et al. (1975a) observed 11 new cases of RE in a population of 52,252 children (age 0–15 years) and calculated an incidence of 0.021 per cent per year. Blom et al. (1972) reported a prevalence of 0.107 per cent in children (age 0–15 years) with at least one seizure in the last three years. For practical reasons these inclusion criteria seem sufficiently robust. However allowing for the fact that 30–50 per cent of patients with RE suffer only from a single seizure per life the complete prevalence for the time period between two and 15 years of age must still be somewhat higher. Blom et al. (1975) estimated a prevalence 0.24 per cent.

The EEG trait is by far more frequent in the general population. Eeg-Olofsson et al. (1971) found 1.6 per cent of FSW carriers in 743 healthy Swedish children age one to 15 years, investigated mostly (80 per cent) by at-rest and sleep recordings. Gerken (1971) found FSW in 1.3 per cent of healthy German children (at rest recordings only). In a large Italian sample of healthy school children Cavazutti et al. (1980) detected 'foci of spikes identical to those found in epileptic children' in 2.4 per cent of 5–14 years old school children. Okubo et al. (1994) found FSW in 4.7 per cent of healthy Japanese school children at six years of age and 1.8 per cent in the seven to 12 years old (no overall prevalence). Therefore, a number of 1.5–2 per cent (point prevalence) can be adopted.

All of these numbers are imperfect for several reasons. Many patients with RE have very few seizures, most of them take place at night. It can be argued therefore that many of these cases will be overlooked for these events are likely to be misinterpreted as parasomnias. The sensitivity to detect FSW in a single EEG recording even if a sleep tracing is included is not known, but is surely incomplete. Also it is important that a prevalence calculated over a period cannot be easily compared to a prevalence obtained by a single EEG recording. However these numbers have been used to show that FSW are by no means very 'epileptogenic' a fact that cannot be overemphasized. Calculating the numbers obtained by Eeg-Olofsson et al. (1971) and by Blom et al. (1972, 1975), Lüders et al. (1987) concluded that only 8.8 per cent of FSW carriers have clinical seizures. For reasons given above this number is debatable but it turns out to be within the same order of magnitude as the 12 per cent and 15 per cent reported by Bray & Wiser (1964) and by Heijbel et al. (1975) respectively. A number of about 10 per cent is frequently used as a rule of thumb. However it has been argued, that this value is still too large because of an ascertainment bias (e.g. Cavazutti, 1980).

The genetics of FSW (and the concept of epilepsy associated EEG traits)

In 1964, Bray and Wiser (Bray & Wiser, 1964, 1965) first recognized the genetic character of RE and claimed that 'temporal-central sharp waves' follow an autosomal dominant mode of inheritance. Even from the title of their paper it becomes clear that they inferred autosomal dominant inheritance from the segregation of the EEG trait and not the epilepsy, which is sometimes incorrectly cited. In common idiopathic epilepsies the monozygotic twin concordance rates are about 65–70 per cent (Berkovic et al., 1990, 1994). This implies that besides the genetic disposition exogenous factors may contribute to disease manifestation, which represents a drawback for genetic analysis. However, it is known that in the absence of disturbing factors the EEG is determined almost completely genetically (e.g. Vogel, 1970). This has also been confirmed by twin studies of monozygotic twins reared apart (Stassen et al., 1988). Therefore in an idiopathic epilepsy with a 'revealing' EEG, the study of the epilepsy associated EEG trait can be advantageous in several respects. First the EEG is closer to the genetic pathogenesis than is the epilepsy itself; secondly it is closer to the origin of the epilepsy than the eye of an observer. It allows carrier detection also in individuals unaffected by the epilepsy. It aids precise phenotype description etc. Pronounced age dependency and the incomplete sensitivity of a single EEG recording to detect the trait are major disadvantages (see Doose, 1997).

In 1964, Bray & Wiser reported that 'the temporal central sharp waves' follow an autosomal dominant mode of inheritance with high but incomplete penetrance. The provided numbers are under debate for it is known that they falsely included a group of (probably five) patients with temporal lobe epilepsy. In 1975 Heijbel et al. applying stricter criteria for phenotype definition tested this hypothesis in the families of 19 children. In the siblings of these children who were investigated by waking and sleep EEG they found that 11 of 32 (34 per cent) showed 'rolandic discharges'. On the basis of these findings they came to the identical conclusion as did Bray and Wiser and claimed that autosomal recessive, x-linked, and polygenous inheritance could be excluded (Heijbel et al., 1975). Again an autosomal dominant mode of inheritance was only reported for the EEG trait, not for the epilepsy. Doose et al. studied 188 siblings of epileptic children with FSW and observed FSW in 14 per cent of siblings (2–10 years). The siblings were investigated mostly by a single waking EEG (Doose et al., 1997). It is well known that sleep recordings are more sensitive than waking EEGs. However no systematic investigation about the sensitivity of a EEG (at rest and sleep) recording at a given age exists. It also has to be considered that several relatives (parents and siblings) with a history of seizures in childhood only could not be investigated by EEG within the appropriate age and therefore were not included in this number. However basically all the remaining probands became seizure free after puberty. Therefore it can be argued that the true number of positive findings must be substantially higher than 14 per cent.

Considering the mode of transmission of FSW we have to face several problems. First of all it is practically impossible to define a truly unaffected individual for it is unknown how many EEG recordings this requires. When we detect the families it is through the children, by definition at a time when the status for the trait can no longer be determined in parents, grandparents etc., therefore no large pedigrees can be ascertained and no segregation analysis of sufficient size can be conducted. The only thing that can possibly be accomplished is a risk calculation for the siblings and this will still be vague. Bray & Wiser (1964, 1965) and Heijbel et al. (1975) based on their large numbers of positive siblings clearly favour an autosomal dominant mode of inheritance. All published twin observations, if conducted at appropriate age, showed concordance (i.e. Doose, 1989; Kajitani et al., 1980). However what if the figures become lower, what if they drop below the 25 per cent limit as in the study of Doose et al. (1997)? In RE there is a well known, however small, male preponderance. In the FSW trait this does not seem to be the case. Therefore no argument exists to support X-linked inheritance. In the face of the fact that the affection status of the parents remains unknown and unaffected individuals can never be determined with certainty we feel that no further assumption can be made that allows us to exclude or disclose an autosomal recessive mode of inheritance. This was also stated by Ottman (1989) who reported that Heijbel et al. did not use the adequate correction function for ascertainment of bias. Autosomal dominant inheritance with reduced penetrance remains as a possibility that allows the explanation of practically any trait that runs in families. Some of these traits might turn out to be autosomal dominantly inherited, but especially when penetrances have to be reduced more and more the probability rises that the trait in question is 'complex', e.g. polygenic.

If this is the case, the risk for the siblings decreases the more genes are involved, but if segregation studies are not feasible no estimate of the number of these genes can be obtained. Unfortunately this holds true for the genetics of FSW. Therefore only quite limited conclusions can be drawn. Heijbel *et al.* (1975) argued against a multifactorial inheritance stating that according to the theory of quasi-continuous traits (Edwards, 1969) the risk of the siblings should be at most the square root of the population prevalence. Assuming a population prevalence for FSW between 1 and 2 per cent a finding of less than 10 to 14 per cent of positive siblings would be required to support the hypothesis of a multifactorial inheritance. Heijbel *et al.* (1975) concluded that autosomal dominant inheritance with age dependant penetrance is most likely responsible for the EEG changes in RE, but that 'the expression of a main gene influenced by a few other genes cannot be ruled out'.

Why does rolandic epilepsy not run in families?

As Lüders *et al.* (1987) wrote in their review on 'benign focal epilepsy of childhood': 'There is sufficient evidence in the literature to conclude that benign focal epilepsy of childhood is a genetic disease'. Since then no data have been brought forward that would allow us to contradict their conclusion. But why then do we find so few family histories positive for RE in the families of our index cases?

Recognition of a simple monogenic mendelian inheritance is usually straightforward and this clearly can be ruled out for RE. Qualitative criteria for a multifactorial inheritance can be based on the concordance rate in twins, on segregation ratios in siblings (plus x minus and minus x minus matings), and sex ratio calculation amongst the affected (e.g. reviewed by Vogel & Motulsky, 1996). In RE twin studies do not exist in a quantity that would allow us to calculate a concordance ratio of significance. Heijbel *et al.* (1975) observed that 15 per cent relatives of his 19 index cases had RE themselves. Phenotype description of the parents rests on the history of 'seizures in childhood only' (four of 38 cases) no EEG performed (at the appropriate age) in all but one case. Determination of the segregation ratio will therefore not result in a reliable number. Ascertainment was performed over the affected children and after correction for ascertainment bias the number of affected individuals will further decrease. Doose *et al.* (1997) recently investigated the families of 147 children with FSW. Doose found that the seizure incidence in first degree relatives ($n = 246$) of probands with classic RE (perioral sensorimotor seizures) was 7 per cent ($n = 16$). Of these 16 individuals only one (6 per cent) showed a classic RE. Again families were ascertained through the affected index case.

In RE a male to female preponderance of about 1.5 to 1 can be observed. A unequal sex ratio, that is still incompatible with sex-linked inheritance is a frequent (and to some extent characteristic) feature of a multifactorial inheritance with a threshold effect. Here the genetic liability is equally distributed between the sexes but the differing threshold is related to physiological differences (for review see Vogel & Motulsky, 1996). In this respect it is of interest that amongst FSW carriers with seizures generalized genetic EEG patterns, are found at a much higher rate than in seizure free FSW carriers – e.g. 66 per cent vs. 23 per cent in the study of Doose *et al.* (1997; reviewed by Doose *et al.*, 1996; Dravet, 1994). The latter additively lowering the seizure threshold and thereby contributing to the manifestation of the epilepsy (Doose, 1997). Therefore it can be said that multi-factorial inheritance with a threshold effect is the most likely model RE can be subsumed under (see also Andermann, 1982; Blandford *et al.*, 1987).

Back to the initial question. Assuming an autosomal dominant mode of inheritance for the EEG trait we still have to take into account that at most 8.8 per cent of those individuals who carry this trait develop seizures. Practically speaking this means that a clinician will have to see at least 20 'sibpair-type' families with an affected index case in order to find one affected sibling.

Symptomatology in children with FSW of genetic origin

It may now seem straightforward to ascertain multiplex families, i.e. with several first degree relatives displaying FSW in the EEG and characterize their clinical symptomatology. The FSW trait is age dependant. (The oldest – seizure free – sibling positive for FSW we detected was 11 years of age.) Therefore parents etc. cannot be investigated, which means that all our hopes rest on the siblings. With an age of onset maximum at 7–9 years (for RE) many older siblings will be too old to display the trait in the EEG. History taking only helps a little because as outlined above the FSW trait is not very 'epileptogenic'. This means that one ends up with the following strategy: families with an individual positive for FSW in the EEG will have to be contacted regularly. As soon as a sibling reaches the appropriate age, EEG recordings have to be carried out at regular intervals until she or he outgrows the age period of manifestation. Even for a reasonably large epilepsy clinic it will take a decade until the first conclusions can be made.

In 1989 H. Doose published first results on the symptomatology in children with FSW of genetic origin (Doose, 1989). Altogether 41 probands (27 boys, 14 girls) and 44 sibs (22 boys, 22 girls) were investigated for clinical and EEG findings; 301 recordings of the probands and 87 of the siblings were evaluated. Table 1a gives a summary of the seizure types observed in the 41 probands, Table 1b of the siblings respectively. Of special interest are four patients with GTCS, atypical absences, nodding, astatic and focal seizure symptomatology. A clinical picture that was designated 'pseudo Lennox syndrome' for its parallels to the Lennox–Gastaut syndrome (Aicardi & Chevrie, 1982; Doose, 1989). Surprisingly two cases of neonatal seizures with benign outcome were observed. Of 36 patients with seizures 18 showed signs of more or less pronounced mental retardation or selective performance deficits respectively. Four patients were found to be severely mentally handicapped. Three of them were normal before onset of seizures and all of them developed 'pseudo Lennox syndrome'.

A second study had different inclusion criteria (Doose *et al.* 1997). These were: (1) at least one EEG with characteristic FSW; (2) at least one sibling investigated by EEG; (3) willingness of the family to be questioned orally or in writing. The collective comprises 147 children (134 with, 13 without seizures). In 188 of 242 siblings an EEG (mostly in the waking state) was performed for scientific reasons, either in the facilities of our department or by an (auto-) mobile EEG unit. In 14 per cent of the siblings (2–10 years) FSW were found. Of 134 probands with seizures 24 per cent showed rolandic seizures in the stricter sense (i.e. perioral somato-sensory partial motor seizures). Again an elevated incidence of neonatal seizures with benign outcome was noted. Seizure symptomatology is illustrated in Table 2.

Table 1a. Seizure symptomatology in 41 probands with FSW of genetic origin

Febrile convulsions	4
Febrile convulsions and absences	1
Febrile convulsions and rolandic seizures	1
Febrile convulsions and GTCS	6
GTCS	10
Focal motor seizures	3
Focal motor seizures, and GTCS	3
Rolandic seizures	2
GTCS, atyp. absences, nodding, astatic, focal seizures	4
Complex partial seizures	1
Unclassifiable seizure	1
No seizures	5

GTCS = generalized tonic–clonic seizures

Table 1b. Symptomatology in 13 probands and their 16 seizure affected siblings

Probands	Siblings
FC	FC
FC	Focal motor seizures
FC	Rolandic seizures
FC and rolandic seizure	FC
Focal motor seizures	FC and absences
Focal motor seizures, and GTCS	Focal motor seizures
GTCS, atypical absences, nodding, astatic and focal seizures	Rolandic seizures (in three siblings)
Rolandic seizures	Rolandic seizures
GTCS	Rolandic seizures
GTCS	GTCS (in two siblings)
GTCS	Complex partial seizures
GTCS	Complex partial seizures
GTCS	Unclassifiable

FC = febrile convulsions; GTCS = generalized tonic–clonic seizures

Table 2. Seizure symptomatology in probands with FSW

Seizure type	n (total = 134)	%
GTCS	66	49
Febrile convulsions	38	28
Rolandic seizures	32	24
Focal seizures (n.r.t.)	50	37
Neonatal seizures	9	6.5

Note that numbers add up to over 100 per cent because 42 per cent of the probands had more than one seizure type.
n = number of probands; GTCS = generalized tonic–clonic seizures, n.r.t. = non-rolandic type

The aggregation of FSW characteristic of idiopathic partial epilepsy of childhood in non-epileptic disorders (like behavioural disorders, specific developmental disabilities etc.) and the age dependency of these features unknown for other genetic EEG patterns as well as their findings in multiplex families, prompted Doose & Baier to formulate a unifying concept. According to this hypothesis the various epileptic and non-epileptic syndromes share a common pathomechanism termed by the authors 'hereditary impairment of brain maturation' (Doose & Baier, 1989; Doose et al., 1996).

Molecular genetic findings

With today´s techniques of molecular biology it is possible to conduct a linkage analysis in order to localize the gene responsible for the FSW trait. Several approaches have been applied. One of the first chromosomal areas reported to harbour a gene predisposing for an idiopathic epilepsy was the HLA locus on chromosome 6p in juvenile myoclonic epilepsy. Linkage of FSW to this locus was excluded (Whitehouse et al., 1993). Several individuals affected by the fragile X syndrome with FSW in the EEG have been reported in the literature. This led Rees et al. to define this locus as a candidate for the FSW trait. However linkage could again be excluded (Rees et al., 1993).

As mentioned above in the series of FSW multiplex families and families of probands with FSW, an overrepresentation of neonatal seizures with benign course (i.e. spontaneously resolving or promptly responding to therapy without relapse after therapy withdrawal) was found. A nation-wide database search confirmed these findings in three further German epilepsy referral centres showing that about 3–5 per cent of probands exhibiting FSW later in life suffer from this seizure type (Hoffmann-Riem et al., 1996). The normal expectation would be about 0.5 per cent (Aicardi, 1992). Other reports – of familial and non familial cases – also are on record (Mami et al., 1993; Roulet et al., 1989; Waltz et al., 1994). To our knowledge all reported pedigrees with benign familial neonatal convulsions map to two distinct loci on chromosome 20q (EBN 1) and 8q (EBN 2) respectively (Leppert et al., 1989; Lewis et al., 1993; Malafosse et al., 1992). However employing a penetrance range of 0.45 to 0.9 linkage for FSW was excluded for autosomal dominant and recessive transmission. This was also true in pedigrees with RE and centro-temporal spikes only (Neubauer et al., 1997).

Vaughn et al. reported on three handicapped children with de novo deletions of 1q43 showing seizures and EEG findings the authors considered similar to those found in 'benign rolandic epilepsy' (Vaughn et al., 1996). Recently, by a combination of candidate locus approach and systematic genome scan linkage in a set of 22 families with FSW and rolandic epilepsy to markers on chromosome 15q44 was demonstrated (Neubauer et al., 1998). Identification of a gene responsible for the FSW trait will aid the determination of the clinical spectrum associated with this EEG trait on a scientific basis.

References

Aicardi, J. & Chevrie, J.J. (1982): Atypical benign partial epilepsy of childhood. *Dev. Med. Child Neurol.* **24**, 281–292.

Andermann, E. (1982): Multifactorial inheritance of generalized and focal epilepsy. In: *Genetic basis of the epilepsies*, Anderson, V.E., Hauser, W.A., Penry, J.K. & Sing, C.F. (eds), pp. 129–145. New York: Raven Press.

Aicardi, J. (1986): *Epilepsy in children*, pp. 39–66. New York: Raven Press.

Beaussart, M. (1972): Benign epilepsy of children with rolandic (centro-temporal) paroxysmal foci. *Epilepsia* **13**, 795–811.

Berkovic, S.F., Howell, R.A., Hopper, J.L., Hay, D.A. & Andermann, E. (1990): A twin study of the epilepsies. *Epilepsia* **31**, 813 (abstract).

Berkovic, S.F., Howell, R.A., Hay, D.A. & Hopper, J.L. (1994): Epilepsy in twins. In: *Epileptic seizures and syndromes*, Wolf, P. (ed.), pp. 157–164. London: John Libbey.

Blandfort, M., Tsuboi, T. & Vogel, F. (1987): Genetic counselling in the epilepsies. *Hum. Genet.* **76**, 303–331.

Blom, S., Heijbel, J. & Bergfors, P.G. (1972): Benign epilepsy of children with centro-temporal EEG foci. Prevalence and follow up study of 40 patients. *Epilepsia* **13**, 609–619.

Blom et al. cited in: Heijbel, J. & Rasmuson, M. (1975): Benign epilepsy of childhood with centro-temporal EEG foci: A genetic study. *Epilepsia* **16**, 285–293.

Bray, P.F. & Wiser, W.C. (1964): Evidence for a genetic etiology of temporal-central abnormalities in focal epilepsy. *N. Engl. J. Med.* **271**, 926–933.

Bray, P.F. & Wiser, W.C. (1965): Hereditary characteristics of familial temporal-central focal epilepsy. *Pediatrics* **36**, 207–211.

Cavazutti, G.B.L., Capella, L. & Nalin, A. (1980): Longitudinal study of epileptiform EEG patterns in normal children. *Epilepsia* **21**, 43–55.

Commission on Classification and Terminology of the International League against Epilepsy (1989): Proposal for revised classification of epilepsies and epileptic syndromes. *Epilepsia* **30**, 389–399.

Doose, H. (1989): Symptomatology in children with focal sharp waves of genetic origin. *Eur. J. Pediatr.* **149**, 210–215.

Doose, H. & Baier, W.K. (1989): Benign partial epilepsy and related conditiones: multifactorial pathogenesis with hereditary impairment of brain matuation. *Eur. J. Pediatr.* **149**, 152–158.

Doose, H., Neubauer, B. & Carlsson, G. (1996): Children with benign focal sharp waves in the EEG – developmental disorders and epilepsy. *Neuropediatrics* **27**, 1–15.

Doose, H., Brigger-Heuer, B. & Neubauer, B.A. (1997): Children with focal sharp waves: clinical and genetic aspects. *Epilepsia* **38**(7), 788–796.

Doose, H. (1997): Genetic traits in the EEG and their significance in the pathogenesis of epilepsy. *J. Epilepsy*, in press

Dravet, Ch. (1994): Benign epilepsy with centro-temporal spikes: do we know all about it? In: *Epileptic seizures and syndromes*, Wolf, P. (ed.), pp. 231–240. London: John Libbey.

Edwards, J.H. (1969): Familial predisposition in man. *Br. Med. Bull.* **25**, 58–64.

Eeg-Olofsson, O., Petersen, I. & Sellden, U. (1971): The development of the electroencephalogram in normal children from age of one through 15 years. *Neuropediatrics* **2**, 375–404.

Gastaut, Y. (1952): Un élément déroutant de la séméiologie électroencéphalographique: les pointes prérolandiques sans signification focale. *Rev. Neurol.* **87**, 488–489.

Gerken, H. (1971): *Über konstitutionelle EEG-Anomalien im Kindesalter*. Habilitationsschrift, Christian-Albrechts-Universität, Kiel.

Gibbs, E.L., Gillen, H.W. & Gibbs, F.A. (1954): Disappearance and migration of epileptic foci in childhood. *Am. J. Dis. Child* **88**, 596–603.

Heijbel, J., Blom, S. & Rasmuson, M. (1975): Benign epilepsy of childhood with centro-temporal EEG foci: a genetic study. *Epilepsia* **16**, 285–293.

Heijbel, J., Blom, S. & Bergfors, P.G. (1975a): Benign epilepsy of children with centro-temporal EEG foci: A study of incidence rate in outpatient care. *Epilepsia* **16**, 657–664.

Kajitani, T., Nakamura, M., Ueoka, K. & Kobuchi, S. (1980): Three pairs of monozygotic twins with rolandic discharges. In: *Advances in epileptology X*, Wada, J.A. & Penry, J.K. (eds), pp. 171–175. New York: Raven Press.

Hoffmann-Riem, M., Diener, W. & Kruse, R. *et al.* (1996): Multicenter retrospective database of epileptic syndromes of childhood. *Epilepsia* **37**, 112 (Suppl. 4, abstract).

Kellaway, P. (1981): The incidence and significance and natural history of spike foci in children. In: *Current clinical neurophysiology. Update on EEG and evoked potentials*, C.E. Henry (ed.). Amsterdam: North Holland, Elsevier.

Leppert, M., Anderson, V.E. & Quattelbaum, T. *et al.* (1989): Benign familial neonatal convulsions linked to genetic markers on chromosome 20. *Nature* **337**, 647–648.

Lerman, P. (1992): Benign partial epilepsy with centro-temporal spikes. In: *Epileptic syndromes in infancy, childhood and adolescence*, Roger, J., Bureau, M., Dravet, Ch., Dreifuss, F.E., Perret, A. & Wolf, P. (eds), 2nd edn., pp.189–200. London: John Libbey.

Lewis, T.B., Leach, R.J., War, K., O'Connel, P. & Ryan, S.G. (1993): Genetic heterogeneity in benign familial neonatal convulsions: Identification of a new locus on chromosome 8q. *Am. J. Hum. Genet.* **53**, 670–675.

Loiseau, P., Cohadon, F. & Mortureux, Y. (1967): A propos d´une forme singulière d'épilepsie de l´enfant. *Rev. Neurol. (Paris)* **116**, 224–248.

Loiseau, P., Duché, B. & Cohadon, S. (1992): The prognosis of benign localized epilepsy of early childhood. In: *Benign localized and generalized epilepsies of early childhood (Epilepsy Res. Suppl. 6)*, Degen, R. & Dreifuss, F.E. (eds), pp. 75–82. Amsterdam: Elsevier.

Lüders, H., Lesser, R.P., Dinner, D.S. & Morris III, H.H. (1987): Benign focal epilepsy of childhood. In: *Epilepsy, electroclincal syndromes*, Lüders, H. & Lesser, R.P. (eds), pp. 303–346. London, Berlin: Springer.

Neubauer, B.A., Moises, H.W., Läβker, U., Waltz, S., Diebold, U. & Stephani, U. (1997): Benign childhood epilepsy with centrotemporal spikes and electroencephalography trait are not linked to EBN1 and EBN2 of benign neonatal familial convulsions. *Epilepsia* **38**, 782–787.

Neubauer, B.A., Fiedler, B., Himmelein, B., Kämpfer, F., Läβker, U., Schwabe, G. *et al.* (1998): Centrotemporal spikes in families with rolandic epilepsy: linkage to chromosome 15q14. *Neurology* (in press).

Malafosse, A., Leboyer, M. & Dulac, O. *et al.* (1992): Confirmation of linkage of benign familial neonatal convulsiones to D20S19 and D20S20. *Hum. Genet.* **89**, 54–58.

Mami, C., Tortorella, G., Manganro, R. & Gemelli, M. (1993): Les convulsiones néonatale familiales bénignes. *Arch. Fr. Pediatr.* **50**, 31–33.

Ottman, R. (1989): Genetics of the partial epilepsies: a review. *Epilepsia* **30**(1), 107–111.

Okubo, Y., Matsuura, M, Asai, T, Asai, K., Kato, M., Kojima, T. & Toru, M. (1994): Epileptiform EEG discharges in healthy children: Prevalence, emotional and behavioral correlates, and genetic influences. *Epilepsia* **35**, 832–841.

Rees, M., Diebold, U., Parker, K. Doose, H., Gardiner, R.M. & Whitehouse, W.P. (1993): Benign childhood epilepsy with centro-temporal spikes and the focal sharp wave trait is not linked to the fragile X region. *Neuropediatrics* **24**, 211–213.

Roulet, E., Deonna, T. & Despland P.A. (1989): Prolonged intermittent drooling and oromotor dyspraxia in benign childhood epilepsy with centro-temporal spikes. *Epilepsia* **30**(5), 564–568.

Stassen, H.H., Lykken, D.T., Propping, P. & Bomben, G. (1988): Genetic determination of human EEG. Survey of recent results on twins reared together and apart. *Hum. Genet.* **80,** 165–176.

van Huffelen, A.C. (1989): A tribute to Martinus Rulandus. A 16th-century description of benign focal epilepsy of childhood. *Arch. Neurol.* **46**(4), 445–447.

Vogel, F. (1970): The genetic basis of the normal human electroencephalogram (EEG). *Hum. Genet.* **10,** 91–114.

Vaughn, B.V., Greenwood, R.S., Aylsworth, A.S. & Tennison, M.B. (1996): Similarities of EEG and seizures in del(1q) and benign rolandic epilepsy. *Pediatric. Neurol.* **15**(3), 261–264.

Vogel, F. & Motulsky, A.G. (1996): Formal genetics in humans: multifactorial inheritance and common diseases. In: *Human genetics – problems and approaches*, 3rd edn, pp. 196–218. Berlin, Heidelberg: Springer

Waltz, St., Neubauer, B., Suttorp, M. & Stephani, U. (1994): Benigne familiäre Neugeborenenkrämpfe und Rolando Epilepsie in einer Familie. *Epilepsieblätter* **7** (Suppl.) 37.

Wirrell, E.C., Camfield, P.R., Gordon, K.E., Doolex, J.M. & Camfield, C.S. (1995): Benign rolandic epilepsy: atypical features are very common. *J. Child. Neurol.* **10,** 455–458.

Whitehouse, W., Diebold, U., Reese, M., Parker, K., Doose, H. & Gardiner, R.M. (1993): Exclusion of linkage of genetic focal sharp waves to the HLA region on chromosome 6p in families with benign partial epilepsy with centro-temporal sharp waves. *Neuropediatrics* **24,** 208–210.

Part III
Idiopathic focal epilepsies in infancy

Chapter 7

Gene mapping for benign infantile familial convulsions

Michel Guipponi,[1] Federico Vigevano,[2] Bernard Echenne[3] and Alain Malafosse[4]

[1]*Laboratory of Experimental Medicine, CNRS ERS 155, INSERM U249, Biology Institute, Boulevard Henry IV, 34000 Montpellier, France;* [2]*Section of Neurophysiology, 'Bambino Gesù' Children's Hospital, National Medical Research Institute, Piazza S. Onofrio 4, 00165 Rome, Italy;* [3]*Section of Neuropediatry, Centre Gui de Chauliac, 34059 Montpellier, France;* [4]*Division of Neuropsychiatry, University Hospital of Geneva, Belle-Idée Hospital, Chemin du Petit-Bel-Air 2, 1225 Chêne-Bourg, Switzerland*

The recent International Classification of Epilepsies and Epileptic Syndromes recognizes three entities with an age of onset within the first year of life: benign familial neonatal convulsions (BFNC), benign neonatal convulsions, and benign myoclonic epilepsy in infancy. The first two appear in the neonatal period, the third at the age of about 1 year. All three are classified generalized forms. The current classification recognizes no other forms of benign idiopathic epilepsy – either partial or generalized – with onset in the first year of life. Indeed, the consensus is that epilepsies arising in the first year of life have an unfavourable prognosis. Benign familial infantile convulsions (BFIC) is a recently recognized idiopathic epileptic syndrome. BFIC was originally described in five Italian families (Vigevano *et al.*, 1990, 1992). The disease has also been reported in other Italian (Dordi *et al.*, 1992) and non-Italian families in Japan (Watanabe *et al.*, 1990), in France (Echenne *et al.*, 1994), Singapore (Lee *et al.*, 1993), Sweden (Lüovigson, personal communication), Germany (Kurlemann, personal communication) and United-States (Ryan, personal communication). BFIC present with onset between 3 and 12 months, seizures of partial type in most cases, no aetiological factors, normal psychomotor development, and normal interictal electroencephalograms (EEGs) (Vigevano *et al.*, 1992). BFIC is inherited in a manner consistent with an autosomal dominant disorder. The specific age of onset of this syndrome could indicate that the corresponding genes play a role in the maturation of regulatory process of cerebral excitability. Some alteration in gene expression may be involved, with the relevant gene being turned on or off too early or too late. Presumably this issue will be resolved when the underlying gene has been mapped and sequenced and the basic gene product is identified.

More recently another familial infantile epileptic syndrome was described. Initially recognized as BFIC (Berquin *et al.*, 1992), the co-existence of paroxysmal choreoathetosis was later identified. This new syndrome was called familial infantile convulsions and choreoathetosis (ICCA) (Szepetowski *et al.*, 1997).

To initiate studies that should lead to the identification of the gene defect responsible for BFIC, genetic linkage analysis was performed in five Italian kindreds with this disorder. As a first step, we have used a candidate gene approach in performing linkage analysis using microsatellite polymorphisms flanking the previously mapped epilepsy genes. We first analysed the BFNC locus on chromosome 20q (EBN1). Although the age of onset is different, the two syndromes are very similar. One question is whether BFIC is simply a late onset form of BFNC or a distinct form of familial convulsions. This region has been excluded. This result demonstrates that the EBN1 gene is not responsible for BFIC (Malafosse et al., 1994) as well as all other candidate regions so far analysed (unpublished data). Consequently, a systematic approach using microsatellite polymorphisms lying in non-excluded regions has been used. We mapped the gene responsible for BFIC in five Italian families to the long arm of the chromosome 19 with a maximum two-point lod-score of 6.36 at D19S114 and a multipoint lod-score 8 were obtained for the interval D19S250 – D19S114 – D19S251 (Guipponi et al., 1997). No evidence of genetic heterogeneity was recognized within our family sample. The main clinical features of BFIC – afebrile seizures between 3 and 12 month of age, normal neurodevelopmental status, normal interictal electroencephalogram and no demonstrable underlying pathology – led us to consider this syndrome as an idiopathic epilepsy. Thus BFIC follows BFNC (Leppert et al., 1989; Malafosse et al., 1992; Lewis et al., 1993), JME (Delgado-Escueta et al., 1994), ADNFLE (Phillips et al., 1995), idiopathic partial epilepsy with auditory symptoms (Ottman et al., 1995), as the fifth form of inherited idiopathic epilepsy that has had its disease locus genetically mapped. These results confirm the genetic basis, the autosomal inheritance of BFIC and the accuracy of the clinical diagnostic. Moreover, the mapping of the BFIC gene on a different chromosome than BFNC definitively demonstrates that these two idiopathic epilepsies are not allelic, and thus confirm our previous results (Malafosse et al., 1994) which indicated that this epileptic syndrome is distinct from the 20q-linked BFNC.

Three pedigrees of benign familial infantile convulsions have been identified in Montpellier (France) since the initial publication by Vigevano et al. (1992). Linkage to DNA markers of chromosome 19q has been rejected in the largest family. The two other families are not large enough to allow to clarify them among 19q-linked or unlinked pedigrees. Our linkage data strongly support the existence of two distinct genetic loci for BFIC. Linkage heterogeneity is highly suspected in BFIC. The genetic heterogeneity is now well established for BFNC, since two families with neonatal onset map to chromosome 8 (EBN2) instead of 20 (EBN1) (Lewis et al., 1993; Steinlein et al., 1993). This kind of genetic heterogeneity occuring at different genetic loci is called non-allelic heterogeneity. Such heterogeneity can also be caused by mutations occurring at the same genetic locus and is referred to allelic heterogeneity, an example is Unverricht-Lundborg disease.

The 19q-unlinked family is the only one which is not from Italian origin. These data suggest that the BFIC subtype linked to chromosome 19 may be associated with an Italian origin. The existence of a founder effect in these Italian 19q-linked BFIC families is possible, and is further supported by the common haplotype found in these pedigrees (Guipponi et al., 1997). However, to confirm this hypothesis a larger number of Italian families and more genealogical information from the pedigrees are required.

Non allelic heterogeneity may also be explained by the type of seizures observed in 19q-linked and 19q-unlinked families. The difference between our French patients and those of Vigevano et al. (1992) concerns the type of seizures. The clinical and EEG features of Vigevano's patients are characteristic of partial seizures, whereas in our patients only generalized seizures of various types (clonic, tonic or atonic) were seen. Ictal or video EEG unfortunately were not performed in our patients, and thus the possibility of secondary generalized seizures cannot be excluded. This observation may indicate that 19q-linked BFIC is a localization-related epilepsy. The implication of this locus in other inherited idiopathic partial epilepsies should be thus tested. Benign occipital epilepsy, which is characterized by an age of onset between the ages of 4 and 8 years and an autosomal dominant mode of inheritance, should be a good candidate for studies.

Additional studies are needed to determine whether there is a consistent relationship between the genetic subtype of BFIC and the clinical features such as ethnicity, partial or generalized seizures and the risk of late epilepsy.

The different kind of seizure types in epilepsies of neonates and infants may be in fact the expression of different 'maturational' factors. Moreover, the specific ages of onset of BFNC and BFIC may indicate that the corresponding genes play a role in the maturation of regulatory processes of cerebral excitability.

The next step will be to identify candidate genes from the region of chromosome 19 that seems to harbour the BFIC mutation. The recent identification of mutations in two new potassium channel genes (*KCNQ2* and *KQT-like*) in families with BFNC (EBN1 and EBN2 respectively) shed light on ion channel genes as new candidate genes for idiopathic epilepsies (Singh *et al.*, 1997; Charlier *et al.*, 1997; Biervert *et al.*, 1998). Interestingly, BFIC was mapped to the long arm of chromosome 19 (Guipponi *et al.*, 1997) where three potassium channel KCNC2, KCNC3, KCNA7 and a sodium voltage-gated channel genes are located on 19q13.3 and 19q13.1 respectively. Moreover, the gene responsible for ICCA was mapped in a 10 cM region around the centromere of human chromosome 16 (Szepetowski *et al.*, 1997), where two subunits of sodium channel SCNN1B-SCNN1G are localized. This could suggest that homologous genes are responsible for BFIC and ICCA, and that ion channel genes are among the best candidates.

The probable presence of heterogeneity in BFIC may complicate efforts to isolate the 19q gene, since a critical step in such a project will be the search for flanking markers. This entails a search for individuals who demonstrate recombination between the disease and the closely linked marker locus. Consequently, the direct and systematic analysis of candidate genes will probably be a more tempting approach.

A familial susceptibility to epilepsy has been recognized, but polygenic inheritance has been implicated for most syndromes (Andermann, 1982). Analysis of rare, single-gene epilepsies such as BFNC, ADNFLE and BFIC may lead to identification of important genes involved in neuronal excitability and may result in a better understanding of the physiopathology of more common epileptic syndromes.

References

Andermann, E. (1992): Multifactorial inheritance of generalized and focal epilepsy. In: *Genetic basis of the epilepsies*, Anderson, V.E., Hauser, W.A., Penry, J.K., Sing, C.F. (eds), pp. 355–374. New York: Raven Press.

Berquin, P., Macron, J.M., Jacquemart, F., Mathieu, M. & Piussan, C. (1992): Les convulsions partielles bénignes du nourrisson d'un an. *Méd. Hyg.* **50**, 425–430.

Biervert, C., Schroeder, B.C., Kudbischm C., Berkovic, S.F., Propping, P., Jentsch, T.J. & Steinlein, O.K. (1998): A potassium channel mutation in neonatal human epilepsy. *Science* **279**, 403–406.

Charlier, C., Singh, N.A., Ryan, S.G., Lewis, T.B., Reus, B.E., Leach, R.J., Leppert, M. (1998): A pore mutation in a novel KQT-like potassium channel gene in an idiopathic epilepsy family. *Nat. Genet.* **18**, 53–56.

Commission on Classification and Terminology of the International League Against Epilepsy (1989): Proposal for revised classification of epilepsies and epileptic syndromes. *Epilepsia* **30**, 389–399.

Delgado-Escueta, A.V., Liu, A., Serratosa, J., Weissbecker, K., Medina, M.T., Gee, M., Treiman, L.J. & Sparkes, R.S. (1994): Juvenile myoclonic epilepsy: is there heterogeneity? In: *Idiopathic generalized epilepsies: Clinical, experimental and genetic aspects*, Malafosse, A., Genton, P., Hirsch, E., Marescaux, C., Broglin, D., Bernasconi, R. (eds), pp. 281–287. London: John Libbey.

Dordi, B., de Marco, P., Biamino, P. & Tiabano, G. (1992): Convulsioni infantili familiari benigne. *Rev. Esp. Epilepsia* **7**, 10.

Echenne, B., Humbertclaude, V., Rivier, F., Malafosse, A. & Cheminal, R. (1994): Benign infantile epilepsy with autosomal dominant inheritance. *Brain Dev.* **16**, 108–111.

Guipponi, M., Rivier, F., Vigevano, F., Beck, C., Crespel, A., Echenne, B., Lucchini, P., Sebastianelli, R., Baldy-Moulinier, M. & Malafosse, A. (1997): Linkage mapping of benign familial infantile convulsions (BFIC) to chromosome 19q. *Hum. Mol. Genet.* **6**, 473–478.

Lee, W.L., Mow, P.S. & Rajan, U. (1993): Benign familial infantile epilepsy. *J. Pediatr.* **123**, 588–590.

Leppert, M., Anderson, V.E., Quattlebaum, T., Stauffer, D., O'Connel, P., Nakamura. Y., Laloue, J.M. & White, R. (1989): Benign familial neonatal convulsions linked to genetic markers on chromosome 20. *Nature* **337**, 647–648.

Lewis, T.B., Leach, R.J., Ward, K., O'Connell, P. & Ryan, S.G. (1993): Genetic heterogeneity in benign familial neonatal convulsions: identification of a new locus on chromosome 8q. *Am. J. Hum. Genet.* **53**, 670–675.

Luovigson, P., Olafsson, E., Rich, S.S., Johannesson, G. & Anderson, V.E. (1993): Benign infantile familial epilepsy: three families with multiple affected members in three generations. *Epilepsia* **34** (S2), 18.

Malafosse, A., Leboyer, M., Dulac, O., Navelet, Y., Plouin, P., Beck, C., Laklou, H., Mouchnino, G., Grandscene, P., Vallee, L., Guilloud-Bataille, M., Samolyk, D., Baldy-Moulinier, M., Feingold, J. & Mallet, J. (1992): Confirmation of linkage of benign convulsions to D20S19 and D20S20. *Hum. Genet.* **89**, 54–58.

Malafosse, A., Beck, C., Bellet, H., D.I., Capua, M., Dulac, O., Echenne, B., Fusco, L., Lucchini, P., Ricci, S., Sebastianelli, R., Feingold, J., Baldy-Moulinier, M. & Vigevano, F. (1994): Benign infantile familial convulsions are not an allelic form of the benign familial neonatal convulsions gene. *Ann. Neurol.* **35**, 479–482.

Ottman, R., Risch, N., Hauser, A., Pedley, T., Lee, J., Baker-Cummings, C., Lustenberg, A., Nagle, K., Lee, K., Scheuer, M., Neystat, M., Susser, M. & Wilhelmsen, K. (1995): Localization of a gene for partial epilepsy to chromosome 10q. *Nat. Genet.* **10**, 56–60.

Phillips, H.A., Scheffer, I.E., Berkovic, S.F., Hollway, G.E., Sutherland, G.R. & Mulley, J.C. (1995): Localization of a gene for dominant nocturnal frontal lobe epilepsy to chromosome 20q13.2. *Nat. Genet.* **10**, 117–118.

Szepetowski, P., Rochette, J., Berquin, P., Piussan, C., Lathrop, G.M. & Monaco, A.P. (1997): Familial infantile convulsions and paroxysmal choreoathetosis : a new neurological syndrome linked to the pericentromeric region of human chromosome 16. *Am. J. Hum. Genet.* **61**, 889–898.

Singh, N.A., Charlier, C., Stauffer, D., DuPont, B.R., Leach, R.J., Melis, R., Ronen, G.M., Bjerre, I., Quattlebaum, T., Murphy, J.V., McHarg, M.L., Gagnon, D., Rosales, T.O., Peiffer, A., Anderson, V.E. & Leppert, M. (1998): A novel potassium channel gene, *KCNQ2*, is mutated in an inherited epilepsy of newborns. *Nat. Genet.* **18**, 25–30.

Vigevano, F., Di Capua, M., Fusco, L., Ricci, S., Sebastianelli, R. & Lucchini, P. (1990): Sixth-month benign familial convulsions. *Epilepsia* **31**, 613.

Vigevano, F., Fusco, L., Di Capua, M., Ricci, S., Sebastianelli, R. & Lucchini, P. (1992): Benign infantile familial convulsions. *Eur. J. Pediatr.* **151**, 608–612.

Watanabe, K., Yamamoto, N., Negoro, T., Takahashi, I., Aso, K. & Machara, M. (1990): Benign infantile epilepsy with complex partial seizures. *J. Clin. Neurophysiol.* **7**, 409–416.

Chapter 8

Benign partial epilepsies in infancy and early childhood: clinical description and genetic background

Kazuyoshi Watanabe

Department of Paediatrics, Nagoya University School of Medicine, 65 Tsurumai, Showa-ku, Nagoya 466-8550 Japan

Summary

Benign partial epilepsies are not rare in infancy and comprise two forms, although both are closely related. One is partial epilepsy with CPS and the other one with SGS. The most frequent site of seizure origin was in the temporal area in the former and central, parietal or occipital area in the latter. The former has not been well recognized because of subtle manifestation and favourable outcome. Benign convulsions are also common in infancy. Most of them may belong to partial epilepsy with SGS, although confirmation with ictal EEG recording is necessary for accurate diagnosis. Some are familial and many of them seem to show an autosomal dominant pattern, but some seem to have autosomal recessive inheritance.

Partial epilepsies in children had been considered as reflecting symptomatic aetiology until benign childhood epilepsy with centro-temporal spikes was delineated. This had also been the case with partial epilepsies in infancy; the prognosis of partial epilepsy in infancy had been considered unfavourable and benign partial epilepsy was reported to be extremely rare or non-existent in infancy (Dulac *et al.*, 1989). In the current International Classification of Epilepsies (Commission, 1989), benign myoclonic epilepsy is only benign epileptic syndrome known in infancy. No syndromes belonging to benign partial epilepsies are mentioned in this age period. This may be because partial seizures are difficult to diagnose in infants unless they show focal motor manifestations and many patients with benign outcome are usually not referred to specialized centres where ictal EEG recordings may be performed for diagnosis. Some infants with benign partial epilepsies may show partial seizures with secondary generalization. Such secondarily generalized seizures are often difficult to diagnose because initial partial seizure manifestations are often missed.

Benign partial epilepsy in infancy with complex partial seizures (CPS)

We previously reported nine infants with CPS who showed an extremely benign course (Watanabe *et al.*, 1987, 1990). Up to the present, we have had 13 infants with this syndrome whose seizure types were confirmed by simultaneous video/EEG monitoring. Six of them were male and seven females. Five of 13 infants had a family history of benign afebrile or febrile seizures. The mother and elder sister of one patient, the mother of one, the father of one, and the elder brother of one, had afebrile seizures only during infancy. Both parents of one patient had febrile seizures during childhood.

Pre-, peri- and postnatal history were not remarkable and psychomotor development prior to the onset was normal in all infants. None of the infants had underlying disorders or demonstrated any signs of acute organic or functional brain insult on physical, neurological and laboratory examinations.

The age of onset was under 1 year in all patients except one and ranged from 3 to 20 months (3 months in three patients, 4 months in three, 5 months in 4, 6 months, 8 months and 20 months in one each).

Seizures occurred in clusters in all cases, 1–10 times a day for 1–3 days, recurring 1–8 weeks later when they did. The duration of seizures, calculated from the first clinical or EEG change until the end of paroxysmal discharges excluding polymorphic delta waves, ranged from 30 to 217 s. Seizures occurred during wakefulness in 11 and during sleep in two. They were characterized by motion arrest, decreased responsiveness, staring or blank eyes mostly with automatisms, and mild convulsive movements. One infant presented with apnea as a chief manifestation. Awakening from sleep and crying were the initial manifestations in infants who had seizures in sleep.

Convulsive movements were observed in 11 patients and consisted of eye deviation or head rotation in 10, mild clonic movements involving face, eyelids, or limbs in seven, and increased limb tone in nine.

Automatisms were noted in six and consisted of simple head, arm, or leg movements in five, oral movements in five, and change in facial expression in two. No complex, semipurposeful automatisms were observed. Eye deviation or head rotation occurred relatively early in the attack, whereas oral automatisms occurred later and one infant experienced them postictally.

Interictal EEGs all were normal. Ictal EEGs usually disclosed focal discharges of low voltage fast waves or rhythmic or repetitive sharp alpha or theta waves of increasing amplitude and decreasing frequency which were followed by theta and delta waves mixed with spikes or sharp waves with gradual or rapid spread to other regions.

The site of initial paroxysmal discharges on the ictal EEGs was in the temporal area in eight patients, in the central area in two, and in the frontal, parietal and occipital areas in one each. Subdivision of temporal foci was not possible because the electrodes were placed in the mid- and posterior temporal areas but not in the anterior temporal area.

Antiepileptic drugs were administered in 13 infants immediately after the ictal EEG and video recordings, resulting in complete seizure control in eight infants. Seizures recurred after the initial dose in five infants. Four of them experienced recurrence 1–2 months after treatment began but seizure control was achieved immediately after an increase in dosage. The dose was unchanged in one infant without further recurrence. Carbamazepine was administered in eight and phenobarbital in three, valproate and zonisamide in one each. All the patients remained seizure-free and demonstrated normal development at the follow-up age of 3 to 10 years. Antiepileptic treatment was withdrawn after 1.5–2.5 years of medication in seven patients and 3–5 years in six.

In summary, benign partial epilepsy in infancy with CPS is characterized by:

(1) Familial or non-familial occurrence
(2) Normal development prior to onset
(3) Onset mostly during the first year of life
(4) No underlying disorders nor neurological abnormalities
(5) Complex partial seizures often occurring in clusters
(6) Normal interictal EEG
(7) Ictal EEG most often showing temporal focus
(8) Excellent response to treatment
(9) Normal developmental outcome

Ictal EEGs and clinical seizure manifestations were not much different from those of infants with refractory seizures reported previously (Yamamoto et al.,1987) But most infants with refractory CPS either were developmentally retarded or often had interictal EEG abnormalities.

Benign partial epilepsy in infancy with secondarily generalized seizures (SGS)

We previously reported seven infants with partial epilepsy who showed SGS confirmed with ictal EEGs and easily controlled with medication (Watanabe *et al.*, 1993). Up to now, we have had 10 such cases diagnosed with ictal EEG recordings.

Five were boys and five girls. Five of 10 infants had a family history of benign afebrile or febrile seizures. The father of two patients had afebrile seizures and the elder brother of one and the elder sister of one had afebrile seizures in infancy. The mother of one patient had febrile convulsions only during infancy.

Pre-, peri- and post-natal histories were not remarkable and psychomotor development before the onset was normal in all infants. Physical, neurological and laboratory examinations including serum chemistry, metabolic screens, serology, and brain CT scans all were normal.

The age of onset ranged from 3 to 20 months, but was under 1 year in eight of 10 patients (3, 4, 5 months in two patients each and 8, 11, 15 and 20 months in one each).

Seizures occurred in clusters in all patients, 2–5 times a day for 1–3 days, recurring 1–3 months later in four infants. Seizures occurred during wakefulness in six and during sleep in three. The clinical seizure manifestation in the former was motion arrest with staring or blank eyes lasting 5–33 s, followed by generalized tonic–clonic convulsions of 40–120 s duration. In the latter, opening of eyes with staring or awakening from sleep with crying lasting 6–13 s was followed by generalized tonic–clonic seizures lasting 40–150 s.

Interictal EEGs revealed no abnormal findings in all patients. Ictal EEG disclosed a focal onset of paroxysmal discharges followed by generalization. The origin of initial focal paroxysmal discharges in 10 recorded seizures was central in three, parietal in two, occipital in five, and posterior temporal in one. In one patient, different foci (occipital and central area) were disclosed at the onset and recurrence.

Antiepileptic medication was started immediately after an ictal EEG was recorded without trying to record another seizure in all cases. Phenobarbital was administered in five, carbamazepine in four and zonisamide in one. In one patient, seizures recurred two months after phenobarbital was administered and carbamazepine was added with complete seizure control. In another, valproate administered by a referring physician was changed to carbamazepine with success. Antiepileptics were withdrawn after the seizure-free period of 3 years in five infants, two years in two and one year in one, without recurrence of seizures.

In summary, benign partial epilepsy in infancy with SGS is characterized by:

(1) Familial or non-familial occurrence
(2) Normal development prior to onset
(3) Onset mostly during the first year of life
(4) No underlying disorders nor neurological abnormalities
(5) Secondarily generalized seizures often occurring in clusters
(6) Foregoing partial seizures consisting of motionless stare or blank eyes
(7) Normal interictal EEG
(8) Ictal EEGs most often showing central, parietal or occipital focus
(9) Excellent response to treatment
(10) Normal developmental outcome

Most of the infants we studied were initially considered to have generalized tonic–clonic convulsions, which turned out to be partial seizures evolving to secondarily generalized seizures with ictal EEG recordings. Initial partial seizure manifestations are easily missed, unless they show localized motor phenomena.

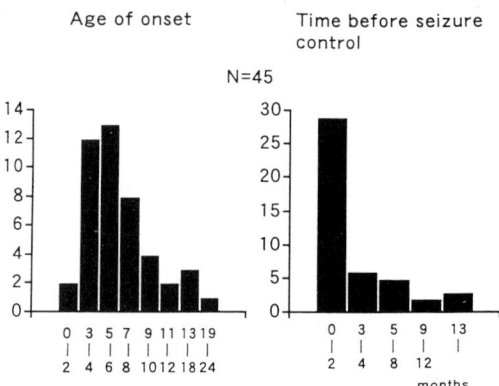

Fig. 1. The age of onset and time before remission in 45 infants with benign partial epilepsy in infancy collected in five affiliated general hospitals. The onset ranged from 1 to 23 months (6.7 months on average) and the last seizure occurred at 1 to 24 months of age (9.9 months on average).

A study of benign partial epilepsy in infancy based on clinical criteria

As mentioned above, benign partial epilepsy had been considered rare in infancy because most infants with this syndrome are usually managed in first-line general hospitals and are not referred to specialized centres. We thus conducted a retrospective survey on this entity in our five affiliated general hospitals, using mainly clinical criteria on the basis of our previous experience.

We defined benign partial epilepsy in infancy as epilepsies meeting the following criteria:

(1) Complex partial seizures (CPS) or secondarily generalized seizures (SGS), or both
(2) Normal development before and after onset
(3) No underlying disorders or neurological abnormalities
(4) Normal interictal EEGs
(5) Good responses to treatment with antiepileptic drugs
(6) Favourable outcome after the follow-up of at least 3 years

CPS were defined as seizures characterized by motion arrest, decreased responsiveness, staring or blank eyes, or mild convulsive movements such as eye deviation, head rotation, clonic movements, or increased limb tone with or without automatisms, cyanosis or foaming from the mouth. A secondarily generalized seizure was one presenting with CPS followed by a generalized tonic–clonic seizure. The duration of seizures was mostly 1–5 min, although it was not measured precisely.

Patients with only neonatal seizures, those having generalized convulsions without preceding CPS features, and those with prolonged seizures lasting more than 30 min were excluded. A cluster of seizures was defined as more than two seizures within 24 h. The age of onset ranged from 1 to 23 months with a mean age at 6.7 months (Fig. 1). Most had onset between between 3 and 8 months. Seizure control was attained within two months in most cases. The age of the last seizure ranged from 1 to 24 months with a mean age of 9.9 months.

The total number of seizures was less than 10 in most cases. A little more than half (53 per cent) of the patients had a cluster of seizures.

Family history was positive in 12 (27 per cent) of 45 patients. Six had siblings with benign partial epilepsy in infancy. The mother of three patients had benign infantile seizures. A sibling of one patient and the father of another had epilepsy of unknown type. A sibling of another had febrile seizures. Eye deviation, cyanosis, staring or blank eyes, motion arrest are clinical manifestations most frequently described. Oral automatisms were infrequent, probably due to the retrospective nature of the study. Secondarily generalized seizures were noted in 69 per cent of patients. Antiepileptic drugs were administered in 91 per cent of the patients. Phenobarbital, zonisamide and carbamazepine were the agents most frequently prescribed and any of them was effective. Part of this study based on patients seen in one of these affiliated hospitals was published elsewhere and reported results similar to the above (Okumura et al., 1996).

Genetic background in benign partial epilepsy in infancy

Seventeen (25 per cent) of 68 patients in our three studies had a positive family history of benign non-febrile seizures only in infancy. Only siblings were affected in nine and parents in eight. Of the latter, the father was affected in three and the mother in five. The mode of inheritance seems to be autosomal dominant or recessive.

Related syndromes and nosological problems

The presence of benign partial epilepsy in infancy with CPS had not been recognized until our first description in 1987, probably because it may be difficult to diagnose CPS in infants and patients with benign seizures are not likely to be referred to specialized centres. Since our first report, there have been a few reports in society meetings and publications in Japan confirming its presence (Yagi et al., 1989; Hanai et al., 1990; Wakai et al., 1991; Ikemoto et al., 1995).

The presence of infantile convulsions with benign outcome had already been noted by Fukuyama (1963), who defined them as having: (1) onset before 2 years of age; (2) generalized, symmetrical convulsion, mainly tonic–clonic, lasting 1–2 min; (3) no family history of epilepsy; (4) past history not remarkable; (5) normal psychomotor development; (6) no aetiology; (7) (EEG normal); (8) (benign course). This variety of infantile convulsions has been a subject of many subsequent studies in Japan and called benign infantile convulsions. As shown above, Fukuyama stressed generalized symmetrical convulsion, and did not consider it partial seizures. Neither did other authors describing benign infantile convulsions (Sugiura et al., 1983). We previously pointed out, however, that ictal EEGs of such patients usually display partial seizures evolving to secondarily generalized tonic–clonic seizures. Tsurui et al. (1989) recently made a similar observation in patients with benign infantile convulsions meeting the criteria of Fukuyama except for positive family history. At least some of the partial seizures they observed were complex. Thus, a considerable number of infants diagnosed as having generalized convulsions in infancy may, in fact, have SGS because of an inability to recognize initial complex seizure manifestations.

The absence of a family history of epilepsy was another criterion of benign infantile convulsions described by Fukuyama but a history of benign convulsions was often elicited. Vigevano et al. (1992, 1994) reported benign infantile familial convulsions characterized by family history of seizures with benign course and similar age of onset, normal development prior to onset, onset between ages 4 months and 8 months, no underlying disorders or neurologic abnormalities, secondarily generalized partial seizures, normal interictal EEGs, benign course, normal developmental outcome. Kubagawa et al. (1976) and Kajiyama et al. (1987) of Japan alluded to familial benign infantile convulsions. Lee et al. (1993) also reported patients with benign familial infantile epilepsy from Singapore. Echenne et al. (1994) of France reported six infants of three families as benign infantile epilepsy with autosomal dominant inheritance. Their clinical characteristics are similar to those of familial or non-familial benign partial epilepsy in infancy with complex partial seizures or secondarily generalized seizures. Ictal EEGs of benign infantile familial convulsions were documented by Vigevano et al. (1992), showing secondary generalization of seizures beginning in the central-occipital areas. They are in general agreement with benign partial epilepsy in infancy with SGS.

Some infants with benign partial epilepsy may have both CPS and SGS. Thus, benign partial epilepsy with CPS and SGS may be closely related with each other and we proposed combining the two syndromes and term them benign partial epilepsy in infancy (Watanabe et al., 1993). One of the differences between these two syndromes is the site of initial paroxysmal discharges on the ictal EEG. The seizure origin was most frequently temporal area in partial epilepsy with CPS, whereas it was central, parietal and occipital area in partial epilepsy with SGS.

Addendum: A recently described syndrome, Familial infantile convulsions and choreoathetosis (ICCA), associates benign familial infantile convulsions and paroxysmal choreoathetosis in the same familioes (Szepetowski *et al.*, 1997).

References

Commission on Classification and Terminology of the International League Against Epilepsy (1989): Proposal for revised classifications epilepsies and epileptic syndromes. *Epilepsia* **30**, 389–399.

Dulac, O., Cusmai, R. & de Oliveira, K. (1989): Is there a partial benign epilepsy in infancy? *Epilepsia* **30**, 798–801.

Echenne, B., Humbertclaude, V., Rivier, F., Malafosse, A. & Cheminal, R. (1994): Benign infantile epilepsy with autosomal dominant inheritance. *Brain Dev. (Tokyo)* **16**, 108–111.

Fukuyama, Y. (1963): Borderland of epilepsy with special reference to febrile convulsions and so called infantile convulsions (in Japanese). *Seishin Igaku (Tokyo)* **5**, 211–213.

Garty, B.Z., Steinberg, T. & Krause, I. (1993): Benign infantile familial convulsions. *Eur. J. Pediatr.* **152**, 701.

Hanai, T., Narasaki, O., Kira, R. & Asahi, T. (1990): Clinical study of benign complex partial seizures in infancy (in Japanese). *Proceeding of 24th Meeting of Japan Epilepsy Society*, p. 166.

Ikematsu, K., Saito, M., Tsuru, T., Yamagata, T., Miyao, M. & Momoi, M. (1995): Clinico-electroencephalographic study of idiopathic complex partial seizures in infancy. *Proceeding of 29th Meeting of Japan Epilepsy Society*, p. 182.

Kajiyama, M., Igei, M., Kusumoto, J. *et al.* (1987): The prognosis of afebrile convulsions in infancy without paroxysmal discharges on the initial EEG (in Japanese). *No to Hattatsu (Tokyo)* **19**, 50–57.

Lee, W.L., Low, P.S. & Rajan, U. (1993): Benign familial infantile epilepsy. *J. Pediatr.***123**, 588–590.

Luovigsson, P., Olafsson, E., Rich, S.S., Johannesson, G. & Anderson, V.E. (1993): Benign infantile familial epilepsy: three families with multiple affected members in three generations. *Epilepsia* **34**(S2), 18.

Okumura, A., Hayakawa, F., Kuno, K. & Watanabe, K. (1996): Benign partial epilepsy in infancy. *Arch. Dis. Childh.* **74**, 19–21.

Sugiura, M., Matsumoto, A., Watanabe, K., Negoro, T., Takaesu, E. & Iwase, K. (1983): Long-term prognosis of generalized convulsions in the first year of life, with special reference to benign infantile convulsions (in Japanese). *Tenkan Kenkyu* **1**, 116–121.

Szepetowski, P., Rochette, J., Berquin, P., Piussan, C., Lathrop, G.M. & Monaco, A.P. (1997): Familial infantile convulsions and paroxysmal choreoathetosis: a new neurological syndrome linked to the pericentromeric region of human chromosome 16. *Am. J. Hum. Genet.* **61**, 889–898.

Tsurui, S., Oguni, H. & Fukuyama, Y. (1989): Analysis of ictal EEG in benign infantile convulsions (in Japanese). *Tenkan Kenkyu (Tokyo)* **7**, 160–168.

Vigevano, F., Fusco, L., di Capua, M., Ricci, S., Sebastianelli, R. & Lucchini, P. (1992): Benign infantile familial convulsions. *Eur. J. Pediatr.* **151**, 608–612.

Vigevano, F., Sebastianelli, R., Fusco, L. *et al.* (1994): Benign infantile familial convulsions. In: *Idiopathic generalized epilepsies: clinical, experimental and genetic aspects*, Malafosse, A., Genton, P., Hirsh, E., Marescaux, C., Broglin, D. & Bernasconi, R. (eds), pp. 45–49. London: John Libbey.

Wakai, S., Youto, Y., Hotsubo, T., Konosita, M., Tachi, N. & Chiba S. (1991): Three cases of benign complex partial epilepsies in infancy (in Japanese). *Shonika Shinryo (Tokyo)* **54**, 348–352.

Watanabe, K., Negoro, T. & Aso, K. (1993): Benign partial epilepsy with secondarily generalized seizures in infancy. *Epilepsia* **34**, 635–638.

Watanabe, K., Negoro, T., Sugiura, T. *et al.* (1981): Ictal EEGs of generalized tonic–clonic seizures in infancy (in Japanese). *Rinsho Noha (Clin. Electroenceph.)* **23**, 445–447.

Watanabe, K., Yamamoto, N., Negoro, T. *et al.* (1987): Benign complex partial epilepsies in infancy. *Pediatr. Neurol.* **3**, 208–211.

Watanabe, K., Yamamoto, N., Negoro T., Takahashi, I., Aso, K. & Maehara, M. (1990): Benign infantile epilepsy with complex partial seizures. *J. Clin. Neurophysiol.* **7**, 409–416.

Yagi, S., Miura, Y., Kobayashi, K., Kataoka, N. & Morita, T. (1989): Two cases of benign complex partial epilepsies in infancy (in Japanese). *Rinsho Noha (Clin. Electroenceph.) (Tokyo)* **31**, 209–213.

Yamamoto, N., Watanabe, K., Negoro, T. *et al.* (1987): Complex partial seizures in children: ictal manifestations and their relation to clinical course. *Neurology* **37**, 1379–1382.

Part IV
Autosomal dominant focal epilepsies

Chapter 9

Autosomal dominant nocturnal frontal lobe epilepsy

Ingrid E Scheffer

Departments of Neurology, Austin and Repatriation Medical Centre, Royal Children's Hospital, Monash Medical Centre; and University of Melbourne, Australia

Since autosomal dominant nocturnal frontal lobe epilepsy (ADNFLE) was first described in 1994 (Scheffer *et al.*, 1994), families have been recognized in Norway (Magnusson *et al.*, 1996), Italy (Oldani *et al.*, 1996), Germany (Khatami *et al.*, 1997), France, Sweden, Scotland and North America (Scheffer *et al.*, 1995) (personal communication). ADNFLE is a relatively common and distinctive epilepsy syndrome which remains a clinical diagnosis. In 1995, we reported linkage of a large Australian family with ADNFLE to chromosome 20q (Phillips *et al.*, 1995) and later that year, reported a mutation in the neuronal nicotinic acetylcholine receptor alpha 4 subunit (Steinlein *et al.*, 1995). A second family with a mutation in this gene was recognized more recently (Steinlein *et al.*, 1997). We have subsequently shown ADNFLE to be a genetically heterogeneous disorder (Berkovic *et al.*, 1995) with a second locus on chromosome 15 (Phillips *et al.*, 1998).

Clinical features

ADNFLE typically begins in the first two decades of life with the mean age of seizure onset 12 years and the median 8 years (Scheffer *et al.*, 1995). There is a wide range of seizure onset from the first year of life to the sixth decade.

ADNFLE is characterized by clusters of brief motor seizures in sleep. Seizures usually occur as the patient dozes within the first hour of falling asleep or in the last few hours before awakening. Seizures may also occur during a daytime nap. Although the occurrence of seizures in sleep is a striking feature, about one quarter of patients have rare attacks while awake. In the more severely affected individuals, this is typically when their seizures are poorly controlled.

Patients are often awakened by an aura which is non-specific. They may vocalise, gasp or grunt, and then have a motor seizure with features which vary from hyperkinetic attacks to tonic seizures which may have clonic components. Some individuals injure themselves during an attack due to non-directed violent motor activity. Retained awareness is common throughout attacks so individuals may find attacks frightening and become fearful of falling asleep. They often have a feeling of difficulty breathing during attacks such as 'the breath is stuck in my throat' and objectively, individuals may hyperventilate. Secondarily generalized tonic–clonic seizures occur in approximately 60 per cent of patients but are infrequent (Scheffer *et al.*, 1995).

Seizures typically occur in a cluster of a mean of eight attacks over a few hours. The most severely affected individuals may have nights of virtually continuous attacks (one individual had 72 attacks documented), while a quarter of individuals are mildly affected with only one attack per night. In general, seizures are brief with a clinically estimated median duration of 74 s (Scheffer *et al.*, 1995), however this figure incorporates secondarily generalized tonic–clonic seizures and probably most partial seizures are even briefer.

There is intrafamilial and interfamilial variation in severity and semiology of the frontal lobe seizures (Scheffer *et al.*, 1995; Hayman *et al.*, 1997). The most mildly affected individuals describe seizures for a few months around puberty which settle spontaneously, or have unrecognized attacks (see misdiagnosis below). By contrast, the most severely affected individuals have onset in infancy with seizures continuing to be refractory throughout adult life. Individuals in their sixth decade describe ongoing milder attacks which they recognize to be fragments of their attacks when younger. Partial seizure semiology within families may vary from thrashing hyperkinetic motor attacks to tonic seizures (Hayman *et al.*, 1997).

Affected individuals are of normal intellect with normal neurological examination. Seizures are often well controlled with carbamazepine and in the more refractory patients, the addition of a benzodiazepine such as clonazepam is often helpful. In the refractory cases, multiple anti-epileptic drugs are often ineffective. Therapy with drugs acting on the cholinergic system has not yielded consistent results.

EEG studies

Interictal EEG studies are usually unhelpful in ADNFLE. Most individuals have a normal interictal EEG although interictal epileptiform discharges may be seen emanating from the anterior quadrants (Scheffer *et al.*, 1995; Oldani *et al.*, 1996).

Ictal EEG studies often show movement artefact. In some cases, bifrontal sharp and slow wave activity may be seen (Scheffer *et al.*, 1995; Oldani *et al.*, 1996) and in others, unilateral frontal onset may be demonstrated (Hayman *et al.*, 1997).

Neuroimaging

Structural neuroimaging (MRI and CT brain scans) is usually normal (Scheffer *et al.*, 1995). SPECT and PET may show unilateral functional defects. We documented unilateral frontal hyperperfusion on ictal SPECT scan when compared with an interictal study in one patient (Hayman *et al.*, 1997). Similarly, interictal PET studies may show unilateral frontal hypometabolism. In two cases reported, one showed a consistent left frontopolar onset while another showed a right parasaggital mid-frontal focus (Hayman *et al.*, 1997). Thus, although individuals have a unilateral frontal lobe focus, heterogeneous locations within the frontal lobe for seizure onset are seen in different individuals.

Misdiagnosis and differential diagnosis

Misdiagnosis in ADNFLE has led to under-recognition of the autosomal dominant inheritance pattern. Common misdiagnoses include a variety of sleep disturbances with some individuals regarding these attacks as 'normal sleep', nightmares, parvor nocturnus or night terrors, and somnambulism. Night terrors can be readily distinguished from ADNFLE as a solitary attack usually occurs 2 h after the child falls asleep. The attacks typically last longer than 5 min and the child is not aware. Attacks are not stereotyped and the child is amnesic of the attack the following morning. Night terrors run a benign course whereas in ADNFLE individuals have multiple brief stereotyped attacks per night with retained awareness, and attacks often persist into adult life.

Retained awareness during attacks has led to a range of psychiatric misdiagnoses including hysteria and hyperactivity. Asthma has also been diagnosed when individuals have respiratory difficulties during the seizures. Other rare neurological conditions such as startle disease and sleep paralysis have been misdiagnosed, as well as more common disorders such as enuresis.

Lugaresi *et al.*, described the condition 'nocturnal paroxysmal dystonia' (NPD) in 1981 (Lugaresi, Cirignotta, 1981) and identified cases with brief and long duration attacks (Lugaresi *et al.*, 1986). Autosomal dominant kindreds were also described (Lee *et al.*, 1985) and although NPD was initially considered a movement disorder, Lugaresi's group later documented that it was epileptic and of probable frontal lobe origin (Tinuper *et al.*, 1990; Montagna, 1992), a finding also concluded by other authors (Meierkord *et al.*, 1992; Bhatia *et al.*, 1992). Thus NPD is a misnomer and familial cases with brief attacks probably represent cases of ADNFLE.

Other familial dyskinesias such as paroxysmal kinesigenic choreoathetoses and paroxysmal dystonic choreoathetoses (Lance, 1977; Mount & Reback, 1940) can be readily distinguished clinically from ADNFLE (Scheffer *et al.*, 1995).

Genetics

ADNFLE follows autosomal dominant inheritance with a penetrance of approximately 70 per cent. This striking inheritance pattern is often overlooked as affected relatives may be undiagnosed, misdiagnosed or only mildly affected. Furthermore, considerable phenotypic variation is seen within families both in terms of seizure semiology and severity which may obscure the inherited nature of the disorder (Hayman *et al.*, 1997).

Future directions

Molecular genetic analysis of ADNFLE has already begun to identify the different genetic mutations causing this condition. These discoveries will definitely lead to a better understanding of the phenotypes of ADNFLE with genotype-phenotype correlations. Other conditions which may be related to ADNFLE include somnambulism where autosomal dominant kindreds are reported, episodic nocturnal wanderings and other sleep disturbances. Whether these conditions represent part of the ADNFLE spectrum or are other, unrelated disorders of sleep will become apparent, but at this time, placing them into one diagnostic basket may be counterproductive to improving our understanding of the neurobiology of ADNFLE.

Sporadic cases of refractory frontal lobe epilepsy are not uncommon and, in those where no lesion has been identified, it may be that they have a similar genetic basis to their attacks, possibly due to somatic mosaicism. The rapid increase in recognition of ADNFLE around the world promises to continue and with that our understanding of the limits of this disorder will expand.

Acknowledgements: The author is indebted to the following colleagues for collaboration in the clinical study of these families: Professor S. Berkovic, Dr K. Bhatia, Dr D. Fish, Professor C. Marsden, Dr E. Andermann, Professor F. Andermann, Dr I. Lopes-Cendes, Dr R. Desbiens, Dr D. Keene, Dr F. Cendes, Dr J. Manson, Dr J. Constantinou and A. McIntosh. Molecular genetic studies were performed by Associate Professor J. Mulley, H. Phillips and Dr O. Steinlein.

References

Berkovic, S.F., Phillips, H.A., Scheffer, I.E., Lopes-Cendes, I., Bhatia, K.P., Fish, D.R. *et al.* (1995): Genetic heterogeneity in autosomal dominant nocturnal frontal lobe epilepsy. *Epilepsia* **36**, 147 (Abstract).

Bhatia, K., Fish, D., Scott, C.A., Wright, G.D.S. & Marsden, C.D. (1992): A family with paroxysmal nocturnal dystonia with evidence of epileptic frontal lobe discharges in one case. *Movement Disord.* **7** (1), 122 (Abstract).

Hayman, M., Scheffer, I.E., Chinvarun, Y., Berlangieri, S.U. & Berkovic, S.F. (1997): Autosomal dominant nocturnal frontal lobe epilepsy: Demonstration of focal frontal onset and intrafamilial variation. *Neurology* **49**, 969–975.

Khatami, R., Neumann, M. & Kolmel, H.W. (1997): A family with frontal lobe epilepsy and mental retardation. *Epilepsia* **38**, 200 (Abstract).

Lance, J.W. (1977): Familial paroxysmal dystonic choreoathetosis and its differentiation from related syndromes. *Ann. Neurol.* **2**, 285–293.

Lee, B.I., Lesser, R.P., Pippenger, C.E., Morris, H.H., Lüders, H., Dinner, D.S. *et al.* (1985): Familial paroxysmal hypnogenic dystonia. *Neurology* **35**, 1357–1360.

Lugaresi, E. & Cirignotta, F. (1981): Hypnogenic paroxysmal dystonia: epileptic seizure or a new syndrome? *Sleep* **4**, 129–138.

Lugaresi, E., Cirignotta, F. & Montagna, P. (1986): Nocturnal paroxysmal dystonia. *J. Neurol. Neurosurg. Psychiat.* **49**, 375–380.

Magnusson, A., Nakken, K.O. & Brubakk, E. (1996): Autosomal dominant frontal epilepsy. *Lancet* **347**, 1191–1192.

Meierkord, H., Fish, D.R., Smith, S.J.M., Scott, C.A., Shorvon, S.D. & Marsden, C.C. (1992): Is nocturnal paroxysmal dystonia a form of frontal lobe epilepsy? *Movement Disord.* **7**, 38–42.

Montagna, P. (1992): Nocturnal paroxysmal dystonia and nocturnal wandering. *Neurology* **42**, 60–67.

Mount, L.A. & Reback, S. (1940): Familial paroxysmal choreoathetosis. *Arch. Neurol.* **44**, 841–847.

Oldani, A., Zucconi, M., Ferini-Strambi, L., Bizzozero, D. & Smirne, S. (1996): Autosomal dominant nocturnal frontal lobe epilepsy: Electroclinical picture. *Epilepsia* **37**, 964–976.

Phillips, H.A., Scheffer, I.E., Berkovic, S.F., Hollway, G.E., Sutherland, G.R. & Mulley, J.C. (1995): Localization of a gene for autosomal dominant nocturnal frontal lobe epilepsy to chromosome 20q13.2. *Nat. Genet.* **10**, 117–118.

Phillips, H.A., Scheffer, I.E., Crossland, K.M., Bhatia, K.P., Fish, D.R., Marsden, C.D., Howell, S.J.L., Stephenson, J.B.P., Tolmie, J., Plazzi, G., Eeg-Olofsson, O., Singh, R., Lopes-Cendes, I., Andermann, E., Andermann, F., Berkovic, S.F. & Mulley, J.C. (1998): Autosomal dominant nocturnal frontal lobe epilepsy: genetic heterogeneity and evidence for a second locus at 15q24. *Am. J. Hum. Genet.* (in press).

Scheffer, I.E., Bhatia, K.P., Lopes-Cendes, I., Fish, D.R., Marsden, C.D., Andermann, F. *et al.* (1994): Autosomal dominant frontal epilepsy misdiagnosed as sleep disorder. *Lancet* **343**, 515–517.

Scheffer, I.E., Bhatia, K.P., Lopes-Cendes, I., Fish, D.R., Marsden, C.D., Andermann, E., *et al.* (1995): Autosomal dominant nocturnal frontal lobe epilepsy. A distinctive clinical disorder. *Brain* **118**, 61–73.

Steinlein, O.K., Mulley, J.C., Propping, P., Wallace, R.H., Phillips, H.A., Sutherland, G.R. *et al.* (1995): A missense mutation in the neuronal nicotinic acetylcholine receptor a4 subunit is associated with autosomal dominant nocturnal frontal lobe epilepsy. *Nat. Genet.* **11**, 201–203.

Steinlein, O.K., Magnusson, A., Stoodt, J., Bertrand, S., Weiland, S., Berkovic, S.F., Nakken, K.O., Propping, P. & Bertrand, D. (1997): An insertion mutation of the CHRNA4 gene in a family with autosomal dominant nocturnal frontal lobe epilepsy. *Hum. Mol. Genet.* **6**, 943–948.

Tinuper, P., Cerullo, A., Cirignotta, F., Cortelli, P., Lugaresi, E. & Montagna, P. (1990): Nocturnal paroxysmal dystonia with short-lasting attacks: Three cases with evidence for an epileptic frontal lobe origin of seizures. *Epilepsia* **31**, 549–556.

Chapter 10

Familial temporal lobe epilepsy

Samuel F. Berkovic

Department of Medicine (Neurology), The University of Melbourne, Austin and Repatriation Medical Centre, Melbourne, Australia

Murray Falconer observed that a family history of seizures was a notable antecedant factor in the history of some of his patients with severe temporal lobe epilepsy (TLE) undergoing epilepsy surgery. These patients typically had a personal history of prolonged febrile seizures in early childhood and hippocampal sclerosis was found in the operative specimen (Falconer *et al.*, 1964; Falconer, 1971). Falconer's observations have been repeatedly confirmed (Loiseau & Beaussart, 1969; Abou-Khalil *et al.*, 1993; Maher & McLachlan, 1995). His hypothesis, that temporal lobe epilepsy associated with hippocampal sclerosis can be caused by a prolonged early childhood convulsion in patients with a familial predisposition to seizures has gained increasing support (Abou-Khalil *et al.*, 1993; Maher & McLachlan, 1995; Jackson *et al.*, 1998). Importantly, the family history of seizures in these patients is *not* that of temporal lobe epilepsy, but rather of febrile seizures or occasionally generalized epilepsy.

Amongst other patients with *severe* temporal lobe epilepsy a family history of seizures is infrequent. Indeed, the general view has been that TLE is essentially an acquired disorder, with only a small genetic contribution. This perspective of the aetiology of TLE has been gained by intensive research on refractory cases, stimulated particularly by interest in surgical treatment. However, approximately 60–70 per cent of new-onset cases of TLE enter remission (Hauser, 1992), yet little is known about the aetiology of these non-refractory cases.

During a twin study of epilepsy based largely on community ascertained twins, five pairs of concordant adult monozygous twins with mild TLE were observed (Berkovic *et al.*, 1994, 1996, 1998). These twins had therapy-responsive TLE with infrequent seizures, no personal history of febrile seizures, and normal neuroimaging without features of hippocampal sclerosis. The pattern of TLE observed was dissimilar to that seen in presurgical evaluation series in terms of severity and impact on quality of life. This observation led to the suspicion that there may be a relatively frequent form of TLE that was inherited. This hypothesis was supported by our description of seven non-twin families with multiple affected individuals with a similar clinical pattern of mild TLE. In contrast to the familial pattern seen in individuals with severe TLE and hippocampal sclerosis, the family history was of mild TLE and not febrile seizures (Berkovic *et al.*, 1996).

These observations have now been confirmed in a number of other centres (Smith *et al.*, 1996; Gambardella *et al.*, 1996; Cendes *et al.*, 1998) and we continue to ascertain new families through routine epilepsy practice. This suggests that familial TLE is a relatively common syndrome. Here we describe the clinical and genetic aspects of this syndrome.

Clinical epileptology

In our study of 13 unrelated caucasian families, there were 38 affected individuals with afebrile seizures from the twin ($n = 14$) and non-twin ($n = 24$) pedigrees (Fig. 1). The mean age of onset was 24 ± 14 years (range 10–63; median 18.5 years; Fig. 2)). recognized antecedent factors for epilepsy were not identified. None had a history of severe pre-natal or peri-natal insult, febrile seizures, meningitis or encephalitis. Five individuals reported post-natal head trauma; in no case was this thought likely to have caused seizures. The intellect and neurological examination were normal in these individuals.

Simple partial seizures occurred in 34 cases (89 per cent); complex partial seizures in 25 (66 per cent) and tonic–clonic seizures in 25 (66 per cent) (Table 1). In 36/38 cases (95 per cent) there was clinical evidence of a focal onset to the seizures including simple partial seizures (34), complex partial seizures preceded by simple partial seizures (20), or tonic–clonic seizures with preceding or associated focal ictal features (23). Two deceased individuals had a history of convulsions only in sleep, and the presence of a focal origin could not be established.

Table 1. Seizure patterns in 38 individuals with familial temporal lobe epilepsy*

Simple partial seizures		34
Psychic[†]		33
déjà vu	18	
cognitive (e.g. slow motion, dreamy perceptions)	13	
affective (e.g. fear, panic)	9	
illusions (e.g. visual, auditory)	8	
structured hallucinations	3	
Autonomic		18
nausea	9	
tachycardia	7	
sweating	3	
flushing	3	
Special sensory		15
somatosensory	8	
gustatory	3	
vertiginous	3	
auditory	3	
Complex partial seizures		25
Preceded by simple partial seizures	20	
Not preceded by simple partial seizures	5	
Tonic–clonic seizures		25

*From Berkovic et al. (1996).
†Most patients had multiple symptoms during simple partial seizures.

The simple partial seizures had psychic (33 cases), autonomic (18) or special-sensory (15) components. Of the psychic symptoms, déjà vu (18) was the most common (Table 1). Other common symptoms were nausea, tachycardia, a sense of slow motion, fear, and complex distortions of vision or sound. Somatosensory auras were not localized to one side, and were reported as diffuse numbness or tingling. There was no obvious intra-family clustering of simple partial seizure symptomatology.

Complex partial seizures were preceded by simple partial seizures in 20/25 cases. On the basis of the history from subjects and observers, the complex partial seizures comprised relatively brief periods

Chapter 10 Familial temporal lobe epilepsy

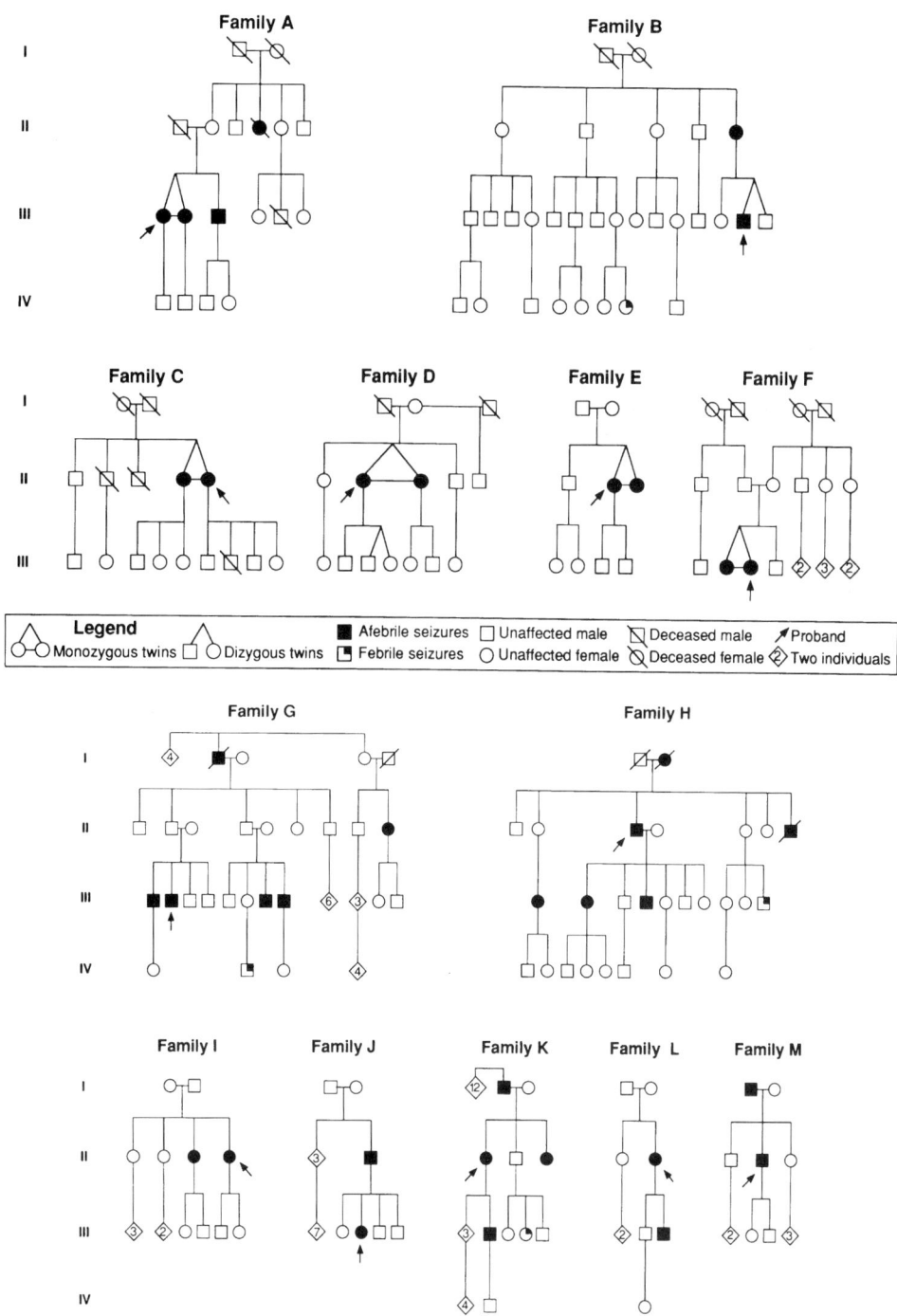

Fig. 1. Pedigrees of twin (A-F) and non-twin (G-M) families.

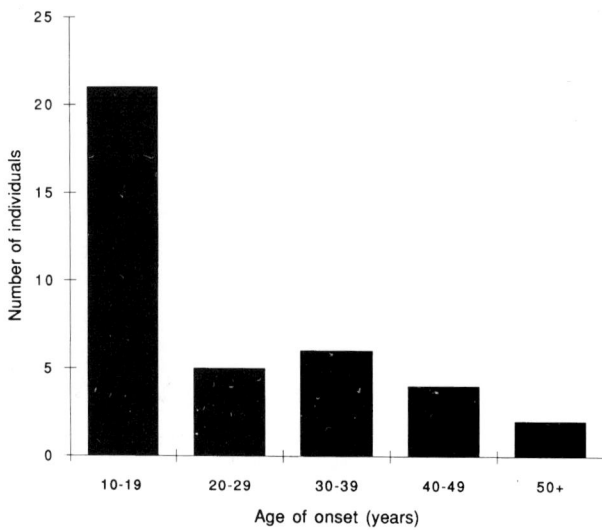

Fig. 2. Age of onset of familial TLE cases.

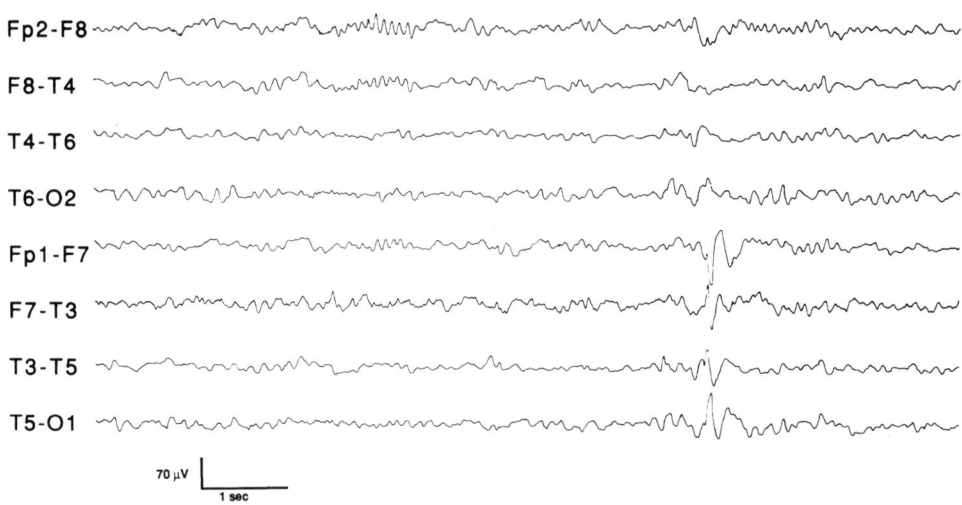

Fig. 3. Interictal epileptiform discharge at F7 recorded on the proband (II–3) from family H.

of impaired consciousness, with subjects being relatively motionless during attacks. In 12/25 cases the subjects claimed that some awareness was maintained. Oro-alimentary automatisms were reported in six cases. None had prominent motor activity unless the seizure became generalized. Post-ictal confusion and amnesia was usually reported as absent, or mild and brief. Only three patients needed to sleep after complex partial seizures.

Of the 38 affected individuals, 29 were known to have epilepsy before the study and nine were diagnosed as a result of the study. A further six individuals had symptoms elicited by seizure questionnaire and confirmed by clinical interview that were compatible but not diagnostic of partial

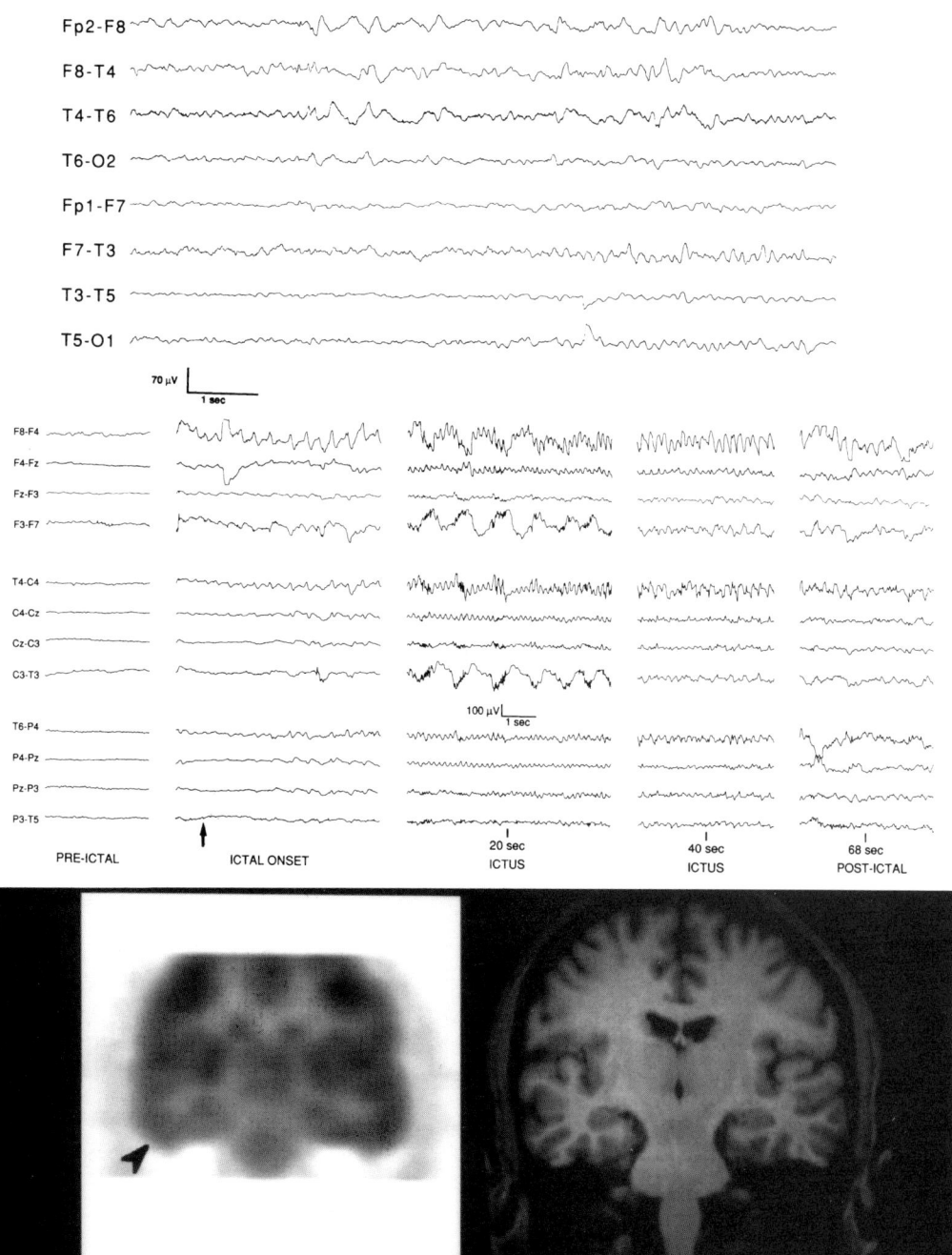

Fig. 4. Right temporal lobe epilepsy in the proband (III–2) of family G. A (above). Interictal EEG showing focal polymorphic slow waves and epileptiform sharp waves maximum at F8 and T4. B (centre). Spontaneous seizure during a routine EEG, recorded on a transverse montage, There is an ictal discharge arising from the right anterior sylvian region (maximum at F8 and T4). C (below). MRI (right) and 18F-FDG PET (left) studies. The MRI is normal but the PET shows right temporal hypometabolism (arrow) (from Berkovic et al., 1996).

seizures (e.g. frequent déjà vu without other features). These individuals were classed as unaffected, but one was an obligate carrier assuming autosomal dominant inheritance.

Electroencephalography and neuroimaging

EEGs were available for 32/38 affected individuals, including multiple records for 20 and sleep recordings in 11 cases. Interictal epileptiform abnormalities were sparse, and only found in 7/32 cases (22 per cent). These comprised focal sharp and slow wave complexes in the temporal regions, usually unilaterally (Figs. 3 and 4). Sleep appeared to activate the focal epileptiform abnormalities in two cases. No generalized epileptiform abnormalities were present. Mild focal slow wave abnormalities, without epileptiform features, were found in an additional nine cases.

Ictal recordings were available in two cases. The proband (case III–2) from family G had a 1 min complex partial seizure recorded during a routine waking EEG without video. There was a right temporal ictal discharge (Fig. 4). The attack was described as beginning with an aura of fear, followed by loss of awareness associated with staring, repeated swallowing and pressing his left hand into his sternum. He was confused and amnestic post-ictally. In family H, case III–2 underwent video-EEG monitoring. Two partial seizures without definitive epileptiform changes were recorded. These comprised an aura of buzzing in the ears, followed on one occasion by definite oral automatisms and impaired awareness. A rapidly secondarily generalized nocturnal partial onset seizure heralded by an aura with early left-sided dystonia did not show lateralized EEG changes.

MRI was available in 17 cases (Fig. 4). No focal mass lesions were detected. None had the features of hippocampal sclerosis (hippocampal atrophy, increased T2 signal, loss of internal hippocampal structure or loss of hippocampal T1 signal on inversion recovery sequences (Jackson *et al.*, 1993a). T2 relaxometry of the hippocampi was normal in all 10 patients studied (mean of 20 hippocampi was 98 ms; range 93–106 ms; normal 1 ms) (Jackson, 1993b). Changes of uncertain significance, such as minor ventricular dilatation or diffuse small high signal areas on T2-weighted images were seen in five cases. Interictal 18F-FDG PET scans were available in two cases. One affected individual (family M, case II–2) who was studied during seizure remission had a normal scan, but case III–2 from family G with ongoing seizures had right temporal hypometabolism (Fig. 4) according with the side of a recorded seizure (Fig. 4).

Evolution and severity

In most cases, seizures were mild, infrequent and responsive to treatment. Six cases had simple partial seizures alone, none had reported their symptoms prior to the study. Seven others had complex partial seizures without tonic–clonic attacks, five of these responded well to medication having no seizures or rare brief attacks.

Of the 25 cases who had tonic–clonic seizures, 13 had them only at the onset of the illness prior to establishment of effective therapy. Twelve of these 13 also had documented simple partial seizures only, or mild complex partial seizures which were well controlled with medication. A further 12 cases had tonic–clonic seizures after establishment of treatment, 11 of these also had simple or complex partial seizures. In five of these cases, tonic–clonic seizures occurred less than once a year.

At the time of the study, five individuals had poorly controlled complex partial or secondarily generalized seizures. Nevertheless, four of these individuals were employed and only one was unable to work due to seizures. Of these five patients, three were either non-compliant or were on inadequate doses of monotherapy and two were undergoing trials of newer anti-epileptic drugs. Only one of these cases was severe enough to consider evaluation for possible surgical therapy.

The effects of different anti-epileptic drugs were not directly evaluated or compared, but carbamazepine, phenytoin and valproate appeared to be effective. The cross-sectional nature of this study precluded accurate determination of remission rates, but the histories of affected individuals suggested that long remissions, with or without therapy, were common.

Genetic analysis

In the non-twin families, four pedigrees had two affected individuals, one had four affected and two had six affected (Fig. 1). Male-to-male transmission occurred in three families excluding X-linked or mitochondrial inheritance. The male to female ratio was 0.71. Clinical anticipation was not present and there was no consanguinity in these pedigrees. Only seven of 18 (39 per cent) of affected sibships had a parent known to be affected. The occurrence of affected individuals in two or more generations in six/seven pedigrees was suggestive of autosomal dominant inheritance with reduced penetrance. The penetrance was estimated at approximately 60 per cent (Berkovic et al., 1996)

Discussion

The clinical features of familial TLE are compared to that of TLE associated with hippocampal sclerosis in Table 2. Onset of familial TLE is typically in teenage or early adult life, with no antecedent factors for epilepsy. No children under the age of 10 years have been identified with this disorder. Although this could be in part due to the subtlety of the symptoms, making recognition of the disorder in children difficult, we did not find any cases of familial TLE in a separate study of new onset TLE in children (Harvey et al., 1997). By contrast, TLE with hippocampal sclerosis usually begins in childhood or adolescence, frequently with antecedents in early childhood. In patients with hippocampal sclerosis a family history of febrile seizures is often found, and occasionally family members with generalized epilepsy are observed, but cases with TLE in other family members are almost unknown (Falconer et al., 1971; Abou-Khalil et al., 1993; French et al., 1993; Wieser et al., 1993). Febrile seizures occurred in only 2.7 per cent of family members of our familial TLE cases, a frequency similar to that reported (3–4 per cent) in the general population (Nelson & Ellenberg, 1978). The seizure patterns in these two syndromes are similar, except that complex partial seizures are less frequent in familial TLE, and the seizure disorder is usually far less severe. The predominant psychic and cognitive features of the simple partial seizures in familial TLE suggests that these seizures originate from limbic structures.

Table 2. *Comparison of familial temporal lobe epilepsy and temporal lobe epilepsy associated with hippocampal sclerosis**

	Familial TLE	TLE with hippocampal sclerosis
Onset of habitual seizures mean (range)	24 years (10–63 yrs)	9 years (9 months–32 yrs)
Antecedent factors	Nil	Febrile seizures (67 per cent)
		Cerebral infection (11 per cent)
Family history		
Febrile seizures	2.5 per cent	6 per cent
Temporal lobe epilepsy	Diagnostic feature	Extremely rare
Seizure patterns		
Simple partial	89 per cent	96 per cent
Complex partial	66 per cent	100 per cent
Secondarily generalized	66 per cent	57 per cent
Focal epileptiform EEG	Uncommon (20 per cent)	Usual (~60 per cent)
MRI	Normal	Hippocampal atrophy
		Increased T2 signal
		Internal hippocampal architecture disrupted
Severity	Usually mild	Often refractory

*From Berkovic et al. (1996).

The benign nature of this disorder was striking, with only one case having more severe socially-disabling attacks leading to loss of employment. The rarity of familial cases of TLE amongst intensively studied surgical series also suggests that familial TLE is rarely difficult to treat.

The occurrence of this disorder in pairs of identical twins brought this entity to our notice. The mild and sometimes subtle nature of this epilepsy in many families members of affected probands has probably obscured recognition of this entity until now. The occurrence of this epilepsy within a family may be more frequent than it initially appears, due to mild symptomatology in some individuals. It is important to stress that in many cases the simple partial seizures, of psychic or autonomic type, were not reported by the patients; these symptoms were often ignored, or regarded as normal phenomena. Only when a careful history was taken directly from other family members was the familial nature of the disorder revealed.

There are previous reports that probably describe the same entity outlined here. Bray & Wiser's (1964, 1965) classic genetic study of temporal-central EEG abnormalities in probands with 'temporal lobe epilepsy' is now recognized as largely describing benign rolandic epilepsy. Five of their subjects had 'psychomotor' seizures persisting into adulthood, however, and some of these might represent familial TLE. Other reports describe the occurrence of 'psychomotor seizures', 'temporal lobe epilepsy', or focal temporal epileptiform abnormalities in family members (Loiseau & Beaussart, 1969; Rodin & Whelan, 1960; Tsuboi & Endo, 1977; Degen *et al.*, 1993). Unfortunately, most of these studies predate the modern classifications of seizures and of epileptic syndromes, which makes interpretation difficult. Since our description (Berkovic *et al.*, 1994, 1996), however, other authors have described a number of families, according with our view that this is a relatively common form of TLE in the community (Smith *et al.*, 1996; Gambardella *et al.*, 1996; Cendes *et al.*, 1998).

The clinical limits of this disorder remains to be fully defined. In the Montreal series, drawn largely from patients considering surgical treatment for epilepsy, a more severe clinical spectrum was observed. Some patients had hippocampal atrophy, including some rare examples of familial hippocampal sclerosis (Cendes *et al.*, 1998). At the other extreme, some subjects have familial déjà vu, without convincing clinical evidence of experiencing attacks with impairment of awareness (F Andermann, personal communication). A number of subjects in our families reported this phenomenon, and we conservatively deemed them as unaffected. Finally, the relationship of familial TLE to partial epilepsy with auditory features needs consideration (Ottman *et al.*, 1995; Ottman, this volume). In that syndrome, auditory disturbances such as ringing or humming were prominent, suggestive of a lateral temporal origin. In our families, auras of probable mesial temporal (limbic) origin were prominent, whereas ringing or humming was reported by only three cases (8 per cent). Ottman *et al.*, (1995) found evidence of linkage to 10q whereas our families do not link to that region (unpublished data).

It appears likely, therefore, that familial temporal lobe epilepsy will be a genetically heterogeneous disorder. Molecular genetic advances in this newly recognized and common syndrome are eagerly awaited.

Acknowledgement: Supported by the National Health and Medical Research Council (NHMRC) of Australia, the Australian NHMRC Twin Registry, and the Austin Hospital Medical Research Foundation.

References

Abou-Khalil, B., Andermann, E., Andermann, F., Olivier, A. & Quesney, L.F. (1993): Temporal lobe epilepsy after prolonged febrile convulsions: excellent outcome after surgical treatment. *Epilepsia* **34**, 878–883

Berkovic, S.F., Howell, R.A., Hay, D.A. & Hopper, J.L. (1998): Epilepsies in twins: genetics of the major epilepsy syndromes. *Ann. Neurol.* (in press).

Berkovic, S.F., Howell, R.A. & Hopper, J.L. (1994): Familial temporal lobe epilepsy: a new syndrome with adolescent/adult onset and a benign course. In: *Epileptic seizures and syndromes*, Wolf, P. (ed.), pp. 257–263. London: John Libbey.

Berkovic, S.F., McIntosh, A.M., Howell, R.A., Mitchell, A., Sheffield, L.J. & Hopper, J.L. (1996): Familial temporal lobe epilepsy: a common disorder identified in twins. *Ann. Neurol.* **40,** 227–235.

Bray, P.F. & Wiser, W.C. (1964): Evidence for a genetic etiology of temporal-central abnormalities in focal epilepsy. *N. Engl. J. Med.* **271,** 926–933.

Bray, P.F. & Wiser, W.C. (1965): Hereditary characteristics of familial temporal-central focal epilepsy. *Pediatrics* **36,** 207–211.

Cendes, F., Lopes-Cendes, I., Andermann, E. & Andermann, F. (1998): Familial temporal lobe epilepsy: a genetically heterogeneous disorder. *Neurology* **50,** 554–557.

Degen, R., Degen, H.E. & Koneke, B. (1993): On the genetics of complex partial seizures: waking and sleep EEGs in siblings. *J. Neurol.* **240,** 151–155.

Falconer, M.A., Serafetinides, E.A. & Corsellis, J.A. (1964): Etiology and pathogenesis of temporal lobe epilepsy. *Arch. Neurol.* **10,** 233–248.

Falconer, M.A. (1971): Genetic and related etiological factors in temporal lobe epilepsy: a review. *Epilepsia* **12,** 13–31.

French, J.A., Williamson, P.D., Thadani, V.M. *et al.* (1993): Characteristics of medial temporal lobe epilepsy: I. Results of history and physical examination. *Ann. Neurol.* **34,** 774–780.

Gambardella, A., Aguglia, U., Le Piane, E., Messina, D. & Quattrone, A. (1996): Autosomal dominant temporal lobe epilepsy: a large family from southern Italy. *Epilepsia* **37** (Suppl. 5): 115.

Gibson, W.C. (1959): Temporal lobe epilepsy in two sisters. *Epilepsia* **1,** 316–324.

Harvey, A.S., Berkovic, S.F., Wrennal, J.A. & Hopkins, I.J. (1997): Temporal lobe epilepsy in childhood: clinical, EEG, and neuroimaging findings and syndrome classification in a cohort with new-onset seizures. *Neurology* **49,** 960–968.

Hauser, W.A. (1992): The natural history of temporal lobe epilepsy. In: *Epilepsy Surgery*, Lüders, H.O. (ed.), pp. 133–141. New York: Raven Press.

Jackson, G.D., McIntosh, A.M., Breillmann, R.S. & Berkovic, S.F. (1998): Hippocampal sclerosis studied in identical twins. *Neurology* (in press).

Loiseau, P. & Beaussart, M. (1969): Hereditary factors in partial epilepsy. *Epilepsia* **10,** 23–31.

Maher, J. & McLachlan, R.S. (1995): Febrile convulsions: is seizure duration the most important predictor of temporal lobe epilepsy? *Brain* **118,** 1521–1528.

Nelson, K.B. & Ellenberg, J.H. (1978): Prognosis in children with febrile seizures. *Pediatrics* **61,** 720–727.

Ottman, R., Risch, N., Hauser, W.A. *et al.* (1995): Localization of a gene for partial epilepsy to chromosome 10q. *Nat. Genet.* **10,** 56–60.

Rodin, E.A. & Whelan, J.L. (1960): Familial occurrence of focal temporal electroencephalographic abnormalities. *Neurology* **10,** 542–545.

Smith, W.B., So, N.K. & Thompson, K. (1996): Familial temporal lobe epilepsy. *Epilepsia* **37** (Suppl. 5), 34.

Tsuboi, T. & Endo, S. (1977): Incidence of seizures and EEG abnormalities among offspring of epileptic patients. *Hum. Genet.* **36,** 173–189.

Wieser, H.G., Engel, J. Jr, Williamson, P.D., Babb, T.L. & Gloor, P. (1993): Surgically remediable temporal lobe syndromes. In: *Surgical treatment of the epilepsies*, 2nd edn., Engel, J. Jr, (ed.), pp. 49–63. New York: Raven Press.

Chapter 11

Genetics of autosomal dominant partial epilepsy with auditory features

Ruth Ottman,[1] Christie Barker-Cummings,[1] Joseph H. Lee[2] and Susanna Ranta[3]

[1]*G. H. Sergievsky Center and School of Public Health (Epidemiology) and* [3]*Department of Psychiatry, Columbia University College of Physicians & Surgeons, 630 W. 168th Street, New York, NY 10032, USA; and* [2]*Department of Psychiatry, University of Pennsylvania School of Medicine, 415 Curie Blvd., Philadelphia, PA 19104, USA*

Summary

In an analysis of a single family containing 11 affected individuals, evidence for linkage on chromosome 10q22–24 was obtained for autosomal dominant partial epilepsy with auditory features (ADPEAF). The clinical manifestations of seizures were quite homogeneous within the family. Age at onset ranged from 8–19 years, epilepsy was clearly localization-related in all of those affected, and more than half affected persons reported nonspecific auditory disturbances as a simple partial component of their seizures. In an additional family containing four individuals with the same syndrome, positive (though nonsignificant) evidence for linkage was also obtained with one of the linked markers on chromosome 10q. In these two families, the similarity in clinical features was as great in persons who were distantly related and geographically dispersed as in those who were more closely related, suggesting that these clinical features resulted from the effects of the causative mutation rather than from the effects of modifying genes or environmental factors. This implies that ADPEAF should be considered separately from other forms of familial temporal lobe epilepsy.

Linkage analysis in localization-related epilepsies: methodological issues

Until recently, most localization-related (partial or focal) epilepsies were presumed to be nongenetic. However, evidence for linkage has been obtained for two forms of localization-related epilepsy. First, we localized a gene for autosomal dominant partial epilepsy with auditory features (ADPEAF) to chromosome 10q (Ottman *et al.*, 1995). Second, autosomal dominant nocturnal frontal lobe epilepsy (ADNFLE) was localized to chromosome 20q (Phillips *et al.*, 1995).

These linkage findings provide powerful evidence of the genetic influences on some forms of localization-related epilepsy. They are derived from analysis of statistical association, within families, between an epilepsy phenotype and a genetic marker allele. Such an association is unlikely to occur because of systematic bias, because most genetic markers have no clinical manifestations or social connotations, and marker information is collected by laboratory analysis of biological samples, independently of disease status. It suggests that a genetic marker allele is being inherited with an epilepsy-causing allele within families, more often than expected by chance. This provides strong evidence both that (1) susceptibility to epilepsy is influenced by a gene (otherwise epilepsy would not be expected to cosegregate with a genetic marker), and (2) the chromosomal location of the susceptibility gene is near that of the marker.

Information obtained from linkage studies about the genomic region likely to contain a susceptibility gene is also a crucial first step in identifying the specific mutation that raises risk for the disorder. In one family with ADNFLE, strong evidence has been obtained that the causal mutation lies within the gene encoding the neuronal nicotinic acetylcholine receptor α4 subunit (Steinlein et al., 1995). Identification of such mutations has great potential importance for public health. It could facilitate early identification of susceptible individuals, early treatment, and perhaps prevention of the disorder in some individuals. It could also provide important basic information about pathogenesis, possibly leading to development of new strategies for treatment and prevention. One of the greatest difficulties in localizing epilepsy susceptibility genes is the extreme clinical heterogeneity of the epilepsies, and the possibility that there are different genetic contributions to different clinically defined subgroups or syndromes. Even in the presence of a strong genetic contribution to a given syndrome, the susceptibility genotype may be present in only a proportion of those affected, while others have a different genetic mechanism or a nongenetic cause. On the other hand, phenotypic expression may be influenced by other genes or environmental exposures, and thus some of those with a given genotype may manifest a different seizure disorder or epilepsy syndrome.

These complexities make it very difficult to decide which phenotypes should be included in the definition of 'affected' in linkage studies of epilepsy. For example, in the families of probands with specific types of epilepsy (e.g. syndromes or seizure types), is risk increased only for the same types, or for all types of epilepsy? This question is best answered by family studies in which risks of specific types of epilepsy can be compared in the relatives of probands with the same specific types. A related question is whether different seizure disorders (epilepsy, isolated unprovoked seizures, febrile convulsions, and other acute symptomatic seizures) are caused by the same, or different genetic susceptibilities. For example, there is a strong basis for assuming a common genetic basis for epilepsy and febrile convulsions (Hauser et al., 1985), and recent studies suggest that epilepsy and alcohol-related seizures may also be genetically related (Schaumann et al., 1994).

Our linkage analysis of ADPEAF involved analysis of a single extended pedigree in which 11 individuals had epilepsy in the absence of a known or suspected exogenous cause (i.e. idiopathic/cryptogenic epilepsy) (Ottman et al., 1995). In this family, the clinical features of epilepsy were very homogeneous. This made it appear more likely that the high incidence of epilepsy in the family was caused by a single gene with a major effect on susceptibility, and greatly simplified assumptions about the phenotype resulting from the susceptibility gene.

The family was ascertained through a large study of the genetic epidemiology of epilepsy (Ottman et al., 1992), whose aims were to evaluate the degree of familial aggregation of various types of epilepsy, test consistency with various models of inheritance, and assess the genetic relationships among different clinically defined subgroups of epilepsy and different seizure disorders. To accomplish these goals, we needed a database of sufficient size to stratify on features of epilepsy in both probands and affected relatives when testing genetic hypotheses. Thus we collected information on seizure disorders in 1,957 probands with epilepsy and more than 10,000 of their first-degree relatives.

The results of our previous investigations with this dataset have indicated that in most families containing multiple individuals with epilepsy, the mode of inheritance is uncertain, and may involve a multigenic (additive or epistatic) model (Ottman et al., 1997). The optimal strategy for investigation of linkage in these families is to use statistical approaches that do not require assumptions about mode of inheritance (i.e. nonparametric methods), such as analysis of marker allele sharing identical-by-descent in affected relative pairs (Risch, 1990).

In a small proportion (fewer than 1.0 per cent) of the families in our previous study, however, the distribution of epilepsy did appear consistent with an autosomal dominant model with high penetrance. The most striking example of this was family 6610, whose pedigree is shown in Fig. 1. In this family,

Chapter 11 Genetics of autosomal dominant partial epilepsy with auditory features

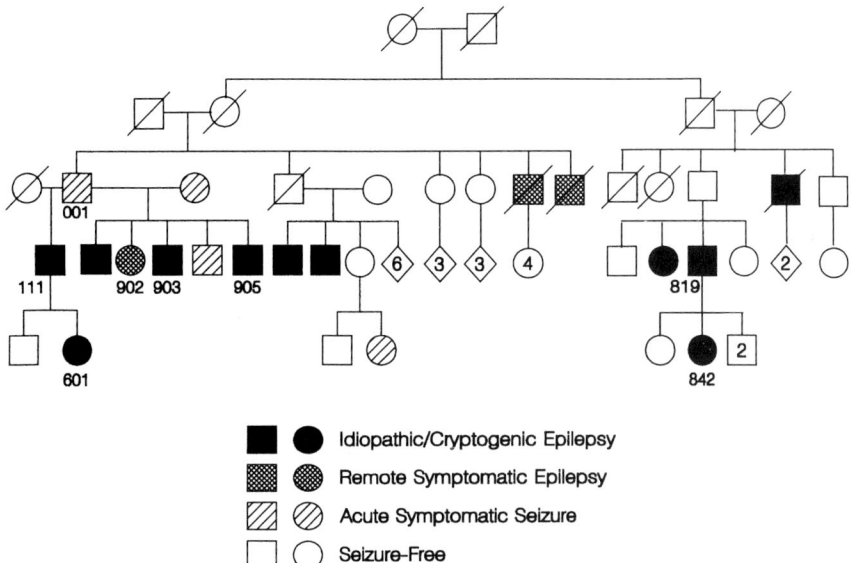

Fig. 1. Pedigree of family 6610.

we proceeded with linkage analysis and localized the susceptibility gene for ADPEAF on chromosome 10q.

Clinical description of ADPEAF in family 6610

Eighteen individuals in family 6610 had seizures, of whom 14 had epilepsy (i.e. recurrent unprovoked seizures), and the remaining four had acute symptomatic seizures (three febrile convulsions, one alcohol-related seizure). Three of those with epilepsy were classified as remote symptomatic (attributed to cerebral palsy, brain tumour, and severe head injury, respectively); the remaining 11 with epilepsy were classified as *idiopathic/cryptogenic*.

As noted above, the clinical manifestations of epilepsy were quite homogeneous within the family. Age at onset of idiopathic/cryptogenic epilepsy ranged from 8 to 19 years. Epilepsy was clearly localization-related in all but one of those with idiopathic/cryptogenic epilepsy; the remaining person had only nocturnal seizures and thus could not be classified. Six (55 per cent) of those with idiopathic/cryptogenic epilepsy, one with posttraumatic epilepsy, and one with alcohol-related seizures reported nonspecific auditory disturbances as a simple partial component of their seizures. Table 1 shows the verbatim descriptions of auditory features taken from our diagnostic interviews.

None of the interictal EEGs showed an epileptiform abnormality. We did not have sufficient data (neuroimaging or depth electrode studies) to localize precisely the epileptogenic abnormality in affected subjects, but the auditory features observed in those affected suggest that the effect of the mutation is localized to a narrowly delimited functional brain region (e.g. neocortical temporal lobe).

All family members had normal intelligence, with the exception of one individual with epilepsy associated with cerebral palsy, who was severely retarded. In family members with epilepsy, seizures occurred infrequently. Seven (64 per cent) of the 11 individuals with idiopathic/cryptogenic epilepsy had been seizure-free for ≥ 3 years prior to interview. Ten of the 11 subjects with idiopathic/cryptogenic epilepsy received phenytoin as a primary anti-seizure medication; the remaining subject received carbamazepine.

Table 1. Verbatim descriptions of auditory symptoms in family 6610.

Subject ID	Verbatim description
111	I get ringing or singing in my ears. It gets louder and louder. I can't hear other people.
601	I had a singing noise in my ears. I knew [the seizure] was coming but it was so quick I couldn't warn my co-workers.
819	It would sound like people were talking backwards or something.
842	I start to hear a humming – like a machine – kind of medium volume. And I can't hear anyone talking.
903	Take a radio and turn it louder ...
905	I hear ringing in my ears, like computer music ... vibrating unbalanced music. Some seizures are triggered by a loud voice.
001*	I started hearing noises, like someone was talking to me. The noises were louder and louder and the next thing I knew, I ended up in the hospital.
902*	I hear a small noise that increases, can't hear normal talking, know that the seizure is coming.

*Subjects who had seizure disorders other than idiopathic/cryptogenic epilepsy (001: alcohol-related seizures, 902: post-traumatic epilepsy).

Linkage analysis in Family 6610

Since the affected individuals in family 6610 did not have a recognized ILAE syndrome, we decided *a priori* to define as affected, for purposes of genetic analysis, anyone in the family who had idiopathic/cryptogenic epilepsy. We classified individuals with remote symptomatic epilepsy, febrile convulsions, or other acute symptomatic seizures as 'unknown'. We assumed an AD model with a susceptibility allele frequency of 0.001, and a risk of 0.01 in non-gene carriers. Lifetime cumulative incidence of idiopathic/cryptogenic epilepsy in gene carriers in this family was estimated to be 71 per cent. All but one of those affected with idiopathic/cryptogenic epilepsy were ≥ 20 years old at observation (current age or age at death), and none of those affected had onset after age 20. Thus we assumed a uniform penetrance of 71 per cent in gene carriers ≥ 20 years, and classified those younger than age 20 who were currently unaffected as unknown.

We genotyped 46 individuals at 200 microsatellite markers spaced at 10–20 centimorgan intervals, and carried out linkage analysis using the 'fast' modification of the LINKAGE computer package (Cottingham *et al.*, 1993; Lathrop & Lalouel, 1984, 1988). After analysing the data for 110 markers, we obtained preliminary evidence for linkage with D10S222 (two-point lod score 2.69 at $\theta = 0.00$) (Table 2). We then explored the region near D10S222 further, by analysing 12 additional tightly linked markers from the 1993–94 Généthon map (Gyapay *et al.*, 1994). We determined genotypes and inferred haplotypes for these additional markers, and obtained a maximum lod score of 3.99 for D10S192. All ten living affected individuals shared a single haplotype for the seven contiguous markers spanning 10 centimorgans from D10S200 to D10S205. Among ten genotyped individuals over age 20 who were classified as unaffected and at 50 per cent risk of being gene carriers, only one carried the haplotype. The two-point lod score for the seven-locus haplotype was 4.83. This figure is a close approximation to the maximum multipoint lod score for these seven loci. The lod score for the haplotype dropped only slightly (from 4.83 to 4.46) when we assumed 50 per cent instead of 71 per cent penetrance, indicating that it was not very sensitive to the penetrance assumption. Key recombination events placed the epilepsy susceptibility locus within the 10 centimorgan region between markers D10S185 and D10S566.

Table 2. Maximum two-point lod scores and maximum likelihood recombination fractions (θs) for 15 chromosome 10q markers in family 6610

Marker locus	Lod score	θ
D10S201	2.79	0.06
D10S583	1.94	0.07
D10S185	3.06	0.06
D10S200	0.97	0.00
D10S574	3.77	0.00
D10S198	2.46	0.00
D10S603	2.35	0.00
D10S192	3.99	0.00
D10S222	2.69	0.00
D10S205	3.01	0.01
D10S566	1.34	0.08
D10S540	1.76	0.08
D10S530	1.46	0.00
D10S597	0.68	0.14
D10S554	0.75	0.18
Haplotype*	4.83	0.00

*Presumed disease allele-bearing haplotype at contiguous loci D10S200 through D10S205 coded as allele '2', all others coded as allele '1'.

Identification of an additional family with ADPEAF

We have recently ascertained one additional family that appears to have ADPEAF (Fig. 2). Four family members have idiopathic localization-related epilepsy. Age at onset was 9–10 years in all of those

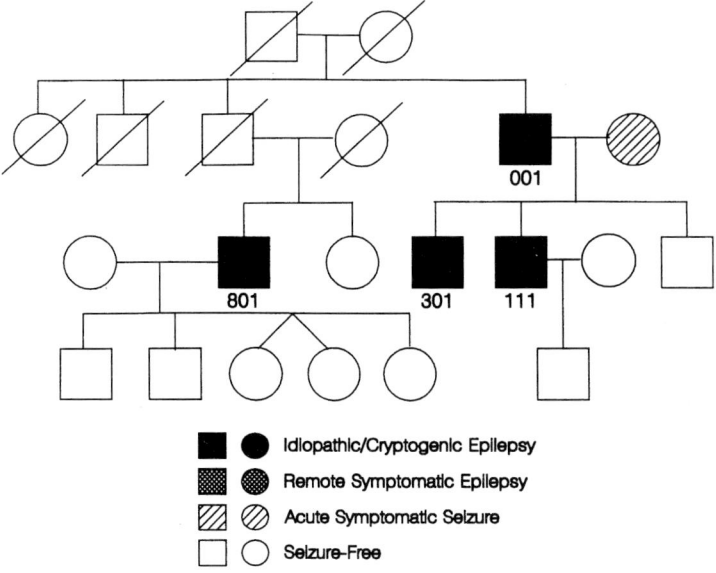

Fig. 2. Pedigree of family 70001.

affected. All four affected individuals had simple or complex partial seizures with secondary generalization, and reported auditory symptoms similar to those in family 6610. The verbatim descriptions of auditory symptoms in these subjects are shown in Table 3.

Table 3. Verbatim descriptions of auditory symptoms in family 70001

Subject ID	Verbatim description
001	All at once, in my left ear, I hear a motor, quite similar to a motor to run a washing machine. First it was a click like valve springs – adink, adink, adink –it started going faster and louder ... a whackety-whack.
111	I usually have a high-pitched whistling in my left ear which would either be preceded or followed by a sound like my heartbeat in my ears ... the intensity of the sound grows as I get close to the big seizure.
301	I hear a very subtle clicking noise, like horses' hooves from left ear, then about 10 s later loss of consciousness ...
801	I would always get ... a popping noise that could get louder and louder until I blacked out. I would have a grand mal seizure if the sound was particularly loud. If it wasn't very loud it might just go away. It sounds like a popgun.

We used the computer program SLINK to estimate the maximum expected lod score for this newly ascertained family (Weeks *et al.*, 1990). We simulated the data under the same genetic model as in our original analysis, i.e. an AD susceptibility gene with 71 per cent penetrance and an allele frequency of 0.001, a risk of 0.01 in non-gene carriers, and tight linkage ($\theta = 0.01$). The results indicated a maximum expected lod score (Z_{max}) of 0.33 for this single family.

After completing clinical data collection (diagnosis and blood sampling) in family 70001, we began molecular analysis of markers on chromosome 10q. As expected from our assessments of statistical power, this individual family was not very informative. However, analysis of four markers found to be linked to ADPEAF in our previous analysis provide positive (though not significant) evidence for linkage to D10S192 (maximum lod score of 0.60 at $\theta = 0.0$).

Estimation of statistical power to replicate linkage

We also used SLINK to estimate power to replicate linkage to chromosome 10q in a dataset of 10 families similar to family 70001. For this purpose we made 10 copies of family 70001 (the 'dataset'), and then simulated 200 replicates of the dataset. The results indicated a maximum expected lod score (Z_{max}) of 3.79 for the 10 families. Power was estimated to be 97.5 per cent for obtaining a lod score ≥ 1.0, and 79.5 per cent for obtaining a lod score ≥ 2.0.

These results indicate that with 10 families similar to family 70001, power will be sufficient for replication of our original linkage finding. Since replication involves testing an established hypothesis, a lower lod score is needed to establish statistical significance in a replication study than in a genome-wide scan used to search for linkage. Lander & Kruglyak (1995) recommend a nominal *P*-value of 0.01 for *confirmation* of linkage, corresponding to a lod score of approximately 1.2 (i.e. lower than their recommended lod score of 3.3 for *detection* of linkage). As noted above, we estimate that with 10 relatively small families similar to family 70001, power is greater than 95 per cent to obtain a lod score ≥ 1.0.

Studies aimed at identifying the mutation

We suspect that this newly identified syndrome is rare. Family 6610 was identified from our database of 1,957 families collected for epidemiological purposes without regard to family history. Very few of the other families in this database appeared to have AD forms of epilepsy, and none appeared to have ADPEAF. However, even if ADPEAF is rare, identification of the causal mutation and study of its pathophysiological effect may help to elucidate basic epileptogenic mechanisms. In order to identify the mutation, we need to refine the localization of the gene by studying additional families.

Study of additional families will also be important for investigating the effects of allelic and locus heterogeneity, and the range of phenotypic manifestations of the susceptibility gene. Some families with ADPEAF may not show linkage to chromosome 10q despite having similar clinical features. On the other hand, mutations at the epilepsy locus on chromosome 10q may raise risk for different types of epilepsy, or even different seizure disorders (e.g. generalized epilepsies, febrile convulsions, or alcohol-related seizures).

In the two families we have studied, the similarity in clinical features is as great in affected family members who are distantly related and geographically dispersed as in those who are more closely related. Thus the specific clinical features we observed, involving temporal lobe epilepsy with onset between 8 and 19 years, with auditory symptoms as a simple partial component of the seizures, probably resulted from the effects of the causative mutation, rather than from the effects of modifying genes or shared environmental exposures. This implies that ADPEAF should be considered separately from other forms of familial temporal lobe epilepsy.

The human genome database (Welch Library, Johns Hopkins University) lists more than 50 genes whose localization overlaps with the cytological localization (10q22-q24) of the epilepsy susceptibility gene on chromosome 10q. This list is probably only a small fraction of the genes residing in this region, and may not include the gene involved in susceptibility to ADPEAF. Several previously identified genes are of potential interest, however. The region contains two neurotransmitter receptors (β-1 and α-2A adrenergic) and several coding sequences with homology to other known receptors. Several genes involved in the metabolism of glutamate, an important excitatory neurotransmitter, also map to this region. Other potentially relevant genes in the region include calcium/calmodulin-dependent protein kinase γ (gamma), which may modulate metabolic and regulatory pathways that affect seizure susceptibility. We will evaluate the relevance of these candidate genes after the ADPEAF locus is more precisely localized.

References

Cottingham, R.W., Jr, Idury, R.M. & Schaffer, A.A. (1993): Faster sequential genetic linkage computations. *Am. J. Hum. Genet.* **53**, 252–263.

Gyapay, G., Morissette, J., Vignal A., Dib, C., Fizames, C., Millasseau, P., Marc, S., Bernardi, G., Lathrop, M. & Weissenbach, J. (1994): The 1993–94 Généthon human genetic linkage map. *Nat. Genet.* **7**, 246–339.

Hauser. W.A., Annegers, J.F. & Kurland, L.T. (1985): The risk of seizure disorders among relatives of children with febrile convulsions. *Neurology* **35**, 1268–1273.

Lander, E. & Kruglyak, L. (1995): Genetic dissection of complex traits: guidelines for interpreting and reporting linkage results. *Nat. Genet.* **11**, 241–247.

Lathrop, G.M. & Lalouel, J.M. (1984): Easy calculations of lod scores and genetic risks on small computers. *Am. J. Hum. Genet.* **36**, 460–465.

Lathrop, G.M. & Lalouel, J.M. (1988): Efficient computations in multilocus linkage analysis. *Am. J. Hum. Genet.* **42**, 498–505.

Ottman, R. & Susser, M. (1992): Data collection strategies in genetic epidemiology: the Epilepsy Family Study of Columbia University. *J. Clin. Epidemiol.* **45**, 721–727.

Ottman, R., Risch, N., Hauser, W.A., Pedley, T.A., Lee, J.H., Barker-Cummings, C., Lustenberger, A., Nagle, K.J., Lee, K.S., Scheuer, M.L., Neystat, M., Susser, M. & Wilhelmsen, K.C. (1995): Localization of a gene for partial epilepsy to chromosome 10q. *Nat. Genet.* **10**, 56–60.

Ottman, R., Hauser, W.A., Barker-Cummings, C., Lee, J.H. & Risch, N. (1997): Segregation analysis of cryptogenic epilepsy and an empirical test of the validity of the results. *Am. J. Hum. Genet.* **60**, 667–675.

Phillips, H.A., Scheffer, I.E., Berkovic, S.F., Holloway, G.E., Sutherland, G.R. & Mulley, J.C. (1995): Localization of a gene for autosomal dominant nocturnal frontal lobe epilepsy to chromosome 20q13.2. *Nat. Genet.* **10**, 117–118.

Risch, N. (1990): Linkage strategies for complex traits. II. The power of affected relative pairs. *Am. J. Hum. Genet.* **46,** 229–241.

Schaumann, B.A., Annegers, J.F., Johnson, S.B., Moore, K.J., Lubozynski, M.F. & Salinsky, M.C. (1994): Family history of seizures in posttraumatic and alcohol-associated seizure disorders. *Epilepsia* **35,** 48–52.

Steinlein, O.K., Mulley, J.C., Propping, P., Wallace, R.H., Phillips, H.A., Sutherland, G.R., Scheffer, I.E. & Berkovic, S.F. (1995): A missense mutation in the neuronal nicotinic acetylcholine receptor alpha 4 subunit is associated with autosomal dominant nocturnal frontal lobe epilepsy. *Nat. Genet.* **11,** 201–203.

Weeks, D.E., Ott, J. & Lathrop, G.M. (1990): SLINK: A general simulation program for linkage analysis [abstract]. *Am. J. Hum. Genet.* **47,** A204.

Chapter 12

Familial partial epilepsy with variable foci

Ingrid E. Scheffer

Departments of Neurology, Austin and Repatriation Medical Centre, Royal Children's Hospital, Monash Medical Centre, and University of Melbourne, Australia

Summary

Familial partial epilepsy with variable foci is an inherited epilepsy syndrome with the novel feature that different family members have partial epilepsy emanating from different cortical regions. To date, one Australian family has been described with partial epilepsies of temporal, frontal, centroparietal and occipital origin. Partial epilepsies vary in severity but the EEG findings are often striking with active focal epileptiform discharges brought out by sleep. Clinically unaffected individuals may have epileptiform EEG recordings. FPEVF appears to follow autosomal dominant inheritance in this kindred with suggestive linkage to chromosome 2q. Ascertainment of similar families has been difficult possibly because they have lower penetrance and less active epileptiform abnormalities on EEG studies.

Familial partial epilepsy with variable foci (FPEVF) joins the recently recognized group of inherited partial epilepsies (Scheffer *et al.*, 1994; Ottman *et al.*, 1995; Scheffer *et al.*, 1995b; Berkovic *et al.*, 1996). All previously described monogenic partial epilepsies have been characterized by seizures arising from the same cortical region in affected family members. For example, although there is a marked range of severity and semiology of autosomal dominant nocturnal frontal lobe epilepsy (ADNFLE), all affected individuals have frontal lobe seizures (Scheffer *et al.*, 1994; Scheffer *et al.*, 1995a; Hayman *et al.*, 1997). Similarly in familial temporal lobe epilepsy (FTLE), individuals have partial seizures with temporal lobe features (Berkovic *et al.*, 1996; Ottman *et al.*, 1995). In FPEVF, all individuals with seizures have either clinical or electrical evidence of partial origin but the region of the cortex involved is variable involving frontal, temporal, centroparietal and occipital lobes in different individuals. FPEVF also stands apart from the other monogenic partial epilepsies in that active epileptiform abnormalities are usually found on EEG studies, including in clinically unaffected individuals.

Clinical features

Epileptology

A single Australian family with FPEVF was reported with 10 individuals with partial seizures over four generations and a further two clinically unaffected individuals with epileptiform EEG abnormalities (Fig. 1) (Scheffer *et al.*, 1998). Two deceased individuals (II–3, II–4) had a clear history of complex partial seizures in the sixth decade of life but more precise characterization was not possible.

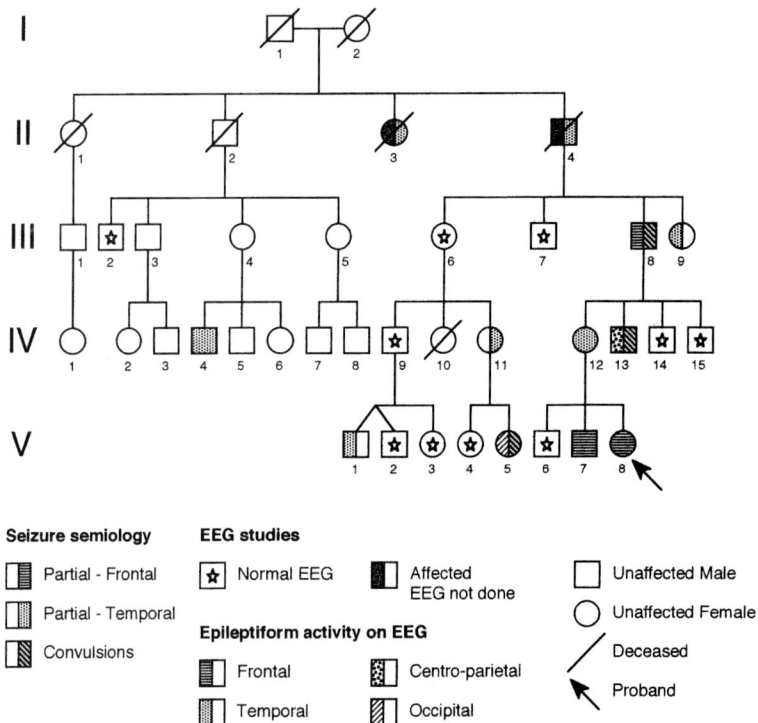

Fig. 1. Pedigree of the family.

For the remaining eight affected family members, mean seizure onset was 13 years with a median age of 10 years (range 9 months to 43 years).

Seizure semiology was heterogeneous with seizures emanating on electroclinical grounds from all four cortical lobes in different individuals (Fig. 1). Five individuals had seizures suggestive of temporal lobe origin. Simple partial seizures occurred in four individuals who described olfactory hallucinations (II–4) and psychic phenomena (IV–4, IV–11, IV–12). Six individuals had complex partial seizures including three of those with simple partial seizures. The typical oral and motor automatisms of temporal lobe seizures were described in the seizures of the two deceased individuals (II–3, II–4). The frontal lobe seizures of the proband (V–8) and her brother (V–7) were characterized by tonic head and eye deviation with altered awareness, as well as asymmetric tonic posturing of the upper limbs in the proband.

Tonic–clonic seizures occurred in six family members. Three individuals had secondarily generalized partial seizures of temporal lobe origin (IV–4, IV–11, IV–12). There were no diagnostic clinical features of partial seizures in the other three cases (III–8, IV–13, V–5) but evidence for a partial origin was obtained from EEG studies (see below).

Seizure frequency varied considerably between individuals with one man (IV–13) having refractory seizures throughout his life while his father (III–8) only had a total of 16 seizures in sleep over 28 years, and his cousin (IV–11) had her first single seizure at 43 years.

EEG features

Interictal focal epileptiform discharges occurred in six of the eight living individuals with seizures.

Each individual had a single focus, remaining constant over time, yet the locations of the epileptiform foci were heterogeneous within the family. Interictal frontal epileptiform abnormalities were found in three individuals (V–8, V–7, III–8) including two children whose later ictal studies confirmed partial seizures of frontal origin. Temporal abnormalities were seen in the three living individuals with temporal lobe seizures, one (IV–12) had interictal epileptiform discharges while the others (IV–4, IV–11) had slowing only. Single individuals had centroparietal (IV–13) and occipital (V–5) epileptiform activity (Fig. 1).

Electroclinical concordance was seen for all four individuals (IV–4, IV–12, V–7, V–8) who had clinical partial seizures and available interictal EEG studies. In three family members (III–8, IV–13, V–5) who only had convulsions without clinical partial seizures, their interictal studies showed focal epileptiform discharges emanating from the left frontal region, left centro-parietal region and the occipital regions suggesting partial onset of their tonic–clonic seizures.

The activity of epileptiform foci varied greatly in different individuals and did not correlate with seizure frequency, but was generally brought out by sleep. For example, the most severely affected family member (IV–13) had such an active focus at 12 years that his EEG was reported as consistent with non-convulsive status epilepticus, whilst at 33 years, it still showed an active discharge in sleep. His father (III–8) who had easily controlled nocturnal convulsions from adolescence, had a very active sleep EEG at 60 years, 15 years after his last seizure. In contrast, two individuals required repeated EEG studies to detect epileptiform abnormalities.

An important finding was that two out of twelve family members who did not have seizures had frontotemporal epileptiform activity (III–9, V–1). Five spouses did not show epileptiform activity on EEG studies.

Other investigations

Neuroimaging in the form of MRI and CT brain scans was performed on five and three individuals respectively and, with one exception, was normal. Widening of the left Sylvian fissure was evident on both CT and MRI of individual IV–11.

The proband (V–8) underwent video-EEG monitoring which captured a brief seizure characterized by asymmetric tonic posturing with extension of the right arm and flexion of the left arm. Ictal EEG showed bi-frontal recruiting rhythm and then bifrontal spike-slow wave activity. Ictal SPECT scan was performed with injection of the ^{99}Tc-HMPAO radioligand 7 s after seizure onset. Hyperperfusion in the left mesial frontal region, the left basal ganglia and right cerebellum was shown consistent with the clinical suspicion of supplementary motor area involvement (Fig. 4 in Harvey et al. (1993)).

Formal neuropsychological assessment was performed on affected and unaffected family members. Although the difference between the mean full scale IQ (FSIQ) in the affected group of 111.8 (range 77–130) versus 124 (range 113–132) in the unaffected group was not significant, there was greater variability in intellect in the affected group. With the exception of the most severely affected individual IV–13 (FSIQ 77), all affected family members were of at least average intelligence.

Genetic analysis

The inheritance of partial epilepsy was consistent with an autosomal dominant pattern with penetrance of 62 per cent for partial seizures and 76 per cent for epileptiform abnormalities on EEG studies. Clinical anticipation was not seen. Male to male transmission excluded sex-linked and mitochondrial inheritance.

Formal linkage studies were performed. Simulation studies predicted a maximum lod score of 4.0 for penetrance of 60 per cent and 4.4 for penetrance of 75 per cent assuming autosomal dominant inheritance and equal marker allele frequencies (four alleles). A total of 224 markers at about 20cM intervals along the genome were tested and a suggestion of linkage was found for markers close to 2qter with a probability of 99.9 per cent for gene assignment to this region using the EXCLUDE analysis (Edwards, 1987). The maximum lod score obtained was 2.74 at recombination fraction of zero with marker *D2S133*. Haplotype analysis indicated that two affected individuals did not carry the appropriate haplotype: individual IV–4 was more distantly related and may have unrelated epilepsy, while V–1 had an epileptiform EEG abnormality alone. Neither individual had an affected sibling or parent which was somewhat different to other parts of the pedigree which were highly suggestive of autosomal dominant inheritance of a major gene.

Discussion

Familial partial epilepsy with variable foci (FPEVF) is a novel condition characterized by partial seizures arising from different cortical regions in different individuals and following autosomal dominant inheritance. It was described in an Australian family with 10 individuals with partial seizures and an additional two clinically unaffected family members had epileptiform activity on EEG studies (Scheffer *et al.*, 1998). Partial seizure semiology was concordant with epileptiform abnormalities on EEG recordings and where convulsions without partial features occurred, focal epileptiform activity was seen on EEG studies. Epileptiform foci were seen in all four cortical lobes yet each focus was constant in each individual. FPEVF is characterized by individuals usually having epileptiform activity on interictal EEG studies, particularly on sleep recordings.

Differentiation from other familial partial epilepsies

FPEVF can be readily differentiated on electroclinical grounds from the other monogenic partial epilepsy syndromes. Although some individuals with FPEVF have frontal lobe epilepsy, they do not have the distinctive clinical pattern of clusters of brief motor seizures arising in sleep seen in the more common disorder ADNFLE (Scheffer *et al.*, 1994; Scheffer *et al.*, 1995a). Indeed, the two children with frontal lobe epilepsy in FPEVF had diurnal seizures characterized by head and eye deviation, whilst their grandfather only had a total of 16 convulsions, one per night, over 28 years. These patterns are completely different to the homogeneous seizure semiology of ADNFLE. Furthermore, the positivity of EEG studies in FPEVF stands in stark contrast to the paucity of interictal and even ictal epileptiform abnormalities of EEG studies in ADNFLE (Scheffer *et al.*, 1995a). (Chapter 9, this volume.)

Two forms of familial temporal lobe epilepsy have been described: the more common is suggestive of mesial temporal origin with psychic and autonomic features (Berkovic *et al.*, 1996) while the other has a lateral temporal flavour with auditory hallucinations (Ottman *et al.*, 1995). Once again, the clinical features in these two disorders are relatively homogeneous distinguishing them from FPEVF where a range of partial epilepsy phenotypes are seen. The EEG is also helpful as the incidence of epileptiform abnormalities is low in both types of familial temporal lobe epilepsy (Berkovic *et al.*, 1996; Ottman *et al.*, 1995). (Chapters 10 and 11, this volume.)

Other single gene partial epilepsies are either rare or do not come in to the differential diagnosis. Autosomal dominant rolandic epilepsy with speech dyspraxia presents in mid childhood with typical rolandic seizures and the classical age-dependent EEG finding of centro-temporal spikes and has been described in one family (Scheffer *et al.*, 1995b). (Chapter 13, this volume.)None of the individuals with FPEVF had either these clinical or electrical features. Benign familial infantile convulsions is an autosomal dominant partial epilepsy presenting with a cluster of seizures at around 6 months (Vigevano *et al.*, 1992). (Chapter 7, this volume.)

Genetic features

FPEVF appears to follow an autosomal dominant inheritance pattern (Fig. 1). The finding of epileptiform abnormalities on routine EEG studies of clinically unaffected individuals is likely to be a marker for the FPEVF trait. There are precedents for this hypothesis in family studies of juvenile myoclonic epilepsy and in siblings of probands with benign rolandic epilepsy, where the EEG trait is considered a genetic marker of the epilepsy syndrome.

Genetic analysis first excluded linkage for FPEVF to the 20q locus found in ADNFLE (Phillips *et al.*, 1995; Scheffer *et al.*, 1995c) where the mutation was later shown to be in a neuronal nicotinic acetylcholine receptor subunit (Steinlein *et al.*, 1995). Subsequent systematic study of the genome found evidence suggestive of linkage to chromosome 2qter but not definitive linkage. This region has not previously been implicated in linkage studies of idiopathic epilepsies. To date, three idiopathic epilepsy genes have been cloned (Steinlein *et al.*, 1995; Steinlein *et al.*, 1997; Biervert *et al.*, 1998; Charlier *et al.*, 1998; Singh *et al.*, 1998; Wallace *et al.*, 1998), all of which are ion channels making any ion channel genes in the linkage region ideal candidate genes for FPEVF.

Identification of other families with FPEVF

Detailed studies of multiplex families with epilepsy in our own material and that of other groups (see Chapter 14, this volume; personal communication, E. Andermann) have identified other families who may have less striking forms of FPEVF. They do not, however, exactly match the phenotypic spectrum of the family described here for a number of possible reasons. First, FPEVF as described here may be extraordinarily rare such that this family has its own 'private syndrome'. Second, this family may be unusual in having such a high penetrance of seizure disorders in the central part of the pedigree which is the feature that originally alerted us to a gene for partial epilepsy. One explanation would be a modifier gene effect. Lower penetrance may be more usual in FPEVF. Third, individuals in other families with FPEVF may have less active EEG studies requiring multiple records to secure epileptiform abnormalities. Identification of the affected status of closer relatives, based on epileptiform EEG activity of clinically unaffected individuals, relies on EEG studies which are not routinely performed. The ultimate answer to the question of whether FPEVF is a common, under-recognized syndrome or a rare, private syndrome lies in identification of the gene for this genetic epilepsy syndrome.

Acknowledgements: The author is grateful to her collaborators for their contribution to the original description of this family: Professor Samuel Berkovic; neuropsychological evaluation performed by Catherine O'Brien with the assistance of Associate Professor Michael Saling, Jacqueline Wrennall and Associate Professor Phillipa Patterson; genetic studies performed by Hilary Phillips, Robyn Wallace and Associate Professor John Mulley. The family was originally referred by Dr Ian Hopkins. Dr Simon Harvey provided SPECT and EEG studies on the proband. Dr Scheffer was supported by the National Health and Medical Research Council of Australia, the Epilepsy Foundation of Victoria, the Royal Children's Hospital Medical Research Foundation, the Austin Hospital Medical Research Foundation, and the Apex Foundation for Research into Intellectual Disability. The family were extremely gracious and helpful in cooperating in this study.

References

Berkovic, S.F., McIntosh, A., Howell, R.A., Mitchell, A., Sheffield, L.J. & Hopper, J.L. (1996): Familial temporal lobe epilepsy: A common disorder identified in twins. *Ann. Neurol.* **40**, 227–235.

Biervert, C., Schroeder, B.C., Kubisch, C., Berkovic, S.F., Propping, P., Jentsch, T.J. *et al.* (1998): A potassium channel mutation in neonatal human epilepsy. *Science* **279**, 403–406.

Charlier, C., Singh, N.A., Ryan, S.G., Lewis, T.B., Revs, B.E., Leach, R.J. *et al.* (1998): A pore mutation in a novel KQT-like potassium channel gene in an idiopathic epilepsy family. *Nat. Genet.* **18**, 53–55.

Edwards, J.H. (1987): Exclusion mapping. *J. Med. Genet.* **24**, 539–543.

Harvey, A.S., Hopkins, I.J., Bowe, J.M., Cook, D.J., Shield, L.K. & Berkovic, S.F. (1993): Frontal lobe epilepsy: clinical seizure characteristics and localization with ictal ^{99m}Tc-HMPAO SPECT. *Neurology* **43**, 1966–1980.

Hayman, M., Scheffer, I.E., Chinvarun, Y., Berlangieri, S.U. & Berkovic, S.F. (1997): Autosomal dominant nocturnal frontal lobe epilepsy: Demonstration of focal frontal onset and intrafamilial variation. *Neurology* **49**, 969–975.

Ottman, R., Risch, N., Hauser, W.A., Pedley, T.A., Lee, J.H., Barker-Cummings, C. *et al.* (1995): Localization of a gene for partial epilepsy to chromosome 10q. *Nat. Genet.* **10**, 56–60.

Phillips, H.A., Scheffer, I.E., Berkovic, S.F., Hollway, G.E., Sutherland, G.R. & Mulley, J.C. (1995): Localization of a gene for autosomal dominant nocturnal frontal lobe epilepsy to chromosome 20q13.2. *Nat. Genet.* **10**, 117–118.

Scheffer, I.E., Bhatia, K.P., Lopes-Cendes, I., Fish, D.R., Marsden, C.D., Andermann, F. *et al.* (1994): Autosomal dominant frontal epilepsy misdiagnosed as sleep disorder. *Lancet* **343,** 515–517.

Scheffer, I.E., Bhatia, K.P., Lopes-Cendes, I., Fish, D.R., Marsden, C.D., Andermann, E. *et al.* (1995a): Autosomal dominant nocturnal frontal lobe epilepsy. A distinctive clinical disorder. *Brain* **118,** 61–73.

Scheffer, I.E., Jones, L., Pozzebon, M., Howell, R.A., Saling, M.M. & Berkovic, S.F. (1995b): Autosomal dominant rolandic epilepsy and speech dyspraxia: A new syndrome with anticipation. *Ann. Neurol.* **38,** 633–642.

Scheffer, I.E., Phillips, H., Mulley, J., Sutherland, G., Harvey, A.S., Hopkins, I.J. *et al.* (1995c): Autosomal dominant partial epilepsy with variable foci is not allelic with autosomal dominant nocturnal frontal lobe epilepsy. *Epilepsia* **36** (3): S28.

Scheffer, I.E., Phillips, H.A., O'Brien, C.E., Saling, M.M., Wrennall, J.A., Wallace, R.H. *et al.* (1998): Familial partial epilepsy with variable foci: A new partial epilepsy syndrome with suggestion of linkage to chromosome 2. *Ann. Neurol.* (in press)

Singh, N.A., Charlier, C., Stauffer, D., DuPont, B.R., Leach, R.J., Melis, R. *et al.* (1998): A novel potassium channel gene, *KCNQ2*, is mutated in an inherited epilepsy of newborns. *Nat. Genet.* **18,** 25–29.

Steinlein, O.K., Mulley, J.C., Propping, P., Wallace, R.H., Phillips, H.A., Sutherland, G.R. *et al.* (1995): A missense mutation in the neuronal nicotinic acetylcholine receptor a4 subunit is associated with autosomal dominant nocturnal frontal lobe epilepsy. *Nat. Genet.* **11,** 201–203.

Steinlein, O.K., Magnusson, A., Stoodt, J., Bertrand, S., Weiland, S., Berkovic, S.F. *et al.* (1997): An insertion mutation of the CHRNA4 gene in a family with autosomal dominant nocturnal frontal lobe epilepsy. *Hum. Mol. Genet.* **6,** 943–948.

Vigevano, F., Fusco, L., Di Capua, M., Ricci, S., Sebastianelli, R. & Lucchini, P. (1992): Benign infantile familial convulsions. *Eur. J. Pediatr.* **151,** 608–612.

Wallace, R.H., Wang, D.W., Singh, N.A., Scheffer, I.E., George, A.L., Phillips, H.A. *et al.* (1998): Febrile seizures and generalized epilepsy associated with a mutation in the Na^+-channel $\beta1$ subunit gene SCN1B. *Nat Genet.* **19,** 366–370.

Chapter 13

Autosomal dominant rolandic epilepsy with speech dyspraxia

Ingrid E. Scheffer

Departments of Neurology, Austin and Repatriation Medical Centre, Royal Children's Hospital, Monash Medical Centre, and University of Melbourne, Australia

Benign rolandic epilepsy (BRE), or benign childhood epilepsy with centro-temporal spikes, accounts for 17 per cent of all childhood epilepsies and is characterized by nocturnal oro-facio-brachial partial seizures in mid-childhood (Commission on Classification and Terminology of the International League Against Epilepsy, 1989). Early studies suggested that the distinctive age-dependent EEG trait of BRE, rather than the seizures themselves, followed autosomal dominant inheritance (Bray & Wiser, 1964; Bray & Wiser, 1965; Heijbel *et al.*, 1975). More recently, BRE has generally been considered to follow polygenic inheritance (Doose & Baier, 1989). (see Chapters 4–6, this volume.)

Autosomal dominant rolandic epilepsy with speech dyspraxia (ADRESD) is a rare condition where affected individuals have childhood rolandic seizures with speech dyspraxia and cognitive impairment. ADRESD was described in an Australian family with nine affected individuals over three generations (Fig. 1). This disorder is related to BRE but shares some features with two rare, more severe childhood syndromes with partial epilepsy, focal epileptiform discharges and speech dysfunction: Landau-Kleffner syndrome (LKS) (Landau & Kleffner, 1957) and Epilepsy with continuous spike and wave during slow wave sleep (CSWS) (Tassinari *et al.*, 1992). Recently, these disorders have been thought to form part of a spectrum with BRE representing the common, benign end of the spectrum, whilst LKS and CSWS are more sinister, rare disorders at the severe end of the spectrum (Deonna, 1991). The fourth related disorder described here may help to clarify these relationships, particularly because of its genetic basis.

Clinical features

Epileptology

All nine affected individuals had a history of childhood seizures except II–3 on whom reliable early information was unavailable. An accurate seizure description could be obtained on six family members as two affected individuals were deceased (Fig. 1).

The mean age of seizure onset was 5.3 years (median 6 years). Seizures occurred exclusively at night in five of six individuals, usually in the first 2 h of falling asleep. Diurnal attacks only occurred in the most severely affected individual, the proband. Seizures had the typical manifestations of rolandic seizures with an aura of perioral or hand paraesthesia or fear in three individuals, difficulty speaking

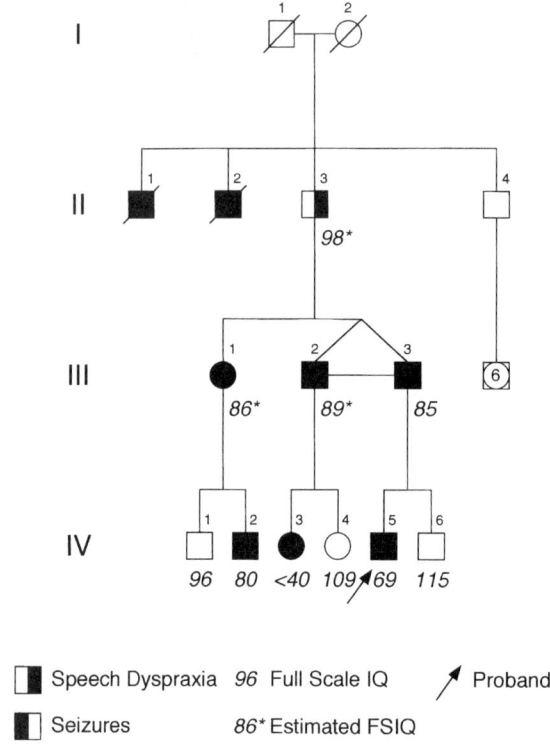

Fig. 1. Pedigree of the family showing affected status for seizures and speech dyspraxia. The figures below each individual indicate the full scale IQ (FSIQ) or an estimate of FSIQ (asterisk). Note the difference in FSIQ between the affected and unaffected children in generation IV.

with stuttering and speech arrest in five, prominent drooling in five, and a variety of motor features including stiffening of the upper limb(s), and unilateral facial and upper limb tonic and clonic activity. Five individuals remained aware through some attacks, however, all six had secondarily generalized tonic–clonic seizures at some time. Seizures were brief-lasting a clinically estimated mean of 2 min and varied in frequency from every 6 months to weekly in different individuals.

The seizure disorder ran the typical course of BRE from 6 to 13 years in all individuals of generation III. A more severe picture occurred in two of the three children in generation IV who had an earlier onset at 1.5 and 2.5 years, while the third child was not diagnosed until she participated in the study although seizures had probably been unrecognized for some time. The proband had a severe seizure disorder with recurrent episodes of non-convulsive status epilepticus characterized by speech regression, drooling and ataxia. A severe exacerbation at 9 years responded to a course of oral steroids.

EEG and neuroimaging

Interictal EEG studies in all affected children showed frequent focal epileptiform abnormalities brought out by sleep. They had centro-temporal discharges which were unilateral in one child and bilateral in two children. The discharges consisted of a sharp wave followed by a prominent aftergoing slow wave and had a field consistent with a horizontal dipole situated in the rolandic sulcus with frontal positivity and centro-temporal negativity (Scheffer et al., 1995).

An ictal video-EEG study on individual IV–3 showed a rapidly secondarily generalized tonic–clonic seizure beginning with contraction of the left side of her face and clenching of her right fist. The preictal EEG showed right centro-temporal discharges during stage 2 sleep with ictal onset over the right central region (C4) associated with reversal of the interictal dipole (Scheffer et al., 1995).

During later episodes of nonconvulsive status epilepticus, the proband had multifocal discharges with evidence of a rolandic horizontal dipole and a tangential dipole around the Sylvian fissure with frontocentral positivity and posterior temporal negativity. EEG studies in all affected adults were normal. Neuroimaging including MRI in four individuals, and CT scan in one of those four individuals, was normal in all cases.

Cognitive function

Full scale IQ testing showed a gradient of worsening cognitive function down the generations. All adults had full scale IQs within the average range, however, case II–3 scored 9 points above his children in generation III. The affected children in generation IV had full scale IQs that were at the lowest limit of the average range (1) or well below average (2), and these values differed markedly from their unaffected siblings who had average scores (Fig. 1). No acquired factors were evident in their clinical histories to account for this difference.

Constructional function was poor in all the affected children in generation IV but was normal in the affected adults. Impairment of high-level language processing was evident in all affected individuals with the exception of the elderly grandfather (II–3) yet was normal in the youngest unaffected child in the family (IV–6). Verbal and nonverbal memory testing was normal in all individuals.

Speech and language

A distinctive pattern of oral and speech disturbance and higher level language impairment was seen in affected family members characterized by oral and speech dyspraxia without evidence of dysarthria. They had difficulty organizing and coordinating the high speed movements necessary to produce fluent and/or intelligible speech. Difficulties with some simple oral movements such as poking out the tongue were also found. Unaffected family members had no abnormalities of speech and language. Poor receptive language processing skills were found in affected individuals and were more prominent in the children than the adults.

Genetic analysis

ADRESD follows autosomal dominant inheritance with high penetrance in this family. The striking feature of the clinical genetics was anticipation, that is, increasing severity of the disorder in subsequent generations. All affected children of the third generation had more severe speech dyspraxia and cognitive impairment than their parents, and two children had a more severe seizure disorder.

Discussion

Relationship to other epilepsy-speech disorders

ADRESD shares many electroclinical features with BRE as both are characterized by nocturnal oro-facio-brachial seizures associated with age-dependent centro-temporal epileptiform activity on interictal EEG studies (Commission on Classification and Terminology of the International League Against Epilepsy, 1989; Lerman, 1992). Only the proband has a more severe seizure disorder than is seen in BRE with recurrent episodes of nonconvulsive status epilepticus. ADRESD differs from BRE in that individuals also have speech dyspraxia and cognitive impairment, whereas children with BRE are defined as being of normal intellect and speech, although minor speech abnormalities have been reported (Roulet *et al.*, 1989; Deonna *et al.*, 1993; Bladin, 1987). The other major difference from BRE is the mode of inheritance as it is rare to see BRE in two generations of one family, let alone such a clear pattern of autosomal dominant inheritance with high penetrance (Neubauer *et al.*, 1997). Where BRE does occur in more than one generation of a family, anticipation has not been described. Neubauer and colleagues have recently excluded linkage of BRE or the BRE EEG trait to the loci for benign familial neonatal convulsions (Neubauer *et al.*, 1997).

LKS is a rare condition where a child who was previously normal or had isolated language impairment, develops aphasia associated with the EEG feature of continuous spike wave in slow wave sleep (Deonna, 1991). Seizures occur in 70 per cent of cases but are generally easily controlled. LKS usually carries a poor prognosis; however, recent reports suggest that oral steroids have met with considerable success. The speech and cognitive impairments seen in ADRESD can be differentiated from LKS as delayed development is evident from birth and, with the exception of the proband, regression does not generally occur. Furthermore, the speech problems are of dyspraxic type with evidence of both a verbal and higher order dyspraxia, and dyspraxia has only been a minor feature of LKS (Deonna *et al.*, 1993). Moreover, in LKS cognitive difficulties influence verbal domains predominantly, whereas in ADRESD, these problems are more widespread with verbal and nonverbal abnormalities apparent.

Although the seizure disorder is more severe in the proband than in LKS, there are some electroclinical similarities. Whilst the proband is in an episode of nonconvulsive status epilepticus, his EEG shows multifocal discharges both awake (atypical for LKS) and asleep. Some discharges have a field consistent with the Sylvian dipole described in LKS. Recently, the proband has shown clinical improvement with oral steroids as described in LKS. The overall picture of ADRESD can, however, be easily distinguished from LKS or the related condition of Worster-Drought syndrome where the onset of aphasia coincides with the seizure disorder (Worster-Drought, 1971).

CSWS is another rare, related epilepsy-speech disorder which occurs in children who may have pre-existing developmental delay. These children may have multiple seizure types which are refractory to medication and they show regression of skills associated with continuous spike wave in slow wave sleep on EEG. Their EEG is striking in the disparity between the awake record which has little epileptiform activity compared to the sleep record which, by definition, has more than 85 per cent continuous epileptiform activity (Tassinari et al., 1992). In ADRESD, the only family member with features suggestive of CSWS is the proband and he can be readily differentiated by his EEG which shows constant epileptiform activity both awake and asleep during periods of nonconvulsive status epilepticus. Moreover the cognitive profile seen in CSWS shows impairment of language-based aspects (Perez et al., 1993) compared with the widespread dysfunction seen in ADRESD.

Another condition where speech disorders and epilepsy are seen is the congenital bilateral perisylvian syndrome (Kuzniecky et al., 1989, 1993, 1994). This condition is associated with major cortical developmental abnormalities on MRI which are not seen in individuals with ADRESD.

Relationship to familial speech disorders

There is no doubt that families with dominantly inherited rolandic seizures are extraordinarily rare. The high frequency of seizures alerted us to study the family described here. In contrast, families with inherited speech problems such as dyspraxias and dysarthrias are common (Bishop et al., 1995). In such children, interest in sleep EEG studies has recently flourished as epileptiform activity may be a marker of an epileptogenic basis to their speech difficulties or perhaps an epiphenomenon associated with their underlying problems (Parry-Fielder et al., 1997).

One family with severe orofacial dyspraxia originally described in 1990 in the UK (Hurst et al., 1990) was subsequently alleged to have a dominantly inherited mutation in a grammar-specific gene (Gopnik, 1990), a claim later refuted (Vargha-Khadem et al., 1995). Some individuals apparently had a history of seizures (personal communication, Graeme Jackson) which was not examined in detail nor were sleep EEG studies performed. There was evidence of anticipation with more severe abnormalities in the third than the second generation (Vargha-Khadem et al., 1995). Molecular genetic studies in this family have recently linked this condition to chromosome 7q31 (Fisher et al., 1997; Fisher et al., 1998).

Molecular genetic studies

Clinical anticipation was observed in our family with ADRESD and the UK kindred with speech dyspraxia (Vargha-Khadem et al., 1995). The basis of anticipation, recognized long ago in a number of neurological disorders, has been clarified by molecular genetic studies (La Spada et al., 1994). Disorders such as myotonic dystrophy and Huntington's disease are associated with expansions of trinucleotide repeats, the size of the expansion correlating with the severity of disease. The family is too small for linkage studies to map the disease locus to define a region of the genome which might contain a repeat expansion responsible for this disorder. The locus recently reported in the British family (see above) on chromosome 7q31 (Fisher et al., 1998) has been excluded from the family in this report by recombination between ADRESD and markers from the 7q31 region (unpublished data). If a gene could be identified in ADRESD, it could provide a valuable tool to aid in identification of the gene for the most common idiopathic partial epilepsy of childhood, benign rolandic epilepsy.

What is the hallmark of this syndrome?

The hallmark of ADRESD may be the dominantly inherited speech dyspraxia, rather than the seizure disorder which could be unusually penetrant in the family described here. EEG sleep studies on children with dominantly inherited speech problems may provide new insights into the relationship between epileptiform activity, seizures and developmental speech and language problems. Indeed, study of families with autosomal dominant speech problems holds the promise of finding genes which are critical for normal development of speech and language, and may unlock the door to understanding the complex interaction in the epilepsy-speech disorders.

Acknowledgement: The author gratefully acknowledges Associate Professor John Mulley and Hilary Phillips for molecular genetic work, Anne Howell and Associate Professor Michael Saling for neuropsychological evaluation of the family, Loretta Jones and Margaret Pozzebon for speech pathology assessments of the family, Professor Samuel Berkovic and Associate Professor John Mulley for critical review of the manuscript. This work was supported by the NHMRC of Australia. The participation of the family was greatly appreciated.

References

Bishop, D.V.M., North, T. & Donlan C. (1995): Genetic basis of specific language impairment: evidence from a twin study. *Dev. Med. Child. Neurol.* **37**, 56–71.

Bladin, P.F. (1987): The association of benign rolandic epilepsy with migraine. In: *Migraine and epilepsy*, Andermann, F. & Lugaresi, E. (eds), pp. 145–152. Boston: Butterworths.

Bray, P.F. & Wiser, W.C. (1964): Evidence for a genetic etiology of temporal-central abnormalities in focal epilepsy. *N. Engl. J. Med.* **271**, 926–933.

Bray, P.F. & Wiser, W.C. (1965): Hereditary characteristics of familial temporal-central focal epilepsy. *Pediatrics* **36**, 207–211.

Commission on Classification and Terminology of the International League Against Epilepsy (1989): Proposal for revised classification of epilepsies and epileptic syndromes. *Epilepsia* **30**, 389–399.

Deonna, T.-W., Roulet, E., Fontan, D. & Marcoz, J.-P. (1993): Speech and oromotor deficits of epileptic origin in benign partial epilepsy of childhood with rolandic spikes. Relationship to the acquired aphasia-epilepsy syndrome. *Neuropediatrics* **24**, 83–87.

Deonna, T.W. (1991): Acquired epileptiform aphasia in children (Landau-Kleffner syndrome). *J. Clin. Neurophysiol.* **8**, 288–298.

Doose, H. & Baier, W.K. (1989): Benign partial epilepsy and related conditions: multifactorial pathogenesis with hereditary impairment of brain maturation. *Eur. J. Pediatr.* **149**, 152–158.

Fisher, S.E., Vargha-Khadem, F., Watkins, K., Monaco, A.P. & Pembrey, M. (1997): Localisation of a gene implicated in a severe speech and language disorder. *Am. J. Hum. Genet.* **61**, A28 (Abstract).

Fisher, S.E., Vargha-Khadem, F., Watkins, K.E., Monaco, A.P. & Pembrey, M.E. (1998): Localisation of a gene implicated in a severe speech and language disorder. *Nat. Genet.* **18**, 168–170.

Gopnik, M. (1990): Feature-blind grammar and dysphasia. *Nature* **344**, 715.

Heijbel, J., Blom, S. & Rasmuson, M. (1975): Benign epilepsy of childhood with centro-temporal EEG foci: A genetic study. *Epilepsia* **16**, 285–293.

Hurst, J.A., Baraitser, M., Auger, E., Graham, F. & Norell, S. (1990): An extended family with a dominantly inherited speech disorder. *Dev. Med. Child Neurol.* **32**, 352–355.

Kuzniecky, R., Andermannm F,, Tampieri, D., Melanson, D., Olivier, A. & Leppik, I. (1989): Bilateral central macrogyria: Epilepsy, pseudobulbar palsy, and mental retardation – A recognizable neuronal migration disorder. *Ann. Neurol.* **25**, 547–554.

Kuzniecky, R., Andermann, F. & Guerrini, R. (1993): CBPS Multicenter Collaborative Study. Congenital bilateral perisylvian syndrome: study of 31 patients. *Lancet* **341**, 608–612.

Kuzniecky, R., Andermann, F. & Guerrini, R. (1994): CBPS Multicenter Collaborative Study . The epileptic spectrum in the congenital bilateral perisylvian syndrome. *Neurology* **44**, 379–385.

La Spada, A.R., Paulson, H.L. & Fischbeck, K.H. (1994): Trinucleotide repeat expansion in neurological disease. *Ann. Neurol.* **36**, 814–822.

Landau, W.M. & Kleffner, F.R. (1957): Syndrome of acquired aphasia with convulsive disorder in children. *Neurology* **7,** 523–530.

Lerman, P. (1992): Benign partial epilepsy with centro-temporal spikes. In: *Epileptic syndromes in infancy, childhood and adolescence*, Roger, J., Bureau, M., Dravet, C., Dreifuss, F.E., Perret, A. & Wolf, P. (eds), pp. 189–200. London: John Libbey.

Neubauer, B.A., Moises, H.W., Lassker, U., Waltz, S., Diebold, U. & Stephani, U. (1997): Benign childhood epilepsy with centro-temporal spikes and electroencephalography trait are not linked to EBN1 and EBN2 of benign neonatal familial convulsions. *Epilepsia* **38,** 782–787.

Parry-Fielder, B., Nolan, T.M., Collins, K.J. & Stojcevski, Z. (1997): Developmental language disorders and epilepsy. *J. Paediatr. Child Hlth.* **33,** 277–280.

Perez, E.R., Davidoff, V., Despland, P.-A. & Deonna, T. (1993): Mental and behavioural deterioration of children with epilepsy and CSWS: acquired epileptic frontal syndrome. *Dev. Med. Child Neurol.* **35,** 661–674.

Roulet, E., Deonna, T. & Despland, P.A. (1989): Prolonged intermittent drooling and oromotor dyspraxia in benign childhood epilepsy with centro-temporal spikes. *Epilepsia* **30,** 564–568.

Scheffer, I.E., Jones, L., Pozzebon, M., Howell, R.A., Saling, M.M. & Berkovic, S.F. (1995): Autosomal dominant rolandic epilepsy and speech dyspraxia: A new syndrome with anticipation. *Ann. Neurol.* **38,** 633–642.

Tassinari, C.A., Bureau, M., Dravet, C., Dalla Bernardina, B. & Roger, J. (1992): Epilepsy with continuous spikes and waves during slow sleep – otherwise described as ESES (epilepsy with electrical status epilepticus during slow sleep). In: *Epileptic syndromes in infancy, childhood and adolescence*, Roger, J., Bureau, M., Dravet, C., Dreifuss, F.E., Perret, A. & Wolf, P. (eds), pp. 245–256. London: John Libbey.

Vargha-Khadem, F., Watkins, K., Alcock, K., Fletcher, P. & Passingham, R. (1995): Praxic and nonverbal cognitive deficits in a large family with a genetically transmitted speech and language disorder. *Proc. Natl. Acad. Sci.* **92,** 930–933.

Worster-Drought, C. (1971): An unusual form of acquired aphasia in children. *Dev. Med. Child Neurol* **13,** 563–571.

Chapter 14

A clinical study of 21 European families with dominant partial epilepsy

F. Picard,[1,2] G. Rudolf,[1] R. Sebastianelli,[3] F. Vigevano,[3] S. Baulac,[4] E. LeGuern,[4] P. Thomas,[5] M. Gavaret,[6] P. Genton,[6] R. Guerrini,[7] C.A. Gericke,[1,2] J.J. Poza,[8] A. Lopez de Munain,[8] I. An,[4] M. Wolff,[9] E. Hirsch,[1] A. Brice [4] and C. Marescaux[1]

[1]*INSERM U 398, Clinique Neurologique, Strasbourg, France;* [2]*Département de Neurologie, Hôpital Cantonal, Geneva, Switzerland;* [3]*Section of Neurophysiology, Bambino Gesù Children's Hospital, Rome, Italy;* [4]*INSERM U 289, Hôpital de la Salpêtrière, Paris, France;* [5]*Service de Neurologie, Hôpital Pasteur, Nice, France;* [6]*Centre Saint Paul, Marseille, France;* [7]*Istituto Neuropsichiatria Infantile, Pisa, Italy;* [8]*Servicio de Neurologia, Hospital Ntra Sra de Aranzazu, San Sebastian, Spain;* [9]*Univ. Kinderklinik, Abt. Neuropädiatrie, Tübingen, Germany*

Different syndromes of autosomal dominant partial epilepsy have been recently identified. They are described under the terms: autosomal dominant nocturnal frontal lobe epilepsy (Scheffer *et al.*, 1995a), familial temporal lobe epilepsy (Berkovic *et al.*, 1994, 1996), autosomal dominant partial epilepsy with auditory hallucinations (Ottman *et al.*, 1995) and autosomal dominant partial epilepsy with variable foci (Scheffer *et al.*, 1995b).

The identification of these new forms of epilepsy has already resulted in the discovery in two families with frontal lobe epilepsy of two different mutations in the α4 subunit of the neuronal nicotinic acetylcholine receptor, localized on chromosome 20q13.2 (Phillips *et al.*, 1995; Steinlein *et al.*, 1995; Steinlein *et al.*, 1997). This is the first time that a gene responsible for a non lesional epilepsy has been identified. Other families with frontal lobe epilepsy did not link to the region 20q (Steinlein *et al.*, 1995). One family with temporal lobe epilepsy described by Ottman *et al.* (1995) was linked to chromosome 10q, whereas other temporal lobe families described by Berkovic *et al.* did not link to this region. A genetic heterogeneity was thus demonstrated in these syndromes. The definition of homogeneous phenotypical sub-groups may facilitate future molecular genetic studies.

We have collected 21 families (20 from Western Europe and one from Algeria) with a non lesional autosomal dominant partial epilepsy, thanks to a collaborative network of epileptologists in France (15 families), Italy (four), Spain (one) and Germany (one) (pedigrees in Fig.1). These families have not been previously reported except for the French family B (Thomas *et al.*, 1998). A detailed clinical and electrophysiological study of these families was performed.

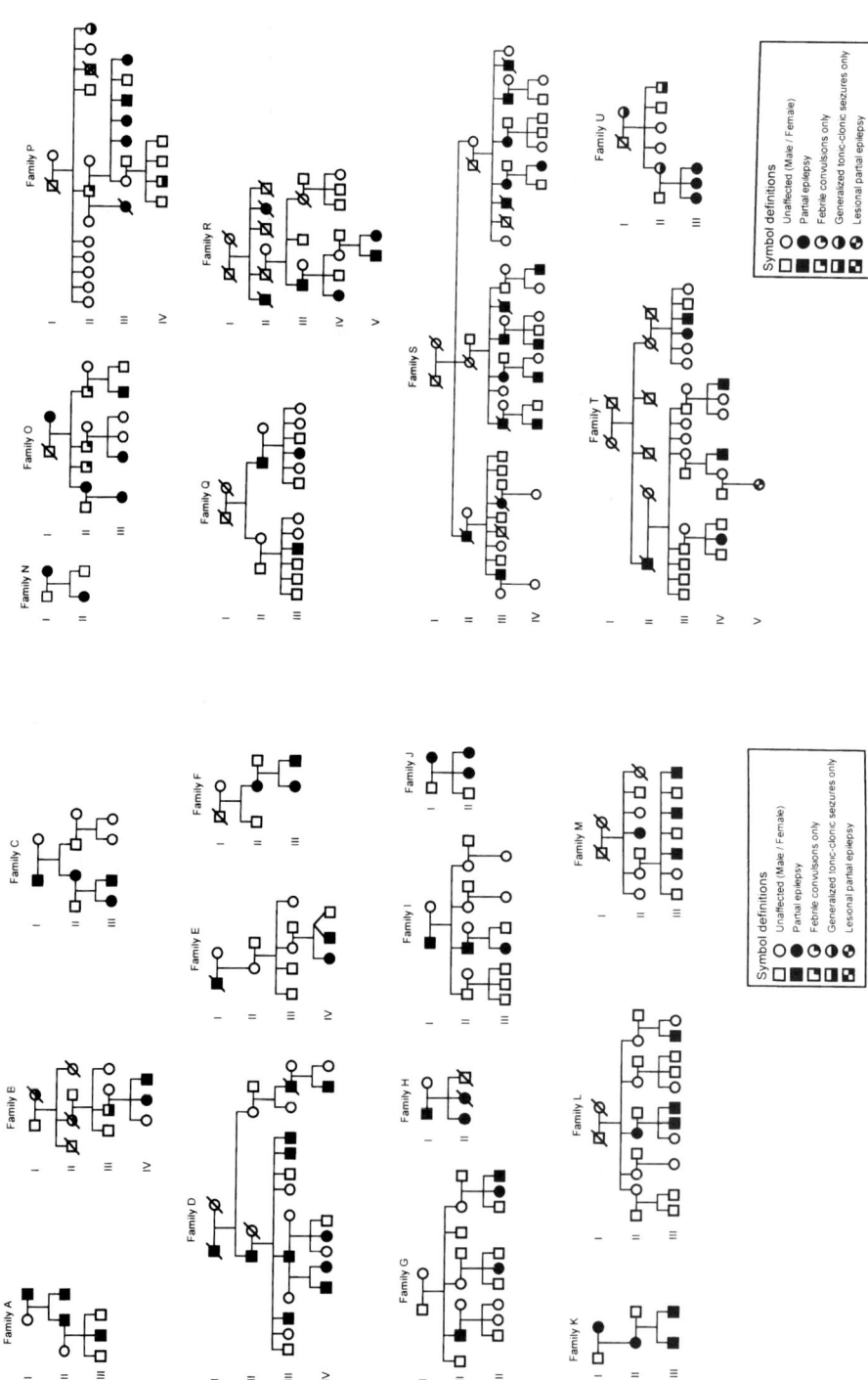

Fig. 1. Pedigrees of the 21 families. Families A to F may correspond to 'autosomal dominant frontal lobe epilepsy', families G to Q to 'familial temporal lobe epilepsy', families R to T to 'autosomal dominant partial epilepsy with variable foci' and family U 'autosomal dominant occipital lobe epilepsy'.

General features

According to the syndromes recently described, the 21 families may be divided into autosomal dominant nocturnal frontal lobe epilepsies, $n = 6$; familial temporal lobe epilepsies, $n = 11$; autosomal dominant partial epilepsies with variable foci, $n = 3$; and familial photosensitive occipital lobe epilepsy (not yet described), $n = 1$. One family (family O) with a familial temporal lobe epilepsy had a history of febrile convulsions in all affected individuals. These 21 families contained 109 epileptic individuals, but we excluded 15 deceased individuals, eight patients who had only nocturnal generalized tonic–clonic seizures, and two patients with a cerebral lesion. Out of the 84 remaining individuals, we obtained detailed data in 75 individuals by means of a clinical examination and/or a questionnaire.

The mean age of onset of the partial epilepsy was 14.2 years (median 11 years, range 2 months–56 years).

The circadian occurrence of seizures was evaluated. In our families with autosomal dominant frontal lobe epilepsy, 33 per cent of the affected individuals had seizures only during sleep, 43 per cent had infrequent attacks when awake in addition to frequent nocturnal seizures, 14 per cent had as many nocturnal as diurnal seizures and 9 per cent had mostly diurnal seizures. Diurnal seizures were also reported in 27 per cent of patients with autosomal dominant nocturnal frontal lobe epilepsy by Scheffer et al. (1995a). The nocturnal incidence of seizures was also high in our 'extra-frontal' familial epilepsies (dominant temporal lobe epilepsies and dominant partial epilepsies with variable foci): 39 per cent of the affected individuals had more nocturnal than diurnal seizures, 41 per cent had as many nocturnal as diurnal seizures and only 20 per cent had mostly diurnal seizures.

The main provocative factors were sleep deprivation and stress. Three women reported an increase of the seizure frequency with menarche or pregnancy. Noise was indicated as a trigger factor by two subjects presenting seizures with auditory hallucinations.

The ictal symptoms of focal seizures were very varied (see 'Level of clinical homogeneity among the dominant partial epilepsies'). Seventy-three per cent of the patients reported rare secondarily generalized seizures. Those who never suffered from generalized tonic–clonic seizure belonged to families with frontal lobe epilepsy.

Affected individuals had no abnormalities on neurological examination. However a detailed neuropsychological study performed in seven epileptic individuals, from six families, showed some moderate specific disturbances, usually concordant with the presumed localization of their epileptogenic focus.

Carbamazepine was the most effective anti-epileptic medication, and suppressed seizures in almost 80 per cent of the patients. Pharmaco-resistance to carbamazepine, and other anti-epileptic drugs, was observed in 12 (18 per cent) subjects, of whom nine presented with frontal lobe epilepsy. Seizures tended to disappear with age, around the fourth or fifth decade, even in refractory patients. At this age, some patients with previously ineffective treatment had a remission of the seizures without any change in medication; in these cases, definitive cessation of drug therapy was not followed by relapse.

Interictal EEGs were performed in 62 patients. Focal EEG abnormalities were observed in 80 per cent of them. In familial frontal lobe epilepsies, abnormalities were observed in 65 per cent of affected individuals, but often only during sleep. Interictal EEG abnormalities consisted in theta or delta slow waves, usually intermingled with sharp waves or sparse spikes. In a few patients, the EEG abnormalities persisted after the disappearance of the clinical seizures.

Ictal video-EEGs were recorded in 16 patients. Nine patients with frontal seizures showed: only artefacts ($n = 1$), unilateral frontal abnormalities ($n = 4$) or bifrontal abnormalities ($n = 4$). The seven extra-frontal seizures were characterized by a classical recruiting pattern with increasing amplitude and decreasing frequency.

EEGs were also performed in 33 asymptomatic (non-epileptic) family members from four families with 'familial temporal lobe epilepsy' or with 'partial epilepsy with variable foci' (families I, M, Q,

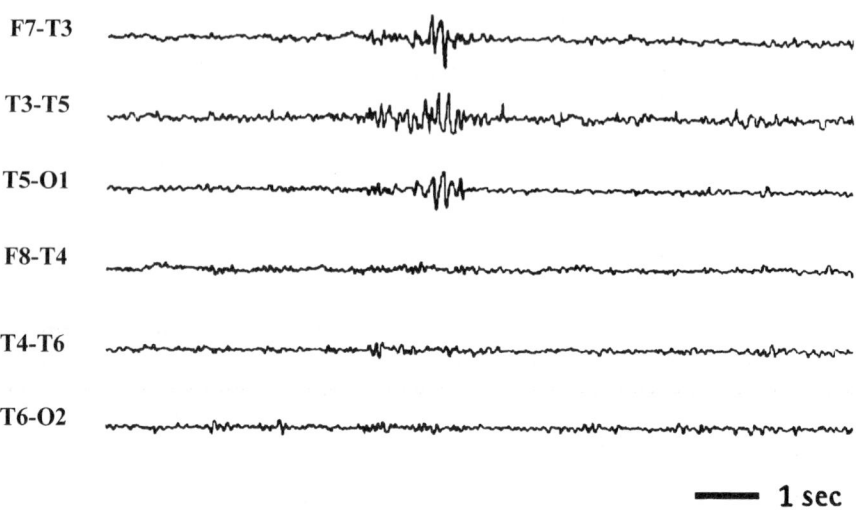

Fig. 2. Epileptiform focal EEG abnormalities recorded during drowsiness in a non-epileptic member of family Q, who was an obligate carrier.

R). Six of them (18 per cent) showed focal spikes, polyspikes or sharp waves appearing several times on a 20 min EEG recording and located consistently over the same area in the same individual. Two out of the three obligate carriers who were tested showed such EEG abnormalities (Fig. 2).

Neuro-imaging was available in 50 patients (39 MRI brain scans, 11 CT scans). Two patients belonging to the same family (I) had a discrete cortical atrophy with a predominance in the left insular and opercular area, which corresponded to the location of their suspected epileptogenic focus. Minor changes (small high-signal areas in right basal ganglia on T2-weighted images, pineal cyst) were seen in three other individuals. No hippocampal sclerosis was observed.

Level of clinical homogeneity among the dominant partial epilepsies

The six families with familial frontal lobe epilepsy showed inter-familial homogeneity: nocturnal occurrence of clusters of seizures, characterized by vegetative symptoms and tonic and dystonic components. Age at onset was similar (1.5–8 years) in the 10 affected individuals of three Italian families (D, E, F). On the contrary, in family A, age at onset was variable, ranging from 5 to 56 years. There was usually an important intra-familial variability in the severity of the disorder. Most of the families with familial frontal lobe epilepsy contained one pharmaco-resistant individual whereas the other affected family members had a good response to the anti-epileptic medication.

In the 15 families with dominant 'extra-frontal' partial epilepsy there was no real shared clinical feature between the families, except the frequent nocturnal occurrence of seizures. There was also intra-familial heterogeneity: age at onset, severity of the disorder and ictal symptoms varied from one individual to another in the same family. The ictal symptomatology was well documented in 29 patients with familial temporal lobe epilepsy. Twenty-four had simple partial seizures, sometimes followed by complex partial seizures, and five had only complex partial seizures. The signal symptoms of the simple partial seizures were: psychic ($n = 13$), autonomic ($n = 1$), somatosensory ($n = 4$), auditory ($n = 7$), aphasic ($n = 1$). However a certain level of intra-familial homogeneity was observed in some, but not all members of a few families. For instance in family I, two individuals presented seizures, consisting of déjà vu followed by a loss of consciousness, and gestural and ambulatory automatisms. In family K, the seizures of a man and his mother were similar, consisting of a shock-like or crackling feeling in the head, followed by the vision of coloured phosphenes. In family R, a man and his sister had similar seizures consisting of a left deviation of the head and then a focal motor seizure limited to the left hemibody with preservation of the consciousness. In family S, four individuals presented visual seizures (loss of vision, flashes, coloured lights, figures), and three individuals auditory seizures (buzzing, humming).

Is the classification based on seizure localization relevant?

The autosomal dominant partial epilepsies current classification is based on seizure localization, even though this localization is only based on the ictal clinical symptoms and on the scalp EEG data. Scalp EEG, even ictal, may be misleading (Rektor *et al.*, 1997). When unilateral EEG abnormalities were observed in the frontal and temporal areas, this led us to consider the use of the term of 'frontotemporal focus'. From a clinical point of view, in the papers individualizing the 'autosomal dominant nocturnal frontal lobe epilepsy' and the 'familial temporal lobe epilepsy', the same auras (déjà vu, fear, auditory symptoms, epigastric discomfort ...) were reported in both syndromes (Scheffer *et al.*, 1995a; Berkovic *et al.*, 1996). Moreover nocturnal occurrence, in clusters and brief duration of seizures, which appear characteristic of 'frontal lobe epilepsy', can be observed in 'temporal lobe epilepsy'.

Thus the current subdivision of autosomal dominant partial epilepsies is often difficult to apply and is often subjective and arbitrary. Classification of these familial partial epilepsies will probably be made possible only by the results of genotypical studies.

Genetics

We selected families with partial epilepsy and a dominant mode of inheritance. The male to female ratio was 1.2. This ratio was 2.0 when taking into account only the families with frontal lobe epilepsy and 1.0 for the families with 'extra-frontal' partial epilepsy. Only 59 per cent of affected sibships had a parent known to be affected. A male to male transmission occurred in nine families, excluding X-linked inheritance.

Familial partial epilepsy expressivity is variable. In the same family, age at onset, ictal symptoms and course of the disease can be very different in affected relatives. The clinical penetrance of the disease varies according to age. As there was no asymptomatic obligate gene carrier in our families with dominant frontal lobe epilepsy, the clinical penetrance may be complete in this syndrome. In contrast, the clinical penetrance is incomplete in the dominant 'extra-frontal' partial epilepsies: asymptomatic obligate carriers were observed in four families with familial temporal lobe epilepsy and in three families with dominant partial epilepsy with variable foci. A 'sub-clinical phenotype' consisting only of EEG abnormalities was discovered in some of our families with dominant 'extra-frontal' partial epilepsy. The EEG study of 33 asymptomatic family members from four families showed clear focal epileptiform EEG abnormalities in six individuals (18 per cent), from three different families. These six asymptomatic individuals with focal EEG abnormalities should be considered as carriers. Indeed, these kind of EEG abnormalities are exceptional in the general population, estimated at less than 0.2 per cent (Trojaborg, 1992). Moreover, such EEG abnormalities were found in two of the three asymptomatic obligate carriers in whom an EEG was carried out. Three asymptomatic individuals with focal EEG abnormalities were adolescents. The follow-up will allow us to see whether the EEG abnormalities may precede the appearance of clinical seizures.

Clinical anticipation may be suggested in four families (A, I, R, T) with three affected generations. Seizures appeared earlier and were more severe in subsequent generations. Based on the 16 clinically affected individuals from these four families, the mean age of onset was 28.5 years in the first affected generation, 13 years in the second one and 7 years in the third one; seizure frequency was greatest in individuals of the last generation.

Genotypical studies were performed in 16 families (all families except J, O, S, T and U). Firstly, the nicotinic receptor α4 subunit gene was assessed. The missense Ser248Phe mutation found in its exon 5 (Steinlein et al., 1995) in one family with autosomal dominant nocturnal frontal lobe epilepsy (Scheffer et al., 1995a) was excluded in all our families. The method included a polymerase chain reaction to amplify a part of the exon 5, then a digestion by a restriction enzyme cutting the normal allele but not the mutated one, and lastly a polyacrylamide gel analysis (Steinlein et al., 1995). Moreover, the six exons of the α4 subunit were studied by SSCP (Single Stranded Conformation Polymorphism) in index cases of each family. In families with frontal lobe epilepsy, two index cases (families B, D) had normal SSCP profiles and three (Families A, C, E) an abnormal pattern for exon 5. In families with temporal lobe epilepsy, five index cases had normal profiles, three an abnormal profile for exon 3 and two an abnormal profile for exon 5. The index case from a family (R) with autosomal dominant partial epilepsy with variable foci had abnormal profiles for both exons 3 and 5. We are now studying if these abnormal profiles correspond to common polymorphisms or not (Steinlein et al., 1996).

Subsequently, linkage to chromosome 10q (Ottman et al., 1995) was assessed, using D10S185, D10S1709, D10S1692 and D10S566 markers. In two families (K, Q) with familial temporal lobe epilepsy, a 10q haplotype cosegregated with the disease, but these families were not informative enough to suggest linkage. In contrast, linkage to 10q was excluded in four families with temporal lobe epilepsy (I, L, M, P) and in one family (R) with partial epilepsy with variable foci. For families with frontal lobe epilepsy, linkage to 10q was excluded in one family (C), but not in two families (A, D).

Nosological position

Up to now, 14 families with autosomal dominant nocturnal frontal lobe epilepsy (Scheffer et al., 1995a; Oldani et al., 1996; Magnusson et al., 1996), 14 families with familial temporal lobe epilepsy (Berkovic et al., 1996; Ottman et al., 1995) and one family with autosomal dominant partial epilepsy with variable foci (Scheffer et al., 1995b) have been reported in the literature. With this present paper there are now 50 reported families with dominant partial epilepsy.

What is the nosological position of familial partial epilepsies in relation to other partial epilepsies? Autosomal dominant partial epilepsies differ from symptomatic familial focal epilepsies related to an inherited central nervous system disorder. All our patients were normal on neurological examination and the neuroradiological images were normal or showed minor abnormalities.

Autosomal dominant partial epilepsies differ also from classical idiopathic focal epilepsies, which have a narrow and homogeneous clinical spectrum, and characteristic EEG abnormalities, clearly activated by sleep. However an idiopathic frontal lobe epilepsy was reported in ten children by Vigevano & Fusco (1993). These cases share many similarities with autosomal dominant nocturnal frontal lobe epilepsy, and now, for these authors, the diagnosis of autosomal dominant nocturnal frontal lobe epilepsy is established for at least two of the children (one is reported in the present paper).

In fact, from an electroclinical point of view familial partial epilepsies are very similar to the 'so-called' cryptogenic focal epilepsies. Thus some isolated cases of cryptogenic partial epilepsy may represent 'sporadic' cases of autosomal dominant partial epilepsy. These cases would correspond to real sporadic cases, related to *de novo* mutations, or to non-identified familial cases, when other affected relatives are not diagnosed because of the variable expressivity (sub-clinical phenotype).

In conclusion, familial forms of cryptogenic partial epilepsy do exist. This leads us to examine the role of genetic factors in all cryptogenic focal epilepsies. The present study of 21 families confirmed that dominant frontal lobe and temporal lobe epilepsies are heterogeneous on both clinical and molecular bases.

References

Berkovic, S.F., Howell, R.A. & Hopper, J.L. (1994): Familial temporal lobe epilepsy: a new syndrome with adolescent/adult onset and a benign course. In: *Epileptic seizures and syndromes*, P. Wolf (ed.), pp. 257–263. London: John Libbey.

Berkovic, S.F., McIntosh, A., Howell, R.A., Mitchell, A., Sheffield, L.J. & Hopper, J.L. (1996): Familial temporal lobe epilepsy: a common disorder identified in twins. *Ann. Neurol.* **40**, 227–235.

Commission on Classification and Terminology of the International League against Epilepsy (1989): Proposal for revised classification of epilepsies and epileptic syndromes. *Epilepsia* **30**, 389–399.

Magnusson, A., Nakken, K.O. & Brubakk, E. (1996): Autosomal dominant frontal lobe epilepsy. *Lancet* **347**, 1191–1192.

Oldani, A., Zucconi, M., Ferini-Strambi, L., Bizzozero, D. & Smirne, S. (1996): Autosomal dominant nocturnal frontal lobe epilepsy: electroclinical picture. *Epilepsia* **37**, 964–976.

Ottman, R., Risch, N., Hauser, W.A., Pedley, T.A., Lee, J.H., Barker-Cummings, C., Lustenberger, A., Nagle, K.J., Lee, K.S., Scheuer, M.L., Neystat, M., Susser, M. & Wilhelmsen, K.C. (1995): Localization of a gene for partial epilepsy to chromosome 10q. *Nat. Genet.* **10**, 56–60.

Phillips, H.A., Scheffer, I.E., Berkovic, S.F., Hollway, G.E., Sutherland, G.R. & Mulley, J.C. (1995): Localization of a gene for autosomal dominant nocturnal frontal lobe epilepsy to chromosome 20q13.2. *Nat. Genet.* **10**, 117–118.

Rektor, I., Svejdova, M., Kanovsky, P., Landré, E., Bancaud, J. & Lamarche, M. (1997): Can epileptologists without access to intracranial EEG use reliably the International League Against Epilepsy Classification of the localization-related epileptic syndromes? *J. Clin. Neurophysiol.* **14**, 250–254.

Scheffer, I.E., Bhatia, K.P., Lopes-Cendes, I., Fish, D.R., Marsden, C.D., Andermann, E., Andermann, F., Desbiens, R., Keene, D., Cendes, F., Manson, J.I., Constantinou, J.E.C., McIntosh, A. & Berkovic, S.F. (1995a): Autosomal dominant nocturnal frontal lobe epilepsy. A distinctive clinical disorder. *Brain* **118**, 61–73.

Scheffer, I.E., Phillips, H., Mulley, J., Sutherland, G., Harvey, A.S., Hopkins, I.J. & Berkovic, S.F. (1995b): Autosomal dominant partial epilepsy with variable foci is not allelic with autosomal dominant nocturnal frontal lobe epilepsy (abstract). *Epilepsia* (Suppl.) **36**, S28.

Steinlein, O.K., Mulley, J.C., Propping, P., Wallace, R.H., Phillips, H.A. & Sutherland, G.R. (1995): A missense mutation in the neuronal nicotinic acetylcholine receptor α4 subunit is associated with autosomal dominant nocturnal frontal lobe epilepsy. *Nat. Genet.* **11**, 201–203.

Steinlein, O., Weiland, S., Stoodt, J. & Propping, P. (1996): Exon-intron structure of the human neuronal nicotinic acetylcholine receptor α4 subunit (CHRNA4). *Genomics* **32**, 289–294.

Steinlein, O.K., Magnusson, A., Stoodt, J., Bertrand, S., Weiland, S., Berkovic, S.F., Nakken, K.O., Propping, P. & Bertrand, D. (1997): An insertion mutation of the CHRNA4 gene in a family with autosomal dominant nocturnal frontal lobe epilepsy. *Hum. Mol. Genet.* **6**, 943–947.

Thomas, P., Picard, F., Hirsch, E., Chatel, M. & Marescaux, C. (1998): Epilepsie frontale nocturne autosomique dominante. *Rev. Neurol.* **154**, 228–235.

Trojaborg, W. (1992): EEG abnormalities in 5,893 jet pilot applicants registered in a 20-year period. *Clin. Electroencephalogr.* **23**, 72–78.

Vigevano, F. & Fusco, L. (1993): Hypnic tonic postural seizures in healthy children provide evidence for a partial epileptic syndrome of frontal lobe origin. *Epilepsia* **39**, 110–119.

Part V
Genetics of other focal epilepsies

Chapter 15

Genetically determined forms of partial symptomatic epilepsies: clinical phenotype, neuropathology and neurogenetic basis of seizures

Renzo Guerrini,[1] William B. Dobyns,[2] Olivier Dulac,[3] Alexis Arzimanoglou,[4] Eva Andermann[5] and Romeo Carrozzo[6]

[1]*Institute of Child Neurology and Psychiatry, University of Pisa-IRCCS Stella Maris Foundation, Pisa, Italy;* [2]*Pediatric Neurology Department, University of Minesota, Minneapolis, USA;* [3]*Neuropédiatrie, Hôpital Saint Vincent de Paul, Paris, France;* [4]*Neuropédiatrie, Hôpital Robert Debré, Paris, France;* [5]*Montreal Neurological Hospital and Institute, Montreal, QC, Canada;* [6]*Department of Medical Genetics, San Raffaele Hospital, Milano, Italy*

Virtually all single gene traits associated with seizures and all known chromosomal abnormalities lead to anatomo-functional impairment of the central nervous system. When seizures are the main manifestation of a genetically determined disorder or present with peculiar electro-clinical patterns, it is extremely important to establish whether these associations result from concomitant structural abnormalities of the CNS due to the genetic changes, a chance fluctuation of the samples studied, or the effect of loci that specifically affect seizure susceptibility. Since brain dysfunction in these disorders is almost always extensive and neuropathological changes are usually complex, it is difficult to understand which of these changes are more directly responsible for epileptogenesis. Furthermore, there are very few genetically determined disorders that are consistently accompanied by epilepsy (Table 1). In most cases, epilepsy appears in a variable percentage of patients, suggesting that seizure susceptibility may be multi-factorial or not merely linked to the genetically determined structural or biochemical abnormalities.

Only those genetic disorders of special importance for their high frequency or association with epilepsy are considered in this chapter.

Aicardi syndrome

Aicardi syndrome (Aicardi *et al.*, 1965, 1969) is exclusively observed in females, with the exception of two reported males with two X chromosomes (Aicardi, 1996) and is therefore thought to be caused by an X-linked gene with lethality in the hemizygous male. Familial occurrence has been reported in one family, in which two sisters were affected (Molina *et al.*, 1989). A possible locus for Aicardi syndrome on the short arm of the X chromosome has been suggested on the basis of numerous reports of the association of eye abnormalities and agenesis of the corpus callosum with translocations involving Xp22.3. Clinical and neuroimaging features include severe mental retardation, infantile spasms, chorioretinal lacunae and agenesis of the corpus callosum. In one study, the estimated survival rate was 75 per cent at 6 years and 40 per cent at 15 years (MacGregor et al., 1993). Neuropathological findings are consistent with a neuronal migration disorder and include: (1) a thin unlayered cortex, (2) diffuse unlayered polymicrogyria with fused molecular layers, (3) nodular heterotopias in the periventricular region and in the centrum semiovale (Billette de Villemeur et al., 1992; Ferrer et al., 1986). The cortical pattern is irregular, with many small cauliflower-like convolutions. No laminar organization is recognizable in the cortex, beyond the molecular layer. Neurons have a radial disposition, but the thickness of the cortex is irregular and difficult to measure because neurons are scattered. As a result of the fusion of the molecular layers the microgyri are packed and not visible at MRI. Additional, less frequent, malformations include agenesis of the anterior commissure, or the fornix, or both, choroid plexus cysts, colobomata, and vertebral and costal abnormalities.

Table 1. Some non-metabolic mendelian disorders associated with epilepsy

Disorder	Gene	Chromosomal mapping	Incidence of epilepsy
Aicardi	Unknown	Xp22	100%
Miller-Dieker/ILS	LIS1	17p13.3	100%
BH/X-linked lissencephaly	doublecortin	Xq22.3	90–100%
Periventricular nodular heterotopia	Unknown	Xq28	80–100%
Angelman	UBE3A	15q11-q13	80–100%
Tuberous sclerosis	TSC1/TSC2	9q24/16p13.3	60–100%
Familial cavernous angiomas	Unknown	7q	69%
Alpha thalassaemia/mental retardation	XH2	Xq13.3	40%
Fragile X	FMR1	Xq27.3	28–45%
Sotos	Unknown	Unknown	25–35%
Lujan-Fryns	Unknown	Unknown	21%
Neurofibromatosis I	NF1	17q11	20%
Kabuki make-up	Unknown	Unknown	16%
Incontinentia pigmenti	Unknown	Xp11.21/Xq28	13%
Huntington disease	HD	4p16	10%
Cockayne	CKN1	5	5–10%
Proteus syndrome	Unknown	Unknown	<5%
Simpson-Golabi-Behmel	GPC3	Xq26	<5%

Specific electroclinical features of Aicardi syndrome include early onset of infantile spasms and partial seizures. Spasms were the only seizure type in 47 per cent of 184 reported patients. In 35 per cent of patients spasms were associated with partial seizures (Chevrie & Aicardi, 1986), involving mainly eyes and face. The partial seizures often begin in the first days of life and precede the onset of spasms. Aicardi syndrome has been reported as one possible cause of 'early infantile epileptic encephalopathy' (Ohtahara et al., 1987). Hypsarrhythmia is observed in a minority of patients (about 18 per cent) (Aicardi, 1996). Interictal EEG abnormalities are typically asymmetric and asynchronous (split brain EEG), with or without suppression bursts during wakefulness and sleep. Seizure and EEG patterns change little, if at all, over time and seizures are almost always resistant. Aicardi syndrome is due to a highly epileptogenic malformation pattern in which multiple cortical areas can originate seizure activity. There is a low tendency to develop seizure types typical of the older child.

Classical lissencephaly and subcortical band heterotopia (agyria-pachygyria-band spectrum)

Classical lissencephaly (smooth brain) is a severe malformation of neuronal migration characterized by absent (agyria) or decreased (pachygyria) surface convolutions, producing a smooth cerebral surface (Fig. 1a) (Matell, 1893; Crome, 1956; Norman *et al.*, 1995; Dobyns & Truwit, 1995). A *forme fruste* of classical lissencephaly known as subcortical band heterotopia (SBH) comprises the mild end of this group of malformations, which may accordingly be called the agyria-pachygyria-band spectrum (Figs. 1b & 2) (Matell, 1893; Barkovich *et al.*, 1994; Dobyns *et al.*, 1996). In SBH, the cerebral convolutions appear normal or mildly broad. Just beneath the cortical ribbon, a thin band of white matter with readily distinguishable U-fibres separates the cortex from symmetric and circumferential bands of gray matter.

Pathological studies of both lissencephaly and SBH demonstrate incomplete neuronal migration. In classical lissencephaly, the cerebral cortex is abnormally thick, usually measuring 10–15 mm compared to the normal width of 2–3 mm. The cytoarchitecture consists of four primitive layers including an outer marginal layer, a superficial cellular layer which corresponds to the true cortex, a variable cell sparse layer, and a deep cellular layer composed of heterotopic neurons, which extends more than half the width of the mantle. The lateral ventricles are usually dysmorphic and mildly enlarged without hydrocephalus, while the corpus callosum is often small or dysmorphic. Additional abnormalities include hypoplasia of the corticospinal tracts, heterotopia of the inferior olives, and mild dysplasia of the cerebellar cortex.

Table 2. Grading system for lissencephaly and SBH (agyria-pachygyria-band spectrum*)

Grade	Description
1	Agyria only
2	Agyria with limited frontotemporal pachygyria
3	Mixed agyria and pachygyria a. frontal pachygyria and posterior agyria b. frontal agyria and posterior pachygyria
4	Pachygyria only a. diffuse pachygyria only b. frontal pachygyria and posterior normal gyri c. frontal normal gyri and posterior pachygyria
5	Mixed pachygyria and subcortical band heterotopia a. pachygyria with subtle band b. pachygyria with clear band c. forme fruste pachygyria with thin cortex and band
6	Subcortical band heterotopia a. thick band b. medium band c. thin band d. thin partial frontal band e. thin partial posterior band

*Scale developed by W.B. Dobyns and C.L. Truwit.

SBH consists of symmetric and circumferential bands of gray matter, which usually extend from the frontal to occipital regions, sparing only the cingulate, striate and medial temporal cortices (Ross *et al.*, 1997; Harding, 1996). The inner margin of the band is usually smooth, while the outer margin may be smooth or follow the interdigitations of the true cortex and white matter. Closer to the ventricle,

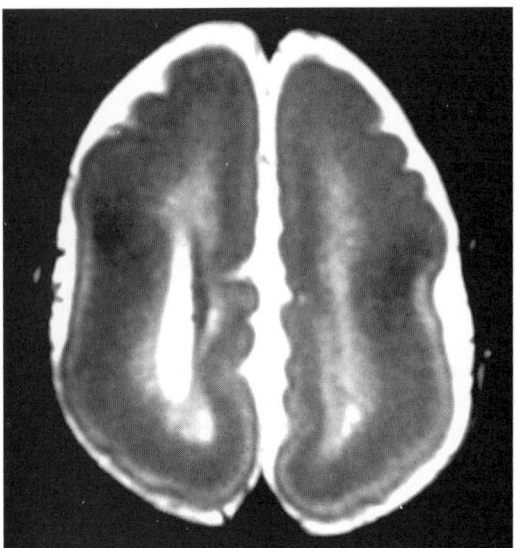

Fig. 1a. Agyria-pachygyria. Brain MR, axial spin-echo T2W image. Agyric pattern of the parietal cortex and mild cortical undulation in frontal lobes. The thin outer cortical layer is separated from a layer of prematurely stopped neurons during their migration, by an hyperintense strip of unmyelinated white matter (cell-sparse zone), more evident in the agyric areas.

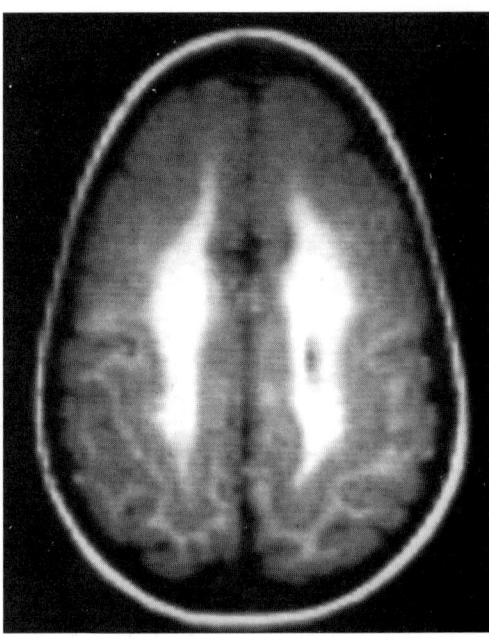

Fig. 1b. Band heterotopia. Axial T1W image. Pachygyria with thick smooth cortex in the frontal lobes and less severe involvement of the posterior cortex where a thick band of heterotopic gray matter is recognizable.

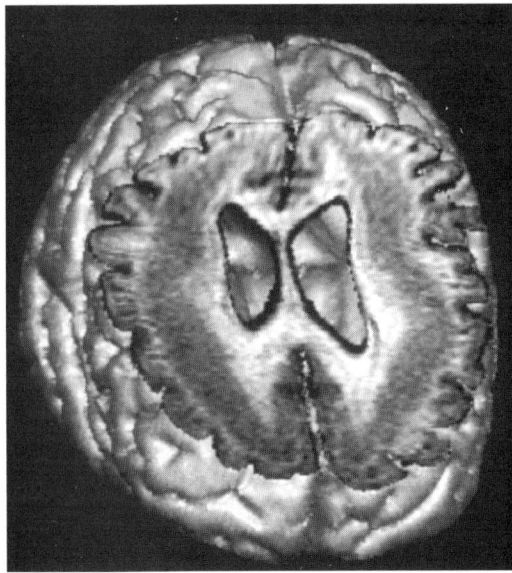

Fig. 2. MRI, 3D reconstruction of the brain; anterior view. 18 year old girl with band heterotopia, severe mental retardation and intractable spasms. Note the shallow sulci, particularly in the frontal lobes, and the thick band of heterotopic gray matter.

the band may become fragmented into islands separated by thick bands of white matter. The band is highly variable in thickness and extent. The cortex overlying the bands usually appears normal, although the gyri may be mildly wide. The band is separated from the cortex by a thin layer of white matter with readily distinguishable U-fibres. Transitional forms have been observed in rare patients, especially frontal pachygyria, which merges with posterior SBH in several patients, and partial frontal or posterior bands in several others (Dobyns & Truwit, 1995). The grading system is shown in Table 2.

On several occasions classical lissencephaly (agyria-pachygyria) and SBH have been observed in different individuals from the same family; rare patients have shown areas of classical lissencephaly (pachygyria with a thick cortex) merging into true subcortical band heterotopia. These observations show that classical lissencephaly and SBH comprise a single malformation spectrum. The most common subtypes are grades 2, 3a and 6, while all the others are relatively rare.

Lissencephaly appears to be quite rare. A case ascertainment study in The Netherlands showed a prevalence of 11.7 per million births (de Rijk-van Andel *et al.*, 1991).

All patients with classical lissencephaly have early developmental delay and eventual profound or severe mental retardation. Rare patients with only partial pachygyria may have only moderate mental retardation. Early feeding problems are common and often improve, only to worsen again as the child grows older. Most have chronic aspiration and gastroesophageal reflux, both of which may be clinically silent. Other neurological manifestations include early diffuse hypotonia, later spastic quadriplegia which is usually mild, and opisthotonus. Some affected children have lived more than 20 years, although anecdotal experience suggests that the lifespan is less than 10 years in most patients.

Seizures occur in over 90 per cent of patients, with onset before 6 months in about 75 per cent, although it may also occur much later (A. Khan & W.B. Dobyns, unpublished data). About 80 per cent of children have infantile spasms in the first year of life, although the EEG may not show typical hypsarrhythmia. Later, most children have mixed seizure disorders including focal motor and generalized tonic seizures (Dulac *et al.*, 1983; Guerrini *et al.*, 1993; Guerrini *et al.*, 1996), partial complex seizures, atypical absences, tonic and atonic seizures causing drop attacks, and even myoclonic seizures. The intractable forms are usually generalized while less severe forms are often partial (Guerrini *et al.*, 1996).

Many children with lissencephaly have characteristic EEG changes, including diffuse fast rhythms which do not react to eye opening (Hakamada *et al.*, 1979; Guerrini *et al.*, 1996) and high amplitude rhythmic activity which has high specificity but low sensitivity (Quirk *et al.*, 1993)

Subcortical band heterotopia – The two major clinical manifestations of SBH consist of cognitive impairment and epilepsy. Mental abilities range from normal to severe mental retardation, and seem to correlate well with MRI parameters, above all band thickness and presence or absence of overlying gyral malformation. When present, the latter consists of mild pachygyria with a thin or normal cortex (Barkovich *et al.*, 1994). Patients with gyral abnormalities have more severe ventricular enlargement and thicker heterotopic bands (Barkovich *et al.*, 1994); patients with pachygyria and more severe ventricular enlargement have significantly earlier seizure onset. The more severe the pachygyria and the thicker the heterotopic band, the higher are the chances of developing Lennox-Gastaut or some other generalized symptomatic epilepsy syndrome (Barkovich *et al.*, 1994). Although almost all reported patients with SBH have had epilepsy, early seizure onset is uncommon. When it occurs, seizure types may include infantile spasms, early Lennox-Gastaut syndrome (Ricci *et al.*, 1992) or partial motor seizures (Palmini *et al.*, 1991; Barkovich *et al.*, 1994). Persistent seizures causing drop attacks have been treated with callosotomy (Palmini *et al.*, 1991; Landy *et al.*, 1993) with worthwhile improvement. Of 42 reported patients with BH (Livingston & Aicardi, 1990; Palmini *et al.*, 1991; Ricci *et al.*, 1992; Morrel *et al.*, 1992; Landy *et al.*, 1993; Barkovich *et al.*, 1994; Ketonen *et al.*, 1994; Guerrini *et al.*, 1996) 40 had epilepsy. Of the 37 patients with epilepsy whose electroclinical data were reported in sufficient detail, 51 per cent had generalized epilepsy; often with the characteristics of Lennox-Gastaut syndrome, and 49 per cent had partial epilepsy. Overall, 65 per cent of the patients studied had intractable seizures.

The correlations between clinical outcome and MRI parameters suggest that only neurons reaching the cortical plate have normal synaptic connections (Barkovich *et al.*, 1994; Caviness, 1989), although neurons in the band are metabolically active since they have the same glucose uptake as the overlying cortex on [18F]fluorodeoxyglucose positron emission tomographic scanning (Miura *et al.*, 1993). Using depth electrodes, Morrell *et al.* (1992) demonstrated that epileptiform activity may originate directly from the heterotopic neurons, independently of the activity of the overlying cortex. Similar findings have been reported by Munari *et al.* (1996) in a patient with a subcortical nodular heterotopia. Therefore, heterotopic neurons are intrinsically epileptogenic and synaptically connected with other neurons. However, it is unclear whether connectivity is exclusively within the heterotopic tissue or also involves normally migrated cortical neurons.

Malformation syndromes with lissencephaly and SBH

Several different malformation syndromes associated with classical lissencephaly have been described. The best known of these is Miller-Dieker syndrome, which is caused by large deletions of the LIS1 gene and contiguous genes primarily telomeric to LIS1. The most recent and least known is Ramer-Lin syndrome. In addition, several different patterns of inheritance have been described as shown in Table 3.

Table 3. Classification of syndromes with classical lissencephaly and subcortical band heterotopia (agyria-pachygyria-band spectrum)

	Inheritance
Chromosome X-linked (XLIS gene)	
Isolated lissencephaly sequence, X-linked (ILSX)	XL
Subcortical band heterotopia, X-linked (SBHX)	XL
Chromosome 17-linked (LIS1 gene)	
Isolated lissencephaly sequence, 17-linked (ILS17)	AD
Miller-Dieker syndrome (MDS)	AD
Unknown gene and gene location	
Isolated lissencephaly sequence, unmapped	AD
Isolated lissencephaly sequence, unmapped (probably includes Norman-Roberts syndrome)	AR
Ramer-Lin syndrome	

Miller-Dieker syndrome and isolated lissencephaly sequence

Children with MDS have characteristic facial abnormalities, and sometimes other birth defects (Dobyns *et al.*, 1991). The facial changes include prominent forehead, bi-temporal hollowing, short nose with upturned nares, low nasal bridge with prominent skin folds leading down and outward to the cheeks, flat midface, thick upper lip with downturned vermillion border, and small jaw. Other common abnormalities include telecanthus, epicanthal folds, low-set and posteriorly rotated ears, malformed ears, high and narrow palate, mild congenital heart malformations, omphalocele, genital hypoplasia, undescended testes (in males), transverse palmar creases, clinodactyly, and mild distal contractures. Almost all have a prominent sacral dimple. Patients with large chromosome deletions or unbalanced derivative chromosomes often have other birth defects, in particular more severe congenital heart malformations. Most children with ILS have either a normal facial appearance or subtle facial changes reminiscent of MDS but not sufficient for diagnosis, such as prominent forehead, low nasal bridge, or slightly short nose (Dobyns *et al.*, 1992; Dobyns & Truwit, 1995). In addition, most have subtle bi-temporal hollowing and somewhat small jaw.

Previous studies identified a lissencephaly critical region in the short arm of chromosome 17 in patients with either MDS or ILS. Chromosome analysis in children with Miller-Dieker syndrome showed visible deletions or other rearrangements in about two-thirds, while the remainder were normal (Dobyns *et al.*, 1991). Chromosome analysis in over 100 children with isolated lissencephaly sequence was normal except for two children with apparently balanced translocations (Dobyns *et al.*, 1992). One of these involved the lissencephaly critical region in chromosome 17p13.3 (Chong *et al.*, 1997), while the other involved the lissencephaly/SBH critical region in chromosome Xq22.3 (Dobyns *et al.*, 1996; Ross *et al.*, 1997).

Molecular genetic studies show a much higher frequency of abnormalities in both MDS and ILS. Fluorescence *in situ* hybridization (FISH) in children with MDS shows deletions in over 90 per cent of patients tested, while FISH in children with ILS shows deletions in 30 per cent or less. The deletions in Miller-Dieker syndrome are consistently larger than in patients with isolated lissencephaly sequence (Dobyns *et al.*, 1993). A candidate gene was isolated from the lissencephaly critical region (Reiner *et al.*, 1993) and has recently been confirmed as the gene responsible for the lissencephaly phenotype (Chong *et al.*, 1997; LoNigro *et al.*, 1997). Point mutations within the LIS1 gene have recently been discovered in three unrelated patients with ILS (LoNigro *et al.*, 1997).

When a deletion is identified in either Miller-Dieker syndrome or in ILS patients, parental studies should be carried out. If the parental studies are normal, indicating a *de novo* event, the recurrence risk is low, probably less than 1 per cent. If one parent carries a balanced structural chromosome rearrangement, the recurrence risk is based on the specific chromosome abnormality identified. If no deletion is identified, the empirical recurrence risk for isolated lissencephaly sequence is about 5 per cent (Dobyns *et al.*, 1992).

X-linked lissencephaly and subcortical band heterotopia

X-linked lissencephaly and SBH consist of classical lissencephaly in hemizygous males and SBH in heterozygous females. Several recent observations have contributed to recognition of this syndrome. First, a striking skew of the sex ratio toward females (51 females and three males) has been reported among patients with SBH (Guerrini *et al.*, 1996; Barkovich *et al.*, 1994; Dobyns *et al.*, 1996; Ricci *et al.*, 1992; Landy *et al.*, 1993; Livingston *et al.*, 1990). At least five families have been reported with X-linked inheritance of ILS in males and SBH in females (Ross *et al.*, 1997; Pinard *et al.*, 1994). In the largest multiplex family with XLIS, a woman with SBH had two daughters with SBH and a son with lissencephaly, each by a different father (Pinard *et al.*, 1994). Finally, one girl has been reported with ILS and a *de novo* balanced translocation involving chromosome Xq22.3 (Dobyns *et al.*, 1996; Ross *et al.*, 1997).

Boys with ILS (or ILSX) due to mutations of the XLIS gene have either a normal facial appearance or subtle facial abnormalities. Based on only a few observations, such abnormalities consist of a low nasal bridge, prominent epicanthal folds, and flat midface (W.B. Dobyns, unpublished observations). Other congenital abnormalities have not been described. Patients with SBH have a normal facial appearance, and generally no other congenital abnormalities. The recurrence risk for carrier females is high; 50 per cent of their sons will have lissencephaly and 50 per cent of their daughters will have subcortical band heterotopia. All female first degree relatives of a girl with subcortical band heterotopia should have a cranial MRI study to determine their carrier status. So far, no known carrier females have had a normal MRI.

The gene responsible for X-linked lissencephaly and subcortical band heterotopia has been mapped to chromosome Xq22.3-q23 by linkage analysis in several families with multiple affected individuals, and physical mapping of an X-autosomal translocation in a girl with classical lissencephaly (Ross *et al.*, 1997) and has recently been cloned (Des Portes *et al.*, 1998; Gleeson *et al.*, 1998).

Other lissencephaly syndromes

Agyria-pachygyria has been observed in other rare syndromes (Dobyns & Truwit, 1995; Ramer *et al.*, 1995). The clinical manifestations, especially severe mental retardation and frequently intractable epilepsy, appear to be similar to those found in children with classical lissencephaly.

Bilateral periventricular nodular heterotopia

This malformation consists of confluent and symmetric subependimal nodules of gray matter located along the supero-lateral walls of the lateral ventricles and extending from the frontal horns to the trigona, particularly along the ventricular body (Fig. 3). There may be hypoplasia of the corpus callosum or cerebellum, especially if the nodules are diffuse and contiguous. A mild abnormality of the gyral pattern is rarely associated (Dobyns *et al.*, 1996). Extent of the heterotopia and associated clinical symptoms are heterogeneous (Di Mario *et al.*, 1993; Kamuro & Tenokuchi, 1993; Huttenlo-

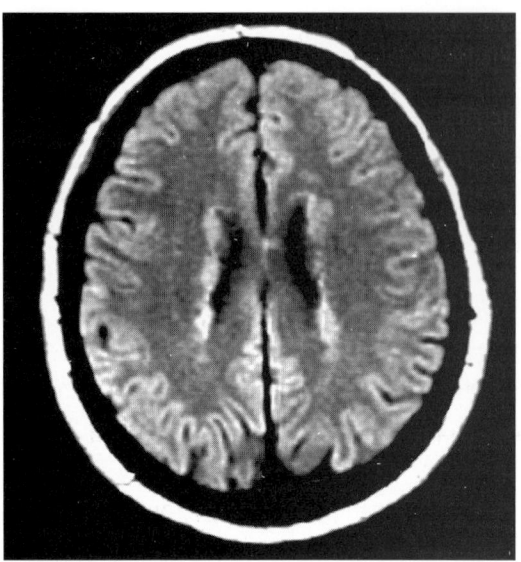

Fig. 3. Bilateral periventricular (subependymal) nodular heterotopia. Brain MR; axial spin-echo PDW image showing nodular strips lining the ventricular walls, isointense with the cortical gray matter.

cher et al., 1994; Dobyns et al., 1996; Dubeau et al., 1996). The malformation is far more frequent in females. It can be either sporadic or show a familial distribution consistent with X-linked transmission.

The syndrome of X-linked bilateral periventricular nodular heterotopia (BPNH) consists of typical BPNH in females and prenatal lethality or a more severe phenotype in males (Dobyns et al., 1996). Several recent observations have contributed to recognition of this syndrome including a striking skew of the sex ratio toward females among patients with BPNH, reports of several families with X-linked inheritance of BPNH in females and a decrease in number of sons born to affected women, and a subtle abnormality of Xq28 in a boy with severe mental retardation, BPNH and other minor anomalies. In the largest multiplex family with BPNH, six females from four generations were affected with no instances of male to male transmission (Huttenlocher et al., 1994). The five women who had reached or passed childbearing age had 12 miscarriages or stillbirths, eight living daughters including five with BPNH, and only two living sons. The rate of pregnancy loss was thus over 50 per cent, while about 20 per cent is considered normal. The ratio of sons to daughters was also skewed, suggesting that most of the miscarriages were males. Thus, the genetic recurrence risk for women with BPNH is 50 per cent for daughters and unknown but presumably much lower for severely affected sons, with an increase in the rate of miscarriages.

The gene responsible for X-linked bilateral periventricular nodular heterotopia (BPNH) was recently mapped to chromosome Xq28 by linkage analysis (Eksioglu et al., 1996) and observation of a small 2.25–3.25 Mb duplication of Xq28 in a boy with BPNH, mental retardation, and syndactyly (Dobyns et al., 1996; Fink et al., 1997).

The clinical phenotype of patients carrying areas of heterotopic cortex ranges from asymptomatic individuals to patients with seizures and normal cognitive level or mild to severe delay (Dobyns et al., 1996; Dubeau et al., 1996; Fink et al., 1997). While interictal EEG of patients with subcortical heterotopias shows focal or lateralized abnormalities correlating with the site of the malformation (Barkovich et al., 1996), the EEG of patients with periventricular heterotopia may show no abnormalities, or interictal discharges often located over the temporal regions (Dubeau et al., 1996). Depth electrodes have been used in a few patients with profound nodules and have demonstrated that seizure activity may originate within the heterotopic cortex (Dubeau et al., 1995; Munari et al., 1996).

The largest patient experience addressing the characteristics of epilepsy associated with periventricular and subcortical nodular heterotopia is that of Dubeau et al. (1995), who studied 33 patients, 29 (88 per cent) of whom had presented seizures, mainly partial attacks with temporo-parieto-occipital auras. Seizures began between the age of 2 months and 33 years and were intractable in 27 patients (82 per cent). BPNH was observed in nine patients. In a second study Dubeau et al. (1996) reviewed surgical outcome in nine patients with periventricular heterotopia, seven of whom with BPNH. Most patients showed clinical and surface EEG findings suggesting temporal lobe seizure onset. In general, however, temporal lobectomy, which in seven patients did not include the area of heterotopia, did not produce a worthwile improvement.

Angelman syndrome

Angelman syndrome (AS) is characterized by microbrachycephaly, severe mental retardation, absent speech or very poor language skills, inappropriate laughter, hyperactivity, seizures, abnormal EEG, and a characteristic 'puppetlike' motor pattern variously described as ataxic gait, jerky limb movements and tremulousness (Angelman, 1965; Bower & Jeavons, 1967; Clayton-Smith, 1993;. Viani *et al.*, 1995; Zori *et al.*, 1992).The tremulous motor pattern is, at least in part, related to quasicontinuous fast-bursting cortical myoclonus (Guerrini *et al.*, 1996). A few individuals with AS develop skills necessary for self-care (Zori *et al.*, 1992).

About 70 per cent of Angelman patients show a deletion involving the maternally inherited chromosome 15q11-q13 (Kaplan *et al.*, 1987; Magenis *et al.*, 1987). This chromosomal region encompasses three $GABA_A$ receptor subunit genes, GABRB3, GABRA5 and GABRG3. The remaining 30 per cent of patients show an apparently normal karyotype. Among these 3–5 per cent show a chromosome 15 uniparental disomy, with both of the homologs being paternal in origin (Malcolm *et al.*, 1991). Uniparental dysomy appears to be associated with a milder phenotype (Bottani *et al.*, 1994; Gillessen-Kaesbach *et al.*, 1995).

This finding has led to the hypothesis that the lack of maternal contribution for the 15q11-q13 region is the main mechanism responsible for AS and that one or more paternally imprinted genes lie within the 15q11–13 region.

About 5 per cent of AS patients show a mutation in the imprinting centre, a large transcriptional regulatory element lying about 1.5 megabases proximal to the GABA receptor cluster. The integrity of the imprinting centre ensures the switch from the paternal to the maternal epigenotype at 15q11-q13 in oogenesis, so that imprinting centre mutations hamper the expression of paternally imprinted genes from the maternal homolog (Dittrich *et al.*, 1996). Recently, a few patients with AS have been shown to harbour intragenic mutations in the UBE3A gene, mapping to 15q12-q13, the expression of which appears to be paternally imprinted in the brain (Kishino *et al.*, 1997; Matsuura *et al.*, 1997). The rare cases of familial recurrence of AS show either mutations in the imprinting centre or in the UBE3A gene. Overall, the molecular mechanism uderlying AS is unknown in about 20 per cent of the cases.

Epilepsy

Several authors have made a detailed analysis of the clinical characteristics of epilepsy in AS. Zori *et al.* (1992) estimated that about 90 per cent of patients have epilepsy. Viani *et al.* (1995) reviewed 155 reported AS patients, of whom 130 (84 per cent) had experienced epileptic seizures. The first seizures occur between the ages of 3 months–20 years (Guerrini *et al.*, 1996; Matsumoto *et al.*, 1992; Sugimoto *et al.*, 1994; Viani *et al.*, 1995; Zori *et al.*, 1992), although onset is in infancy or early childhood in most patients. It is not unusual for the first convulsive seizure to be precipitated by fever (Matsumoto *et al.*, 1992; Sugimoto *et al.*, 1994; Viani *et al.*, 1995). Infantile spasms with hypsarrhythmia are exceptional. Complex partial seizures with eye deviation and vomiting, possibly indicating occipital lobe origin were estimated to occur quite frequently by Viani *et al.* (1995). Atypical absences, myoclonic seizures, GTC and clonic unilateral seizures are among the main ictal patterns (Guerrini, *et al.*, 1996; Matsumoto *et al.*, 1992; Sugimoto *et al.*, 1994; Viani *et al.*, 1995). Over half the patients present episodes of decreased alertness and hypotonia lasting days or weeks, described as nonconvulsive status epilepticus (Matsumoto *et al.*, 1992; Sugimoto *et al.*, 1994). Most often, however, there is concomitant mild jerking, rhythmic or not (Dalla Bernardina *et al.*, 1992; Guerrini *et al.*, 1996; Viani *et al.*, 1995), typical of myoclonic status. Polygraphic recordings during myoclonic status or during short myoclonic seizures presenting as fragments of myoclonic absences reveal diffuse, slow irregular spike and wave complexes at about 2 Hz. In some patients each spike is accompanied by a myoclonic potential (Fig. 4) (Dalla Bernardina *et al.*, 1992; Guerrini *et al.*, 1996). Myoclonus shows a rostrocaudal pattern of activation, indicating cortical rather than brainstem origin (Guerrini *et al.*, 1996). In

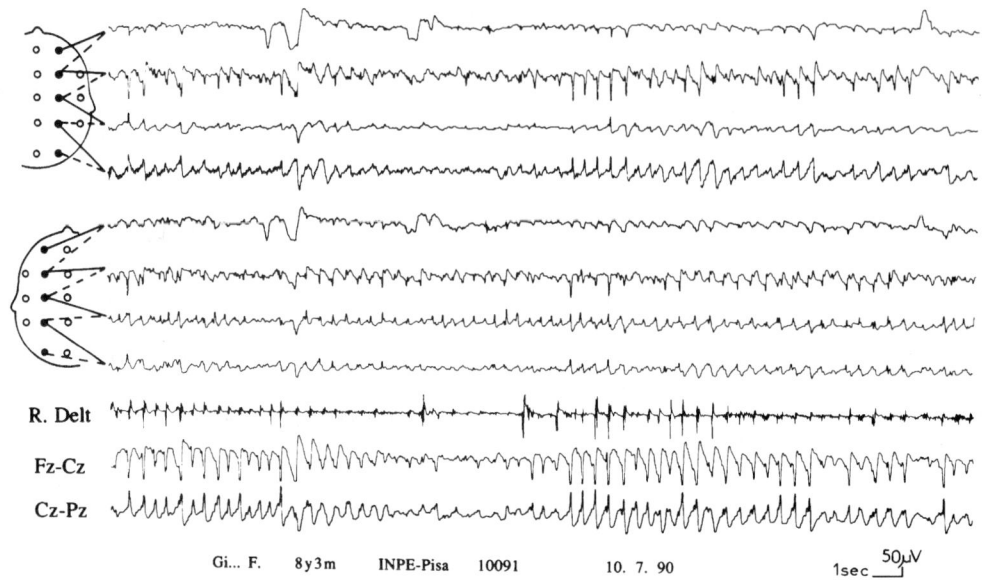

Fig. 4. Polygraphic recording. 8-year-old girl with Angelman syndrome. The patient has long lasting myoclonic status, characterized by reduced responsiveness and jerky movements. The EMG channel (R. Delt = right deltoid) shows continuous rhythmic jerks. Each jerk is accompanied on the EEG by a spike which is bilateral and synchronous, with phase reversal over the C3, C4 and CZ electrodes.

other patients, myoclonus may remain erratic, showing no apparent relation with the observed EEG abnormalities (Viani et al., 1995). Myoclonus typically ceases during sleep (Guerrini et al., 1996; Viani et al., 1995). Occurrence of myoclonic status is rare after the age of six. In addition to myoclonic seizures, or manifest myoclonic status, almost all AS patients exhibit a quasicontinuous focal or multifocal rhythmic myoclonus at about 11 Hz, mainly involving the hands and face, producing a mild jerking or twitching, easily mistaken for tremor (Fig. 5) (Guerrini et al., 1996). A cortical origin of this fast-bursting myoclonus has been demonstrated using burst-locked EEG averaging (Fig. 6) (Guerrini et al., 1996). The clinical and electrographic pattern of this form of myoclonus suggests that small distinct areas within an hyperexcitable motor cortex are spontaneously able to originate rhythmic hypersynchronous neuronal activity, leading to myoclonic muscle activity. It has been documented that in the *pcp* mouse, a deletion eliminating a cluster of $GABA_A$ receptor genes in a region syntenic to the one deleted in AS produces a 60–80 per cent reduction in benzodiazepine binding in most brain regions. It is possible that the rhythmic 8–12 Hz neuronal bursting responsible for the rhythmic myoclonus of AS may be originated by excitatory networks of neurons of cortical layer V in the presence of reduced $GABA_A$-receptor mediated inhibition (Flint & Connors, 1996).

In a recent study addressing electroclinical-phenotypic differences in 20 patients representing all genetic classes of AS (Minassian et al., 1998), was observed that while anteriorly predominant slow spike and wave complexes or notched slow waves were present irrespective of the genetic mechanism involved, patients with large deletions had much more severe epilepsies, in which generalized seizure types were largely predominant. On the other hand, the epilepsy phenotype was relatively milder in patients with loss-of-function mutations or methylation imprint abnormalities. It was concluded that involvement of the GABRB3 may detemine the more severe epilepsy phenotype.

Neuroimaging does not disclose conspicuous CNS anomalies (Guerrini et al., 1996; Zori et al., 1992).

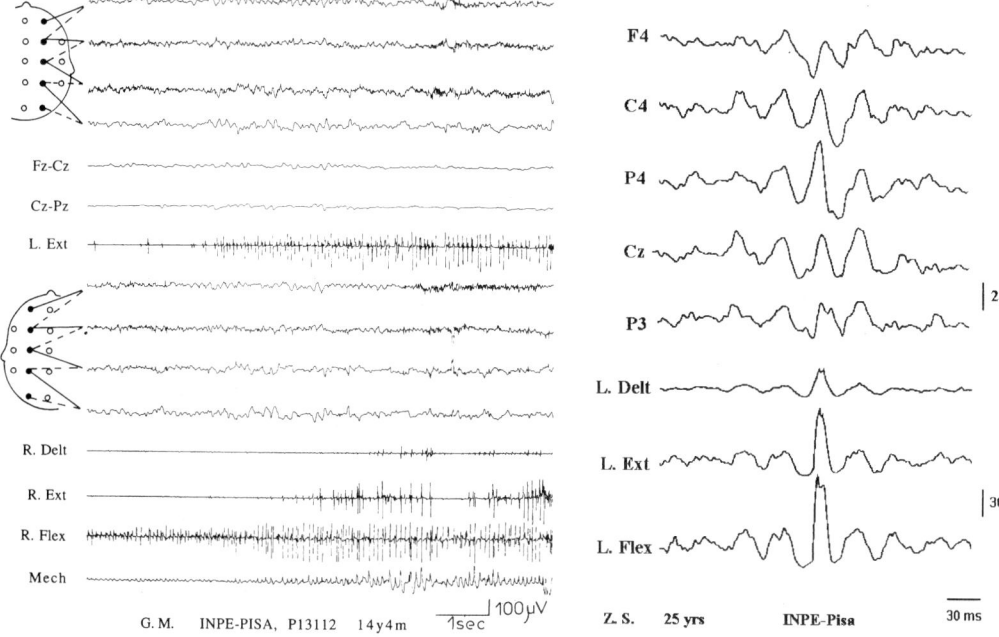

Fig. 5. Polygraphic recording. 14 year old boy with Angelman syndrome. The patient presents a continuous tremulous jerking of both hands, with fluctuating amplitude. The EMG shows rhythmic fast myoclonic potentials at about 10 Hz, over the wrist extensor and flexor muscles (L. Ext = left extensor; R. Ext = right extensor; R. Flex = right flexors) which translate in a tremulous movement of both hands, as documented in the mechanogram (Mech). The EEG shows rhythmic 5 – 7 Hz activity, well recognizable over the frontocentral regions. EEG and EMG are apparently not time locked.

Fig. 6. Same patient as in Fig. 5. Jerk locked back averaging shows that each myoclonic jerk is preceded by a premyoclonic EEG potential, with maximum amplitude over the contralateral centro-parietal areas. Average = 100.

Available neuropathological data derive from the study of the brains in two AS patients in whom the syndrome had not been confirmed by genetic analysis. Jay et al. (1991) found cerebellar atrophy with loss of Purkinje and granule cells and extensive Bergman's gliosis. Neurochemical study of the cerebellar cortex demonstrated markedly reduced GABA content, possibly suggesting failure to develop or a loss of Purkinje cells and inhibitory GABAergic interneurons. Kyriakides et al. (1992), reported small temporal and frontal lobes with disorganized and irregular gyri, irregular distribution of neurons in layer 3, and minor cell heterotopia in both the cerebrum and cerebellum. As indicated above, there is some evidence that in AS the motor cortex is hyperexcitable. Since the deletion involving the maternal 15q11–13 chromosome eliminates a cluster of $GABA_A$ receptor genes (b3, a5, g3), it has been suggested that cortical hyperexcitability could result from reduced GABAergic inhibition (Guerrini et al., 1996). The antiabsence and antimyoclonic action of BDZs, which is based on their GABAergic properties, seems to be confirmed in AS.

While seizures are generally difficult to treat in infancy and early childhood, the severity of epilepsy shows marked attenuation from later childhood on (Zori et al., 1992). The percentage of patients continuing to suffer seizures as adults is so far unknown.

Episodes of status myoclonicus or nonconvulsive status epilepticus are usually controlled with intravenous injection of BDZs (Guerrini et al., 1996; Viani et al., 1995), although showing a frequent tendency to relapse or occasionally become intractable (Matsumoto et al., 1992). Chronic treatment with BDZs also achieves fairly effective control of myoclonus; particularly effective is the association BDZ-VPA for long-term treatment of epilepsy (Guerrini et al., 1996; Viani et al., 1995). VPA and ESM in association are also effective in patients presenting recurrent status myoclonicus (Dalla Bernardina et al., 1992). Worsening of myoclonus and absence seizures may be produced by CBZ treatment (Viani et al., 1995). Cortical myoclonus in AS patients may be improved by generous doses of piracetam (up to 400 mg/kg/day), in addition to conventional antimyoclonic drugs.

Tuberous sclerosis

Tuberous sclerosis or tuberous sclerosis complex (TSC) is a multisystemic disorder involving primarily the central nervous system, the skin, and the kidney (Gomez, 1979). A prevalence of 1:30,000–50,000 has been reported. The classical clinical triad of mental retardation, epilepsy and 'adenosum sebaceum' (facial angiofibromas) is present in only one-third of the cases. Cutaneous findings include hypopigmented macules and facial angiofibromas occurring in up to 90 per cent of cases, shagreen patches in 20–40 per cent, and ungueal fibromas in up to 50 per cent. Half of the patients show dental enamel pits. Renal involvement includes mainly angiomyolipomas (that are present in up to two-thirds of adults with TSC) and renal cysts (present in 10 per cent of cases). Radiological abnormality of the bones (sclerotic patches, pseudocysts, periosteal new bone formation) are present in 60 per cent. About one half of the children with TSC show single or multiple rhabdomyomas detectable on cardiac ultrasound. These lesions are rarely symptomatic and tend to regress with time in number and size. A consensus for the diagnostic criteria of TSC has been reached by the US National Tuberous Sclerosis Association (Roach et al., 1992).

In the brain, the characteristic features are cortical tubers, subependymal nodules and giant cell tumours. The *cortical tubers* are the lesions that are more directly related to epileptogenesis. They are identified by their nodular appearance, firm texture, and variability in site, number and size. Microscopically, the tubers consist of subpial glial proliferation with orientation of the glial processes perpendicular to the pial surface, and an irregular neuronal lamination with giant multinucleated cells that are not clearly neuronal or astrocytic. The pathological changes observed in cortical tubers are remarkably similar to those seen in focal cortical dysplasia (Taylor et al., 1972; Robain, 1996), and consist of a highly epileptogenic lesion, without familial distribution. The junction between grey and white matter is indistinct and maybe partly demyelinated. The cerebral cortex intervening between tubers has normal architecture, both by examination with routine cell stains and with the Golgi method (Huttenlocher & Wollman, 1980).

TSC is transmitted as an autosomal dominant trait, with variable expression seen among families and reported among patients within the same family. Recurrence in sibship of non-affected parents has rarely been reported and is thought to be related to low expressivity or gonadal mosaicism. There is no clear evidence of nonpenetrance for TSC. Therefore careful clinical and diagnostic evaluation of apparently 'unaffected' parents is indicated before counseling the families. Between 50 to 75 per cent of all cases are sporadic.

Linkage studies on TSC families have allowed the identification of two loci for TSC, mapping to chromosome 9q34 (TSC1) and 16p13.3 (TSC2) (Povey et al., 1994). About 40 per cent of the families are linked to TSC1, the remaining being linked to TSC2. No obvious phenotypic differences have been found in the families linked to the TSC1 or TSC2 region. The existence of two additional loci as suggested by previous studies has not been subsequently confirmed.

A classical positional cloning approach has led to the isolation of the TSC1 gene (van Slegtenhorst et al., 1997). This gene consists of 23 exons and encodes for a predicted protein of 1,164 amino acids, named 'hamartin'. A mutation in the TSC1 gene has so far been identified in about 40 per cent of the families linked to chromosome 9q34. The predicted amino acid sequence does not show an overt homology to other known proteins.

The identification of the gene mapping to 16p13.3 has been facilitated by the identification of interstitial deletions in five unrelated TSC patients. A gene (TSC2) was found to be disrupted by all the deletions and was demonstrated to harbour intragenic mutations in other non-deleted TSC patients (European Chromosome 16 Tuberous Sclerosis Consortium, 1993). This gene comprises 40 exons and encodes for a predicted protein of 1,784 amino acids (tuberin). Subcellular fractionation studies have shown that tuberin is associated with a membrane/particulate fraction, indicating that tuberin is prevalently associated with cellular or intracellular membranes. The mouse protein shows a region of homology with the catalytic domain of the GTPase activating protein Rap1GAP, which is involved in cell proliferation and differentiation (Wienecke *et al.*, 1995).

Somatic deletions of 9q24 and 16p13.3 have been found in hamartomas from TS patients, involving either TSC gene. This observation fits the 'two-hit' hypothesis proposed by Knudson for retinoblastoma and indicates that both TSC genes act as tumour suppressor (Carbonara *et al.*, 1994; Sepp *et al.*, 1996).

Epileptic seizures are frequent in TS. They usually begin before the age of 15, mostly in the first 2 years of life: 63.4 per cent before 1 year (Gomez, 1979), 70 per cent before 2 years (Abo *et al.*, 1983). Infantile spasms are the commonest seizure type in the first year of life, sometimes preceded by partial seizures (Dulac *et al.*, 1984). However other types of epilepsy are not infrequent in infants and young children. In their study of 126 patients, Roger *et al.* (1984) found 63 (50 per cent) with West syndrome and 63 (50 per cent) with other types (35 partial epilepsies, 11 Lennox-Gastaut syndromes, four symptomatic generalized epilepsies, six occasional seizures and seven unclassifiable cases). Forty two of the latter 63 patients had their first seizure before 2 years (22 (28 per cent) partial epilepsies, 22 (28 per cent) other types) and the prognosis was strongly related to this early onset. In the group of partial epilepsies, initial seizures were mainly simple partial motor and unilateral seizures, often associated with generalized seizures (tonic, atonic). The course of epilepsy was severe in about one third of patients (three deaths). Almost all patients were mentally impaired.

MRI studies have established a rather good correspondence between tubers and epilepsy. In the study by Curatolo & Cusmai (1988) the largest tuber was found in the cortical area corresponding to the main EEG focus, in patients with partial epilepsy as well as in those with infantile spasms. Parasagittal frontal lesions were linked to more severe epilepsy with diffuse EEG discharges. However, MRI may fail to show all the tubers in infants because the myelination is not complete (Curatolo, 1996), and the EEG may likewise fail to show frontal paroxysmal discharges at this age.

Diffuse SW discharges are frequent in partial epilepsies in childhood TS and are related to secondary bilateral synchrony. This phenomenon has therapeutic implications. Anterior callosotomy can markedly reduce drop attacks associated with partial seizures (Garcia-Flores, 1987). Patients with partial epilepsy and TS must be carefully investigated in order to determine whether there is a single epileptogenic area responsible for the seizures despite multifocal EEG abnormalities and multiple lesions on MRI. In these patients, surgical removal of one epileptogenic lesion has allowed good control of seizures (Bebin *et al.*, 1993; Sivelle *et al.*, 1995).

The most striking finding to emerge from the study by Roger *et al.* (1984) was the strong influence of age at the onset of epilepsy on the outcome, regardless of epilepsy type: the earlier the onset, the more severe the epilepsy and the mental deficit. These results have been confirmed by other authors (Gomez, 1988; Webb *et al.*, 1991). A further important finding is the frequency of psychiatric manifestations in children with TS and early seizure onset. Several authors have demonstrated a correlation between the number and size of tubers and the severity of epilepsy and mental disturbances (Roach *et al.*, 1987; Jambaqué *et al.*, 1991). It is crucial for future research to assess whether the epilepsy phenotype of TSC1 patients is different from that of TSC2 patients.

Fragile X syndrome

Fragile X syndrome has an approximate incidence of 1:1500 males (Webb et al., 1986) and is the most common chromosomal abnormality associated with heritable mental retardation. Both males and females may be affected, but in agreement with X-linked inheritance, the phenotype is notably more severe in males. It is estimated that one in 1000 females are carriers (Blomquist et al., 1983). The chromosome analysis shows a 'fragile' site at Xq27.3, when cells are grown in a folic-deprived medium. The condition results from a dynamic mutation in heritable unstable DNA (Richards & Sutherland, 1992), due to variation in the copy number of a trinucleotide repeat p(CGG)n within the FMR–1 gene. This fragile site is termed FRAXA. The number of (CGG) repeats is less than 50 in the general population and greater than 200 in the affected individuals (full mutation). In this case, a methylation event occurs at the promoter region of the FMR–1 gene, so that its expression is impaired. Subjects with a number of repeats between 60 and 200 (premutation) show a normal expression of the FMR–1 gene, but they are at risk to pass on to their offspring an expanded allele. Males who carry a premutation are clinically and cytogenetically normal (normal transmitting males), and about 30 per cent of females who carry a full mutation have mental impairment. Transmission through families is consistent with an X-linked semidominant condition. The main clinical features include moderate mental retardation, hypotonia, poor language, behaviour and social skills, growth retardation, macrocephaly, prominent forehead, long narrow facies, large ears, macro-orchidism, pectus excavatum, a floppy mitral valve, hyperactive or autistic behaviour (Finelli et al., 1985; Wisniewski et al., 1985).

Two additional fragile sites reside in the distal Xq, termed FRAXE and FRAXF. While FRAXF is not clearly associated with a specific phenotype, subjects with FRAXE show mental impairment, usually milder than that observed for patients bearing a mutation at the FRAXA locus.

The prevalence of epileptic seizures varies in the different series but is thought to be roughly 25 per cent (Wisniewski et al., 1991). According to Wisniewski et al. (1991), seizures usually appear before the age of 15 and tend to disappear during the second decade of life. Epilepsy is usually not severe. In most patients seizures are fairly rare or are controllable with simple drug regimens (Guerrini et al., 1992; Guerrini et al., 1993b; Musumeci et al., 1991; Wisniewski et al., 1991). One individual with West syndrome followed by Lennox-Gastaut syndrome has been reported (Musumeci et al., 1988). The most frequently mentioned seizure types are GTC seizures (Finelli et al., 1985; Wisniewski et al., 1985). In a study attempting a classification of epilepsy, 13 patients, aged 7 to 29 years, experienced the first seizure between ages 2 and 12 years. Two patients had experienced an isolated seizure, while the other 11 had only rare seizures, mainly GTC and complex partial, or unilateral motor in a minority (Guerrini et al., 1993b). Background EEG activity is slow (Musumeci et al., 1991; Wisniewski et al., 1991). An EEG pattern of mid-temporal spikes, possibly age-related, similar to the waveform of benign rolandic epilepsy, has been described in affected males, with or without seizures (Musumeci et al., 1988). This EEG pattern has been confirmed by other investigators (Guerrini et al., 1993b; Wisniewski et al., 1991). However, although a 44 per cent frequency was estimated in the 18 patients described by Musumeci et al. (1991), occurring mainly in the age range 8–16 years, in another study (Guerrini et al., 1993b) rolandic spikes were observed in only 9 per cent of 33 patients (13 with epilepsy) studied within the same age range with at least one EEG while awake and asleep. Using linkage analysis, the fragile-X locus has been excluded as the candidate gene for benign rolandic epilepsy (Rees et al., 1993).

The variety in seizure types in the fragile-X syndrome may reflect the extreme clinical polymorphism associated with this syndrome (Menini et al., 1996). Its clinical polymorphism is related to the variability of amplification of the trinucleotide repeat among patients (Fu et al., 1991). A somatic variation in DNA amplification during development is also possible (Wöhrle et al., 1992). Very little is known of the pathology. Rudelli et al. (1985) have described anomalous synapses, using Golgi impregnation and electron microscopy. Wisniewski et al. (1991) carried out a neuropathological study on the brain of a 6-year-old patient, detecting mild brain atrophy, abnormal development of dendritic spines at Golgi impregnation and marked reduction in the length of synapses, as determined by EPTA-postfixed tissue. Several neuroimaging studies have shown hypoplasia of the cerebellar vermis in adult patients (Reiss *et al.*, 1991). This means that the FMR–1 gene has an early effect on embryonic brain development. Such a role has been confirmed by Menini *et al.* (1996) through *in situ* hybridization study in fetal tissue sections. The latter authors also hypothesized an interference with neuronal proliferation and migration processes as a cause of the microdysgenetic changes.

Neurofibromatosis type 1

Neurofibromatosis type 1 (NF1) is an autosomal dominant disorder characterized by café-au-lait spots, peripheral neurofibromas and hamartomas of the iris (Lisch nodules) (Riccardi, 1982; Riccardi & Eichner, 1986). The prevalence of the disease is estimated to be 1:3000.

Café-au-lait spots may be present at birth and increase in number and size with age. After puberty, virtually all of the patients have at least six such spots with a diameter greater than 15 mm. Cutaneous neurofibromas tend to appear in the second decade and are present in more that 90 per cent of patients above the age of forty. Lisch nodules are uncommon before the age of three, but are present in nearly all of the adult patients and can easily be recognized by slit lamp examination. Macrocephaly and short stature are common. Plexiform neurofibromas occur in about 25 per cent of affected persons, scoliosis in 17 per cent, epilepsy in 10 per cent, and optic gliomas in 13 per cent. About 25 per cent of patients require educational assistance because of learning disabilities. Risk of malignant degeneration of neurofibromas is calculated to lie between 2 per cent and 4 per cent for patients older than twenty. Infrequent manifestations include aqueductal stenosis, interstitial pulmonary fibrosis, vascular changes such as renal artery stenosis leading to renovascular hypertension, tibial pseudoarthrosis, pheochromocytoma, duodenal carcinoid and congenital glaucoma. Clinical criteria for diagnosis have been established (NIH Consensus Development Conference, 1988).

NF1 is transmitted as an autosomal dominant disease, with variable expressivity and full penetrance by the age of five. Careful clinical and ophthalmological evaluation should be performed on the parents of an affected child before counselling the family. About half of the cases are due to a new mutation (Littler & Morton, 1990).

The NF1 gene maps to chromosome 17q11 and contains a putative translated sequence of 2,818 amino acids. The gene spans about 350 kb and consists of at least 59 exons. It is widely expressed in a variety of human tissues (Viskochil *et al.*, 1990; Wallace *et al.*, 1990; Xu *et al.*, 1990; Marchuk *et al.*, 1991). About 100 different mutations have been so far reported in the NF1 gene, including splice mutations, insertions, deletions, and point changes (Upadhyaya *et al.*, 1995; Abernathy *et al.*, 1997). Over 80 per cent of these mutations are predicted to result in a truncated protein (Heim *et al.*, 1994). A few cases due to a large deletion encompassing the entire NF1 gene have been reported. The phenotype in these cases appears to be more severe (Wu *et al.*, 1989). Prenatal diagnosis is feasible only in familial cases, when either a direct detection of the mutation or a linkage analysis can be performed.

The protein encoded by the NF1 gene, neurofibromin, contains a domain homologous to the catalytic domain of the GTPase-activating protein (GAP) family. All of these proteins downregulate RAS activity, and this finding, together with the evidence of loss of heterozygosity at the NF1 locus in neurofibrosarcoma, supports the hypothesis of NF1 as a tumour suppressor gene (De Clue, 1992; Li *et al.*, 1992; Legius *et al.*, 1993). Expression studies of the NF1 gene in neurofibrosarcoma and cutaneous neurofibroma suggest that mRNA editing could play a role in NF1 tumorigenesis and may account for the phenotypic intrafamiliar variability of the disease (Cappione *et al.*, 1997).

Estimates of the frequency of epilepsy in NF1 have varied, depending on patient recruitment procedures. Riccardi (1974) reported a frequency of 3 per cent in 139 cases. Other estimates have given higher values, although never exceeding 20 per cent (Bird, 1987; Pou Serradell, 1984) despite the finding of migration abnormalities. To date, little research has addressed the characterization of epilepsy. All seizure types have been reported, with the exception of typical absences (Pou Serradell,

1984). No seizure type appears to predominate over others, nor has a developmental profile been observed apart from a slightly higher frequency of infantile spasms, which appear to have a benign prognosis (Motte, 1993).

Other genetic disorders associated with epilepsy

The progressive myoclonus epilepsies have been the object of intensive genetic investigations in the last years. Although virtually all of them are accompanied by generalized seizures and multifocal and generalized myoclonus, some forms may be accompanied by partial seizures. In particular, both spontaneous and IPS induced occipital lobe seizures have been reported in Lafora disease (Tinuper et al., 1983) and in Gaucher disease type III (Guerrini et al., 1989). The gene for Lafora disease, an autosomal recessive disorder, has been mapped to chromosome 6q (Serratosa et al., 1995).

Familial cavernous angiomatosis is an autosomal dominant disorder characterized by multiple cavernous angioma affecting the central nervous system and the retina (Dobyns et al., 1987;. Rigamonti et al., 1988). The cavernomas, located in most cases in the cerebral hemispheres, may remain clinically silent or give rise to various neurological manifestations. Seizures represent the most frequent manifestation, occurring in 69 per cent of affected patients and 64 per cent of symptomatic first degree relatives (Rigamonti et al., 1988). In most individuals with epilepsy, seizures were the presenting symptom. The cavernomas are formed by communicating cavities, and may contain circulating blood or be completely thrombosed. Cavernoma walls show no arterial or venous differentiation. Calcifications are frequently observed, and the surrounding tissue is often gliotic and rich in hemosiderin. A locus for familial cavernous angiomatosis maps to chromosome 7q (Marchuk et al., 1995).

Summary and conclusions

Some genetically determined disorders are associated with a risk of developing seizures equal to or only slightly exceeding that of the general population, others with a risk close to 100 per cent. Susceptibility to development of seizures is not necessarily correlated with severity of structural impairment of the central nervous system or with the extent of chromosomal derangement or the type of mutation. It may on the other hand be strongly influenced by imbalance in neurotransmitter activity, or abnormal cortical connectivity if specific genes are involved. This is clearly demonstrated by the finding that with certain disorders, some epilepsy types or syndromes occur more frequently, or at times are so closely associated that they become part of the phenotype. Some genetically determined disorders are accompanied by intractable partial or generalized seizures, while others may be complicated by epilepsies with a favourable prognosis. Awareness of these associations may help to detect specific genes affecting seizure susceptibility

References

Abernathy, C.R., Rasmussen, S.A., Stalker, H.J., Zori, R., Driscoll, D.J., Williams, C.A., Kousseff, B.G. & Wallace, M.R. (1997): NF1 mutation analysis using a combined heteroduplex/SSCP approach. *Hum. Mutat.* **9**, 548–554.

Abo, K., Morikawa, T., Fujiwara, T. & Ishida, S. (1983): Tuberous sclerosis and epilepsy. *Advances in epileptology, XIVth Epilepsy International Symposium*, pp. 105–111. New York: Raven Press.

Aicardi J., Chevrie J.J. & Rousselie F. (1969): Le syndrome agénésie calleuse, spasmes en flexion, lacunes choriorétiniennes. *Arch. Franc. Pédiatr.* **26**, 1103–1120.

Aicardi, J. (1996): Aicardi syndrome. In: *Dysplasias of cerebral cortex and epilepsy*, Guerrini, R., Andermann, F., Canapicchi, R., Roger, J., Zifkin, B.G. & Pfanner, P. (eds), pp. 211–216. Philadelphia, New York: Lippincott-Raven.

Aicardi, J., Lefebvre, J. & Lerique-Koechlin, A. (1965): A new syndrome: spasms in flexion, callosal agenesis, ocular abnormalities. *Electroencephalogr. Clin. Neurophysiol.* **19**, 609–610.

Angelman, H. (1965): 'Puppet' children: a report on three cases. *Dev. Med. Child. Neurol.* **7**, 681–683.

Barkovich, A.J., Guerrini, R., Battaglia, G., Kalifa, G., N'Guyen, T.N., Parmeggiani, A., Santucci, M., Giovanardi-Rossi, P., Granata, T., D' Incerti, L. (1994). Band heterotopia: correlation of outcome with MR imaging parameters. *Ann. Neurol.* **36**, 609–617.

Barkovich, A.J. (1996): Subcortical heterotopia: a distinct clinicoradiologic entity. *AJNR* **17**, 1315–1322.

Bebin, E.M., Kelly, P.J. & Gomez, M. (1993): Surgical treatment in cerebral tuberous sclerosis. *Epilepsia* **34**, 651–657.

Billette de Villemeur, T., Chiron, C. & Robain, O. (1992): Unlayered polymicrogyria and agenesis of the corpus callosum: a relevant association? *Acta Neuropathol.* **83**, 265–270.

Bird, T.D. (1987): Genetic considerations in childhood epilepsies. *Epilepsia* **29**, (Suppl.), 71–81.

Blomquist, H.K., Gustavson, K.H., Holmgren, G., Nordenson, I. & Palsson-Strae, U. (1983): Fragile X syndrome in mildly retarded children in a northern Swedish country. *Clin. Genet.* **24**, 393–398.

Bottani, A., Robinson, W.P, DeLozier-Blanchet, C.D, Engel, E., Morris, M.A., Schmitt, B., Thun-Hohestein, L. & Schinzel, A. (1994): Angelman syndrome due to paternal uniparental disomy of chromosome 15: a milder phenotype? *Am. J. Med. Genet.* **51**, 35–40.

Bower, B.D. & Jeavons, P.M. (1967): The 'happy puppet' syndrome. *Arch. Dis. Child.* **42**, 298–302.

Cappione, A.J., French, B.L. & Skuse, G.R. (1997): A potential role for NF1 mRNA editing in the pathogenesis of NF1 tumors. *Am. J. Hum. Genet.* **60**, 305–312.

Carbonara, C., Longa, L., Grosso, E., Borrone, C., Garre, M.G., Brisigotti, M. & Migone, N. (1994): 9q34 loss of heterozygosity in a tuberous sclerosis astrocytoma suggests a growth suppressor-like activity also for the TSC1 gene. *Hum. Mol. Genet.* **3**, 1829–1832.

Caviness, V.S., Jr. (1989): Normal development of the cerebral neocortex. In: *Developmental neurobiology*, Evrard, P. & Minkowski, A. (eds), pp. 1–10. New York: Raven Press.

Chevrie, J.J. & Aicardi, J. (1986): The Aicardi syndrome. In: *Recent advances in epilpesy*. Vol 3, Pedley, T.A. & Meldrum, B.S. (eds), pp. 189–210. Edinburgh: Churchill Livingston.

Chong, S.S., Pack, S.D., Roschke, A.V., Tanigami, A., Carrozzo, R., Smith, A.C.M., Dobyns, W.B. & Ledbetter, D.H. (1997): A revision of the lissencephaly and Miller-Dieker syndrome critical regions in chromosome 17p13.3. *Hum. Mol. Genet.* **6**, 147–155.

Clayton-Smith, J. (1993): Clinical research on Angelman Syndrome in the United Kingdom: observations on 82 affected individuals. *Am. J. Genet.* **46**, 12–15.

Crome, L. (1956): Pachygyria. *J. Pathol. Bacteriol.* **71**, 335–352.

Curatolo, P. (1996): Tuberous sclerosis: relationships between clinical and EEG findings and magnetic resonance imaging. In: *Dysplasias of cerebral cortex and epilepsy*, Guerrini, R., Andermann, F., Canapicchi, R., Roger, J., Zifkin, B. & Pfanner, P. (eds), pp. 191–198. Philadelphia: Lippincott-Raven.

Curatolo, P. & Cusmai, R. (1988): MRI in Bourneville disease: relationship with EEG findings. *Neurophysiol Clin* **18**, 149–157.

Cusmai, R., Curatolo, P., Mangano, S., Cheminal, R. & Echenne, B. (1990): Hemimegalencephaly and neurofibromatosis. *Neuropediatrics* **21**, 179–182.

Dalla Bernardina, B., Zullini, E., Fontana, E., Colamaria, V., Cappellaro, O. & Avesani, E. (1992): Sindrome di Angelman: studio EEG-poligrafico di 8 casi. *Boll.Lega It.Epil.* **79/80**, 257–259.

de Rijk-van Andel, J.F, Arts, W.F.M., Hofman, A., Staal, A. & Niermeijer, M.F. (1991): Epidemiology of lissencephaly type I. *Neuroepidemiology* **10**, 200–204.

DeClue, J.E., Papageorge, A.G., Fletcher, J.A., Diehl, S.R., Ratner, N., Vass, W.C. & Lowy, D.R. (1992): Abnormal regulation of mammalian p21(ras) contributes to malignant tumor growth in von Recklinghausen (type 1) neurofibromatosis. *Cell* **69**, 265–273.

Delach, J.A, Rosengren, S.S, Kaplan, L., Greenstein, R.M., Cassidy, S.B. & Benn, P.A. (1994): Comparison of high resolution chromosome banding and fluorescent *in situ* hybridization (FISH) for the laboratory evaluation of Prader-Willi syndrome and Angelman syndrome. *Am. J. Med. Genet.* **52**, 85–91.

Des Portes, V., Pinard, J.-M., Billuart, P., Vinet, M.-C., Koulakoff, A., Carrié, A., Gelot, A., Dupuis, E., Motte, J., Berwald-Netter, Y., Catala, M., Kahn, A., Beldjord, C. & Chelly, A. (1998): A novel CNS gene required for neuronal migration and involved in X-linked subcortical laminar heterotopia and lissencephaly syndrome. *Cell* **92**, 51–61.

Di Mario, F.J., Cobb, R.J., Ramsby, G.R. & Leicher, C. (1993): Familiar band heterotopias simulating tuberous sclerosis. *Neurology* **43**, 1424–1426.

Dittrich, B., Buiting, K., Korn, B., Rickard, S., Buxton, J., Saitoh, S., Nicholls, R.D., Poustka, A., Winterpacht, A., Zabel, B. & Horsthemke, B. (1996): Imprint switching on human chromosome 15 may involve alternative transcripts of the SNRPN gene. *Nat. Genet.* **14,** 163–170.

Dobyns, W.B., Andermann, E., Andermann, F., Czapansky-Beilman, D., Dubeau, F., Dulac, O., Guerrini, R., Hirsch, B., Ledbetter, D.H., Lee, N.S, Motte, J., Pinard, J.M., Radtke, R.A., Ross, M.E., Tampieri, D., Walsh, C.A. & Truwit, C.L. (1996): X-linked malformations of neuronal migration. *Neurology* **47,** 331–339.

Dobyns, W.B. & Truwit, C.L. (1995): Lissencephaly and other malformations of cortical development: 1995 update. *Neuropediatrics* **26,** 132–147.

Dobyns, W.B., Curry, C.J.R., Hoyme, H.E., Turlington, L. & Ledbetter, D.H. (1991): Clinical and molecular diagnosis of Miller-Dieker syndrome. *Am. J. Hum. Genet.* **48,** 584–594.

Dobyns, W.B., Guerrini, R., Czapansky-Beilman, D.K., Pierpoint, M.E.M., Breningstall, G, Yock, D.H., Bonanni, P. & Truwit, C.L. (1997): Bilateral periventricular nodular heterotopia (BPNH) with mental retardation and syndactyly in boys: a new X-linked mental retardation syndrome. *Neurology* **49,** 1042–1047.

Dobyns, W.B., Reiner, O., Carrozzo, R. & Ledbetter, D.H. (1993): Lissencephaly: a human brain malformation associated with deletion of the LIS1 gene located at chromosome 17p13. *JAMA* **270,** 2838–2842.

Dobyns, W.B. & Truwit, C.L. (1995): Lissencephaly and other malformations of cortical development: 1995 update. *Neuropediatrics* **26,** 132–147.

Dobyns, W.B., Curry, C.J.R., Hoyme, H.E., Turlington, L. & Ledbetter, D.H. (1991): Clinical and molecular diagnosis of Miller-Dieker syndrome. *Am. J. Hum. Genet.* **48,** 584–594.

Dobyns, W.B., Elias, E.R., Newlin, A.C., Pagon, R.A. & Ledbetter, D.H. (1992): Causal heterogeneity in isolated lissencephaly. *Neurology* **42,** 1375–1388.

Dobyns, W.B., Michels, V.V., Groover, R.V., Mokri, B., Trautmann, J.C., Forbes, G.S. & Laws, E.R., Jr. (1987): Familial cavernous malformations of the central nervous system and retina. *Ann. Neurol.* **21,** 578–583.

Dubeau, F., Tampieri, D., Andermann, E., Lee, N., Radtke, R., Carpenter, S., Leblanc, R., Villemure, J.C., Olivier, A. & Andermann, F. (1996): Periventricular and subcortical nodular heterotopia: comparison of clinical findings and results of surgical treatment. In: *Dysplasias of Cerebral Cortex and Epilepsy,* Guerrini, R., Andermann, F., Canapicchi, R., Roger, J., Zifkin, B.G. & Pfanner, P. (eds), pp. 395–406. Philadelphia, New York: Lippincott-Raven.

Dubeau, F., Tampieri, D., Lee, N., Andermann, E., Carpenter, S., Leblanc, R., Olivier, A., Radtke, R., Villemure, J.C. & Andermann, F. (1995): Periventricular and subcortical nodular heterotopia. A study of 33 patients. *Brain* **118,** 1273–1287.

Dulac, O., Lemaitre, A. & Plouin, P. (1984): Maladie de Bourneville : aspects cliniques et électroencéphalographiques de l'épilepsie dans la première année. *Boll. Lega It. Epil.* **45/46,** 39–42.

Dulac, O., Plouin, P., Perulli, L., Diebler, C., Arthuis, M. & Jalin, C. (1983): Aspects électroencéphalographiques de l'agyrie-pachygyrie classique. *Rev. EEG Neurophysiol. Clin.* **13,** 232–239.

Eksioglu, Y.Z., Scheffer, I.E., Cardenas, P., Knoll, J., Di Mario, F., Ramsby, G., Berg, M., Kamuro, K., Berkovic, S.F., Duyk, G.M., Parisi, J., Huttenlocher, P.R. & Walsh, C.A. (1996): Periventricular heterotopia: an X-linked dominant epilepsy locus causing aberrant cerebral cortical development. *Neuron* **16,** 77–78.

European Chromosome 16 Tuberous Sclerosis Consortium (1993): Identification and characterization of the tuberous sclerosis gene on chromosome 16. *Cell* **75,** 1305–1315.

Ferrer, I., Cusi, M.V., Liarte, A. & Campistol, J. (1986): A Golgi study of the polymicrogyric cortex in Aicardi syndrome. *Brain Dev.* **8,** 518–525.

Finelli, P.F., Pueschel, S.M., Padre-Mendoza, T., O'Brien, M.M. (1985): Neurological findings in patients with fragile-X syndrome. *J. Neurol. Neurosurg. Psychiatry* **48,** 150–153.

Fink, J.M., Dobyns, W.B., Guerrini, R. & Hirsch, B.A. (1997): Identification of a duplication of Xq28 associated with bilateral periventricular nodular heterotopia. *Am. J . Hum. Genet.* **61,** 379–387.

Flint, A.C. & Connors, B.W. (1996): Two types of network oscillations in neocortex mediated by distinct glutamate receptor subtypes and neuronal populations. *J. Neurophysiol.* **75,** 951–956.

Fu, Y.H., Kuhl, D.P.A., Pizzuti, A., Pieretti, M., Sutcliffe, J.S., Richards, S., Verkerk, A.J., Holden, J.J., Fenwick, R.G., Jr., Warren, S.T. *et al.* (1991): Variation of the CGG repeat at the fragile X site results in genetic instability: resolution of the Sherman paradox. *Cell* **67,** 1047–1059.

Garcia-Flores, E. (1987): Corpus callosum section for patients with intractable epilepsy. *Appl. Neurophysiol* **50,** 390–397.

Gillesen-Kaesbach, G., Gross, S., Kaya-Westerloh, S., Passarge, E. & Horsthemke, B. (1995): DNA methylation based testing of 450 patients suspected of having Prader-Willi syndrome. *J. Med. Genet.* **32**, 88–92.

Gillessen-Kaesbach, G., Albrecht, B., Passarge, E. & Horsthemke, B. (1995): Further patients with Angelman syndrome due to paternal disomy of chromosome 15 and a milder phenotype. *Am. J. Med. Genet.* **56**, 328–329.

Gleeson, J.G., Allen, K.M., Fox, J.W., LAmperti, E.D., Berkovic, S., Scheffer, I., Cooper, E.C., Dobyns, W.B., Minnerath, S.R., Ross, M.E. & Walsh, C.A. (1998): Doublecortin, a brain-specific gene mutated in human X-linked lissencephaly and double cortex syndrome, encodes a putative signaling protein. *Cell* **92**, 63–72.

Gomez, M.R. (1979): *Tuberous Sclerosis*. New York: Raven Press.

Gomez, M.R. (1988): *Tuberous Sclerosis* (2nd edn). New York: Raven Press.

Guerrini, R., Dravet, Ch., Bureau, M., Farnarier, G., Gatti, R., Veneselli, E. & Tassinari, C.A. (1989): Epilepsie myoclonique progressive dans la maladie de Gaucher (Type III). Etude neurophysiologique. In: *IVème Congrès de la Société Européenne de Neurologie Pédiatrique; Barcellone*, 167.

Guerrini, R., Battaglia, A., Stagi, P., Bureau, M., Dravet, C., Camara-Silva, A., Santanelli, P., Vigliano, P., Livet, M.O. & Pinsard, N. (1989): Caratteristiche elettrocliniche dell'epilessia nella Sindrome di Down. *Boll. Lega It. Epil.* **66/67**, 317–319.

Guerrini, R., De Lorey, T.M., Bonanni, P., Moncla, A., Dravet, C., Suisse, G., Livet, M.O., Bureau, M., Malzac, P., Genton, P., Thomas, P., Sartucci, F., Simi, P. & Serratosa, J.M. (1996): Cortical myoclonus in Angelman syndrome. *Ann. Neurol.* **40**, 39–48.

Guerrini, R., Battaglia, A., Mattei, M.G., Genton, P., Dravet, C., Montoya-Murcia, M.C., Medina, M., Salvadori, P. & Dellacasa, P. (1992): Epilessia e crisi epilettiche nella sindrome del cromosoma X fragile. *Boll. Lega It. Epil.* **79/80**, 73–74.

Guerrini, R., Bonanni, P., De Lorey, T.M.T., Moncla, A., Dravet, C., Livet, M.O., Bureau, M., Malzac, P. & Serratosa, J.M. (1996): Fast bursting cortical myoclonus of Angelman syndrome. *Mov. Dis.* **11** (Suppl. 1), 101.

Guerrini, R., Dravet, C., Bureau, M., Mancini, J., Canapicchi, R., Livet, M.O. & Belmonte, A. (1996): Diffuse and localized dysplasias of cerebral cortex: clinical presentation, outcome, and proposal for a morphologic MRI classification based on a study of 90 patients. In: *Dysplasias of cerebral cortex and epilepsy*, Guerrini, R., Andermann, F., Canapicchi, R., Roger, J., Zifkin, B.G. & Pfanner, P. (eds), pp. 255–269. Philadelphia, New York: Lippincott-Raven.

Guerrini, R., Robain, O., Dravet, C., Canapicchi R. & Roger, J. (1993a): Clinical, electrographic and pathological findings in the gyral disorders. In: *New Trends in Pediatric Neurology*, Fejerman, N. & Chamoles, N.A. (eds), pp. 101–107. Amsterdam: Elsevier.

Guerrini, R., Dravet, C., Ferrari, A.R., Battaglia, A., Mattei, M.G., Salvadori, P., Genton, P. & Pfanner, P. (1993b): Evoluzione dell'epilessia nelle più frequenti forme genetiche con ritardo mentale (sindrome di Down e sindrome dell'X fragile). *Ped. Med. Chir.* **15**, 19–22.

Hakamada, S., Watanabe, K., Hara, K. & Miyazaki, S. (1979): The evolution of electroencephalographic features in lissencephaly syndrome. *Brain Dev.* **4**, 277–283.

Harding, B. (1996): Gray matter heterotopia. In: *Dysplasias of cerebral cortex and epilepsy*, Guerrini, R., Andermann, F., Canapicchi, R., Roger, J., Zifkin, B.G. & Pfanner, P., pp. 81–88. Philadelphia-New York: Lippincott-Raven.

Heim, R.A., Silverman, L.M., Farber, R.A., Kam-Morgan, L.N.W. & Luce, M.C. (1994): Screening for truncated NF1 proteins. (Letter) *Nat. Genet.* **8**, 218–219.

Heitz, D., Devys, D., Imbert, G., Kretz, C., Mandel, J.L. (1992): Inheritance of the fragile X premutation is a major determinant of the transition to full mutation. *J. Med. Genet.* **29**, 794–801.

Huttenlocher, P.R., Taravath, S. & Mojtahedi, S. (1994): Periventricular heterotopia and epilepsy. *Neurology* **44**, 51–55.

Jambaqué, I., Cusmai, R., Curatolo, P., Cortesi, F., Perrot, C. & Dulac, O. (1991): Neuropsychological aspects of tuberous sclerosis in relation to epilepsy and MRI findings. *Dev. Med. Child Neurol.* **33**, 698–705.

Jay, V., Becker, L.E, Chan, F.-W. & Perry, T.L. (1991): Puppet-like syndrome of Angelman: a pathologic and neurochemical study. *Neurology* **41**, 416–422.

Kamuro, K. & Tenokuchi, Y. (1993): Familial periventricular nodular heterotopia. *Brain Dev.* **15**, 237–241.

Kaplan, L.C., Wharton, R., Elias, E., Mandell, F., Donlon, T. & Latt, S.A. (1987): Clinical heterogeneity associated with deletions in the long arm of chromosome 15: report of three new cases and their possible genetic significance. *Am. J. Med. Genet.* **28**, 45–53.

Ketonen, L., Roddy, S. & Lannan, M. (1994): Band heterotopia. *J. Child Neurol.* **9**, 384–385.

Kishino, T., Lalande, M. & Wagstaff, J. (1997): UBE3A/E6-AP mutations cause Angelman Syndrome. *Nat. Genet.* **15**, 70–73.

Kyriakides, T., Hallam, L.A, Hockey, A., Silberstein, P. & Kakulas, B.A. (1992): Angelman's syndrome: a neuropathological study. *Acta Neuropathol. (Berl)* **83**, 675–678.

Landy, H.J., Curless, R.G., Ramsay, R.E., Slater, J., Ajmone-Marsan, C. & Quencer, R.M. (1993): Corpus callosotomy for seizures associated with band heterotopia. *Epilepsia* **34**, 79–83.

Legius, E., Marchuk, D.A., Collins, F.S. & Glover, T.W. (1993): Somatic deletion of the neurofibromatosis type 1 gene in a neurofibrosarcoma supports a tumour suppressor gene hypothesis. *Nat. Genet.* **3**, 122–125.

Li, Y., Bollag, G., Clark, R., Stevens, J., Conroy, L., Fults, D., Ward, K., Friedman, E., Samowitz, W., Robertson, M., Bradley, P., McCormick, F., White, R. & Cawthon, R. (1992): Somatic mutations in the neurofibromatosis 1 gene in human tumors. *Cell* **69**, 275–281.

Littler, M. & Morton, N.E. (1990): Segregation analysis of peripheral neurofibromatosis (NF1). *J. Med. Genet.* **27**, 307–310.

Livingston, J. & Aicardi, J. (1990): Unusual MRI appearance of diffuse subcortical heterotopia or 'double cortex' in two children. *J. Neurol. Neurosurg. Psychiatry* **53**, 617–620.

LoNigro, C., Chong, S.S, Smith, A.C.M., Dobyns, W.B., Carrozzo, R. & Ledbetter, D.H. (1997): Point mutations and an intragenic deletion in LIS1, the lissencephaly causative gene in isolated lissencephaly sequence and Miller-Dieker syndrome. *Hum. Mol. Genet.* **6**, 157–164.

MacGregor, D.L, Menezes, A. & Buncic, J.R. (1993): Aicardi syndrome (AS): – natural history and predictors of severity. *Can. J. Neurol. Sci.* **20** (Suppl. 2), S36.

Magenis, R.E., Brown, M.G., Lacy, D.A., Budden, S. & LaFranchi, S. (1987): Is Angelman syndrome an alternate result of del (15)(q11-q13)? *Am. J. Med.Genet.* **28**, 829–838.

Malcolm, S., Clayton-Smith, J., Nicholls, M., Robb, S., Webb, T., Armour, J., Jeffreys, A.J. & Pembrey, M.E. (1991): Uniparental paternal disomy in Angelman's syndrome. *Lancet* **337**, 694–697.

Marchuk, D.A., Gallione, C.J., Morrison, L.A., Clericuzio, C.L., Harts, B.L., Kosofsky, B.E., Louis, D.N., Gusella, J.F., Davis, L.E. & Prenger, V.L. (1995): A locus for cerebral cavernous malformations maps to chromosome 7q in two families. *Genomics* **28**, 311–314.

Marchuk, D.A., Saulino, A.M., Tavakkol, R., Swaroop, M., Wallace, M.R., Andersen, L.B., Mitchell, A.L., Gutmann, D.H., Boguski, M. & Collins, F.S. (1991): cDNA cloning of the type 1 neurofibromatosis gene: complete sequence of the NF1 gene product. *Genomics* **11**, 931–940.

Matell, M. (1893): Ein fall von heterotopie der frauen substanz in den beiden hemispheren des grosshirns. *Arch. Psychiatr. Nervenkr.* **25**, 124–136.

Matsumoto, A., Kumagai, T., Miura, K., Miyazaki, S., Hayakawa, C. & Yamanaka, T. (1992): Epilepsy in Angelman syndrome associated with chromosome 15q deletion. *Epilepsia* **33**, 1083–1090.

Matsuura, T., Sutcliffe, J.S., Fang, P., Jan Galjaard, R., Jiang, Y-H., Benton, C.S., Rommens, J.M. & Beaudet, A.L. (1997): De novo truncating mutations in E6-AP ubiquitin-protein ligase gene (UBE3A) in Angelman Syndrome. *Nat. Genet.* **15**, 74–77.

Menini, C., Abitol, M. & Mallet, J. (1996): A possible role for FMR–1 gene expression in neuronal migration and differentiation. In: *Dysplasias of cerebral cortex and epilepsy*, Guerrini, R., Andermann, F., Canapicchi, R., Roger, J., Zifkin, B. & Pfanner, P. (eds), pp. 17–26. Philadelphia-New York: Lippincott-Raven.

Minassian, B., DeLorey, T., Olsen, R.W., Philippart, M., Zhang, Q., Bronstein, Y., Guerrini, R., Van Ness, P., Livet, M.O. & Delgado-Escueta, A.V. (1998): The epilepsy of Angelman syndrome due to deletion, disomy, imprinting center and UB3A mutations. *Ann. Neurol.* **43**, 485–493.

Miura, K., Watanabe, K., Maeda, N., Matsumoto, A., Kumagai, T., Ito, K. & Kato, T. (1993): MR imaging and positron emission tomography of band heterotopia. *Brain Dev.* **15**, 288–290.

Molina, J.A., Mateos, F., Merino, M., Epifanio, J.L. & Gorrono, M. (1989): Aicardi syndrome in two sisters. *J. Pediatr.* **115**, 282–283.

Morrell, F., Whisler, W.W., Hoeppner, T.J., Smith, M.C., Kanner, A.M., Pierre-Louis, S. J-C., Chez, M.G. & Hasegawa, H. (1992): Electrophysiology of heterotopic gray matter in the 'double cortex' syndrome. *Epilepsia* **33** (Suppl. 3), 76.

Motte, J., Billard, C., Fejerman, N., Sfaello, Z., Arroyo, H. & Dulac, O. (1993) Neurofibromatosis type 1 and West syndrome: a relatively benign asociation. *Epilepsia* **34**, 723–726.

Munari, C., Francione, S., Kahane, P., Tassi, L., Hoffmann, D., Garrel, S. & Pasquier, B. (1996): Usefulness of stereo EEG investigations in partial epilepsy associated with cortical dysplastic lesions and gray matter heterotopia. In: *Dysplasias of cerebral cortex and epilepsy*, Guerrini, R., Andermann, F., Canapicchi, R., Roger, J., Zifkin, B.G. & Pfanner, P. (eds), pp. 383–394. Philadelphia-New York: Lippincott-Raven.

Musumeci, S.A., Ferri, R., Elia, M., Cologna, R.M., Bergonzi, P. & Tassinari, C.A. (1991): Epilepsy and fragile X syndrome: a follow-up study. *Am. J. Med. Genet.* **38**, 511–513.

Musumeci, S.A., Colognola, R.M., Ferri, R., Gigli, G.L., Petrella, M.A., Sanfilippo, S., Bergonzi, P. & Tassinari, C.A. (1988): Fragile-X syndrome: A particular epileptogenic EEG pattern. *Epilepsia* **29**, 41–47.

Mutirangura, A., Greenberg, F., Butler, M.G., Malcom, S., Nicholls, R.D, Chakravarti, A. & Ledbetter, D.H. (1993): Multiplex PCR of three dinucleotide repeats in the Prader-Willi/Angelman critical region (15q11-q13): molecular diagnosis and mechanism of uniparental disomy. *Hum. Mol. Genet.* **2**, 143–151.

Nakatsu, Y., Tyndale, R.F, DeLorey, T.M., Deonna, D.P., Gardner, J.M., McDanel, H.J., Nguyen, Q., Wagstaff, J., Lalande, M., Sikela, J.M., Olsen, R.W., Tobin, A.J. & Brilliant, M.H. (1993): A cluster of three GABA$_A$ receptor subunit genes is deleted in a neurological mutant of the mouse p locus. *Nature* **364**, 448–450.

National Institutes of Health Consensus Development Conference (1988): Neurofibromatosis: conference statement. *Arch. Neurol.* **45**, 575–578,

Norman, M.G., McGillivray, B.C., Kalousek, D.K., Hill, A. & Poskitt, K.J. (1995): *Congenital malformations of the brain: pathological, embryological, clinical, radiological and genetic aspects.* New York: Oxford University Press.

Ohtahara, S., Ohtsuka, Y., Yamatogi, Y. & Oka, E. (1987). The early infantile epileptic encephalopathy with suppression burst: developmental aspects. *Brain Dev.* **9**, 371–376.

Palmini, A., Andermann, F., Aicardi, J., Dulac, O., Chaves, F., Ponsot, G., Pinard, J.M., Goutières, F., Livingston, J., Tampieri, D., Andermann, E. & Robitaille, Y. (1991): Diffuse cortical dysplasia, or the double cortex syndrome: the clinical and epileptic spectrum in 10 patients. *Neurology* **41**, 1656–1662.

Pieretti, M., Zhang, F.P., Fu, Y.H., Warren, S.T., Oostra, B.A., Caskey, C.T. & Nelson, D.L. (1991): Absence of expression of the FMR–1 gene in fragile X syndrme. *Cell* **66**, 817–822.

Pinard, J.M., Motte, J., Chiron, C., Brian, R, Andermann, E. & Dulac, O. (1994): Subcortical laminar heterotopia and lissencephaly in two families: a single X linked dominant gene. *J. Neurol. Neurosurg. Psychiatry* **7**, 914–920.

Pou Serradell, A. (1984): Epilepsia y neurofibromatosis. *Boll. Lega It. Epil.* **45/46**, 47–49.

Povey, S., Burley, M.W., Attwood, J., Benham, F., Hunt, D., Jeremiah, S. J., Franklin, D., Gillett, G., Malas, S., Robson, E.B.,Tippett, P., Edwards, J.H., Kwiatkowski, D.J., Super, M., Mueller, R., Fryer, A., Clarke, A., Webb, D. & Osborne, J. (1994): Two loci for tuberous sclerosis: one on 9q34 and one on 16p13. *Ann. Hum. Genet.* **58**, 107–127.

Quan, F., Zonana, J., Gunter, K., Peterson, K.L., Magenis, R.E. & Popovich, B.W. (1995): An atypical case of fragile X syndrome caused by a deletion that includes the FMR1 gene. *Am. J. Hum. Genet.* **56**, 1042–1051.

Quirk, J.A., Kendall, B., Kingsley, D.P.E. & Boyd, S.G. & Pitt, M.C. (1993): EEG features of cortical dysplasia in children. *Neuropediatrics* **24**, 193–199.

Ramer, J.C., Lin, A.E, Dobyns, W.B, Aymè, S., Pallotta, R. & Ladda, R. (1995): Previously apparently undescribed syndrome: shallow orbits, ptosis, coloboma, trigonocephaly, gyral malformations, mental and growth retardation. *Am. J. Med. Genet.* **57**, 403–409.

Rees, M., Diebold, U., Parker, K., Doose, H., Gardiner, R.M. & Whitehouse, W.P. (1993): Benign childhood epilepsy with centro-temporal spikes and the focal sharp wave trait is not linked to the Fragile X region. *Neuropediatrics* **24**, 211–213.

Reiner, O., Carrozzo, R., Shen, Y., Wehnert, M., Faustinella, F., Dobyns, W.B., Caskey, C.T. & Ledbetter, D.H. (1993): Isolation of a Miller-Dieker lissencephaly gene containing G protein β-subunit-like repeats. *Nature* **364**, 717–721.

Reiss, A.L., Aylward, E., Freund, L.S, Joshi, P.K. & Bryan, N. (1991): Neuroanatomy of fragile X syndrome: the posterior fossa. *Ann. Neurol.* **29**, 26–32.

Riccardi, V.M. & Eichner, J.E. (1986): *Neurofibromatosis: Phenotype, natural history and pathogenesis.* Baltimore: Johns Hopkins University Press.

Riccardi, V.M. (1974): Neurofibromatosis (Von Recklinghausen disease). *Advances in Neurology*, vol.29. New York: Raven Press.

Riccardi, V.M. (1981): Von Recklinghausen neurofibromatosis. *N.. Eng. J. Med.* **305**, 1617–1626.

Ricci, S., Cusmai, R., Fariello, G., Fusco, L. & Vigevano, F. (1992): Double cortex. A neuronal migration disorder as a possible cause of Lennox-Gastaut syndrome. *Arch. Neurol.* **49**, 61–64.

Richards, R.I. & Sutherland, G.R. (1992): Dynamic mutations: a new class of mutations causing human disease. *Cell* **70,** 709–712.

Rigamonti, D., Hadley, M.N., Drayer, B.P., Johnson, P.C., Hoenig-Rigamonti, K., Knight, J.T. & Spetzer, R.F. (1988): Cerebral cavernous malformations: Incidence and familial occurrence. *N. Engl. J. Med.* **319,** 343–347.

Roach, E.S., Smith, M., Huttenlocher, P., Bhat, M., Alcorn, D. & Hawley, L. (1992): Diagnostic criteria: tuberous sclerosis complex. Report of the Diagnostic Criteria Committee of the National Tuberous Sclerosis Association. *J. Child Neurol.* **7,** 221–224.

Roach, E.S., William, D.P. & Laster, D.W. (1987): Magnetic resonance imaging in tuberous sclerosis. *Arch. Neurol.* **44,** 301–303.

Roger, J., Dravet, Ch., Boniver, C. *et al.* (1984): L'épilepsie dans la Sclérose Tubéreuse de Bourneville. *Boll Lega It. Epil.* **45/46,** 33–38.

Ross, M.E, Allen, K.M., Srivastava, A.K., Featherstone, T., Gleeson, J.G., Hirsch, B., Harding, B.N., Andermann, E., Abdullah, R., Berg, M., Czapansky-Bielman, D., Flanders, D.J., Guerrini, R., Motte, J., Puche Mira, A., Scheffer, I., Berkovic, S., Scaravilli, F., King, R.A., Ledbetter, D.H., Schlessinger, D., Dobyns, W.B. & Walsh, C.A. (1997): Linkage and physical mapping X-linked lissencephaly/SBH (XLIS): a novel gene causing neuronal migration defects in human brain. *Hum. Mol. Genet.* **6,** 555–562.

Rudelli, R.D., Brown, W.T., Wisniewski, K., Jenkins, E.C., Lauren-Kamionowska, M., Connell, F. & Wisniewski, H.M. (1985): Adult fragile X syndrome: clinico-neuropathologic findings. *Acta Neuropathol. (Berl)* **67,** 289–295.

Sepp, T., Yates, J.R.W. & Green, A.J. (1996): Loss of heterozygosity in tuberous sclerosis hamartomas. *J. Med. Genet.* **33,** 962–964.

Serratosa, J.M., Delgado-Escueta, A.V., Posada, I., Shih, S., Drury, I., Berciano, J., Zabala, J.A., Antunez, M.C. & Sparkes, R.S. (1995): The gene for progressive myoclonus epilepsy of the Lafora type maps to chromosome 6q. *Hum. Mol. Genet.* **4,** 1657–1664.

Sivelle, G., Kahane, P., de Saint-Martin, A., Hirsch, E., Hoffmann, D. & Munari, C. (1995): La multilocalité des lésions dans la sclérose tubéreuse de Bourneville contre-indique-t-elle une approche chirurgicale? *Epilepsies* **7,** 451–464.

Sugimoto, T., Araki, A., Yasuhara, A., Woo, M., Nishida, N. & Sasaki, T. (1994): Angelman syndrome in three siblings: genetic model of epilepsy associated with chromosomal DNA deletion of the $GABA_A$ receptor. *Jpn. J. Psychiatry Neurol.* **42,** 271–273.

Tarleton, J., Richie, R., Schwartz, C., Rao, K., Aylsworth, A.S. & Lachiewicz, A. (1993): An extensive *de novo* deletion removing FMR1 in a patient with mental retardation and the fragile X syndrome phenotype. *Hum. Mol. Genet.* **2,** 1973–1974.

Tinuper, P., Aguglia, P., Pellissier, J.F. & Gastaut, H. (1983): Visual ictal phenomena in a case of Lafora disease proven by skin biopsy. *Epilepsia* **24,** 214–8.

Upadhyaya, M., Maynard, J., Osborn, M., Huson, S.M., Ponder, M., Ponder, B.A.J. & Harper, P.S. (1995): Characterisation of germline mutations in the neurofibromatosis type 1 (NF1) gene. *J. Med. Genet.* **32,** 706–710.

van Slegtenhorst, M., de Hoogt, R., Hermans, C., Nellist, M., Janssen, B., Verhoef, S., Lindhout, D., van den Ouweland, A., Halley, D., Young, J., Burley, M., Jeremiah, S. and 29 others (1997): Identification of the tuberous sclerosis gene TSC1 on chromosome 9q34. *Science* **277,** 805–808.

Verheij, C., Bakker, C.E., de-Graaf, E., Keulemans, J., Willemsen, R., Verkerk, A.J., Galjaard, H., Reuser, A.J., Hoogeven, A.T. & Oostra, B.A. (1993): Characterization and localization of the FMR–1 gene product associated with fragile X syndrome. *Nature* **363,** 722–724.

Viani, F., Romeo, A., Viri, M., Mastrangelo, M., Lalatta F., Selicorni, A., Gobbi, G., Lanzi, G., Bettio, D., Briscioli, V., Di Segni, M., Parini, R. & Terzoli, G. (1995): Seizure and EEG patterns in Angelman's syndrome. *J. Child Neurol.* **10,** 467–471.

Viskochil, D., Buchberg, A.M., Xu, G., Cawthon, R.M., Stevens, J., Wolff, R.K., Culver, M., Carey, J.C., Copeland, N.G., Jenkins, N.A., White, R. & O'Connell, P. (1990): Deletions and a translocation interrupt a cloned gene at the neurofibromatosis type 1 locus. *Cell* **62,** 187–192.

Wallace, M.R., Marchuk, D.A., Andersen, L.B., Letcher, R., Odeh, H.M., Saulino, A.M., Fountain, J.W., Brereton, A., Nicholson, J., Mitchell, A.L., Brownstein, B.H. & Collins, F.S. (1990): Type 1 neurofibromatosis gene: identification of a large transcript disrupted in three NF1 patients. *Science* **249,** 181–186.

Webb, D.W., Fryer, A.E, Osborne, J.P. (1991): On the incidence of fits and mental retardation in tuberous sclerosis. *J. Med. Genet.* **28,** 395–397.

Webb, T.P., Bundey, S.E., Thacke, A.I. & Todd, J. (1986): Population incidence and segregation ratios in the Martin-Bell syndrome. *Am. J. Med. Genet.* **23,** 573–580.

Wienecke, R., Konig, A. & DeClue, J.E. (1995): Identification of tuberin, the tuberous sclerosis-2 product: tuberin possesses specific Rap1GAP activity. *J. Biol. Chem.* **270,** 16409–16414.

Wisniewski, K.E., French, J.H., Fernando, S., Brown, W.T., Jenkins, E.C., Friedman, E., Hill, A.L. & Miezejeski, C.M. (1985): Fragile X syndrome; associated neurological abnormalities and developmental disabilities. *Ann. Neurol.* **18,** 665–669.

Wisniewski, K.E., Segan, S.M., Miezejesji, E.A., Sersen, E.A. & Rudelli, R.D. (1991): The Fra (X) syndrome: neurological, electrophysiological, and neuropathological abnormalities. *Am. J. Med. Genet.* **38,** 476–480.

Wöhrle, D., Kotzot, D., Hirst, M.C., Manca, A., Korn, B., Schmidt, A., Barbi, G., Rott, H.D., Poustka, A., Davies, K.E. et al. (1992): A microdeletion of less than 250 kb, including the proximal part of the FMR–1 gene and the fragile -X site, in a male with the clinical phenotype of fragile-X syndrome. *Am. J. Hum. Genet.* **51,** 299–306.

Wu, B.-L., Austin, M.A., Schneider, G.H., Boles, R.G. & Korf, B.R. (1995): Deletion of the entire NF1 gene detected by FISH: four deletion patients associated with severe manifestations. *Am. J. Med. Genet.* **59,** 528–535.

Xu, G., O'Connell, P., Viskochil, D., Cawthon, R., Robertson, M., Culver, M., Dunn, D., Stevens, J., Gesteland, R., White, R. & Weiss, R. (1990): The neurofibromatosis type 1 gene encodes a protein related to GAP. *Cell* **62,** 599–608.

Zori, R.T, Hendrickson, J., Woolven, S. Whidden, E.M., Gray, B. & Williams, C.A. (1992): Angelman syndrome: clinical profile. *J. Child. Neurol.* **7,** 270–280.

Chapter 16

The genetics of febrile convulsions and temporal lobe epilepsy

Richard S. McLachlan[1] and Dennis E. Bulman[2]

[1]*Professor, Department of Clinical Neurological Sciences, University of Western Ontario, London, Canada;*
[2]*Research Scientist, Ottawa General Hospital Research Institute; Assistant Professor, Division of Neurology, Department of Medicine, University of Ottawa, Ottawa, Canada*

'Of these various factors [which contribute to the pathogenesis of temporal lobe epilepsy] *two stand out, namely a positive family history of epilepsy and febrile convulsions. These two factors are often linked and are not easily separated.'*
Murray Falconer, 1971

Febrile convulsions occur as clonic, tonic–clonic or atonic seizures associated with fever in 2–5 per cent of children age 6 months to 6 years (Schuman & Miller, 1966; VandenBerg & Yerushalmy, 1969; Hauser, 1981; Verity *et al.*, 1985; Berg, 1992). This is usually a benign, self-limited disorder which is not associated with any longterm sequelae. However, a small percentage of children with febrile convulsions do develop epilepsy later in life, most studies reporting an incidence of 2–7 per cent depending on the duration of follow-up (VandenBerg & Yerushalmy, 1969; Nelson & Ellenberg, 1976, 1978; Annegers *et al.*, 1979, 1987; Berg & Shinnar, 1996). This is some 2–10 times higher than the expected rate of 0.7 per cent in the general population (Hauser & Kurland, 1975). Although generalized epilepsy following febrile convulsions is widely accepted, it is still controversial as to whether there is a relationship between febrile convulsions and focal epilepsy, particularly temporal lobe epilepsy. In this chapter, evidence is presented which supports such a relationship followed by a discussion of the influence of hereditary factors on what are commonly considered to be acquired conditions, the syndromes of febrile convulsions and temporal lobe epilepsy.

Are febrile convulsions and temporal lobe epilepsy related?

Many studies have supported an association between febrile convulsions and the subsequent development of temporal lobe epilepsy (Nelson & Ellenberg, 1976; Annegers *et al.*, 1987; Kuks *et al.*, 1993; Maher & McLachlan, 1995) but others have disputed such a relationship (Lee *et al.*, 1981; Sofijanov *et al.*, 1983), particularly the role of febrile convulsions in the pathogenesis of mesial temporal sclerosis, the most common cause of temporal lobe epilepsy. Reports of the surgical treatment of complex partial seizures of temporal lobe origin have described antecedent febrile convulsions in 9–67 per cent of patients (Table 1) and a population-based controlled study of patients with complex partial seizures reported that 20 per cent of 82 patients with temporal lobe epilepsy but only 2 per cent of 150 unaffected controls had febrile convulsions (Rocca et al., 1987). In another population-based study of 504 children with epilepsy, Camfield et al. (1994) found a history of febrile convulsions in 13 per cent of patients with complex partial seizures which was lower than the 22 per cent occurrence in those with generalized epilepsy. Of 100 children with temporal lobe epilepsy followed into adult life by Lindsay et al. (1980), 59 per cent had a history of febrile convulsions.

Table 1. Febrile convulsions in patients with temporal lobe epilepsy or complex partial seizures

	n	Febrile convulsions	Prolonged febrile convulsions
Jensen et al., 1976	74	9%	–
Camfield et al., 1994	326[1]	13%	–
Rocca et al., 1987	82[1]	20%	–
Falconer, 1971	100	20%	–
Blume et al., 1995	125	35%	–
Abou Khalil et al., 1993	47	40%	28%
Kanemoto et al., 1996	111	55%	22%
Lindsay et al., 1980	100	59%	–
French et al., 1993	67	67%	50%[2]

[1]complex partial seizures; [2]complicated febrile convulsions.

Although most studies have looked at the occurrence of febrile convulsions in patients with temporal lobe epilepsy in general, some have attempted to narrow the focus by assessing only those with evidence of mesial temporal sclerosis. Falconer (1971) in his series of 100 pathologically proven cases of mesial temporal sclerosis found a prior history of febrile convulsions in 35 per cent, however, recent studies suggest this was an under estimate. Kanemoto et al. (1996) found antecedent febrile convulsions in 64 per cent of 111 patients with mesial temporal sclerosis demonstrated by MRI and in an even purer culture of temporal lobe epilepsy, French et al. (1993) found febrile convulsions in 67 per cent of 67 operated patients with temporal lobe epilepsy who not only had mesial temporal sclerosis but were also seizure free after surgery.

Temporal lobe epilepsy has been associated specifically with long duration, focal or recurrent febrile convulsions, particularly in association with a neurologic deficit. Ounsted et al. (1966) found that 32 per cent of their 100 patients with childhood temporal lobe epilepsy had prolonged febrile convulsions and the same figure of 32 per cent with prolonged febrile convulsions was cited in the study by Kanemoto et al. (1996). French et al. (1993) indicated that 50 per cent of their patients had what they called 'complicated' febrile seizures. Annegers et al. (1987) suggested that febrile convulsions lasting longer than 30 min were strongly associated with the development of partial seizures, a concept supported by Abou Khalil et al. (1993) who reported a mean duration of febrile convulsions of 4 h in 17 of 18 selected patients with temporal lobe epilepsy.

In a study of six large multiplex families with febrile convulsions and other seizure disorders, we found a rate of temporal lobe epilepsy after febrile convulsions of 13 per cent during a mean follow-up of 32 years, strongly supporting an association between temporal lobe epilepsy and febrile convulsions in the families (Maher & McLachlan, 1996). Figure 1 identifies 59 family members affected by febrile convulsions of whom eight progressed to temporal lobe epilepsy. Of 213 family members with no febrile convulsions, one developed temporal lobe epilepsy. Partial seizures from the temporal lobe started an average of 12 years after the first febrile convulsion. Five patients had temporal lobectomies and the pathology was mesial temporal sclerosis in each case. The only factor which distinguished

Chapter 16 The genetics of febrile convulsions and temporal lobe epilepsy

those with febrile convulsions who progressed on to temporal lobe epilepsy from those who did not was duration of febrile seizure. In those with temporal lobe epilepsy, febrile convulsions averaged 100 min in duration compared to 9 min in those who did not develop later epilepsy ($P = 0.02$) and temporal lobe epilepsy did not occur if duration of febrile convulsion was less than 30 min. Our finding that prolonged febrile convulsions are significantly associated with subsequent temporal lobe epilepsy

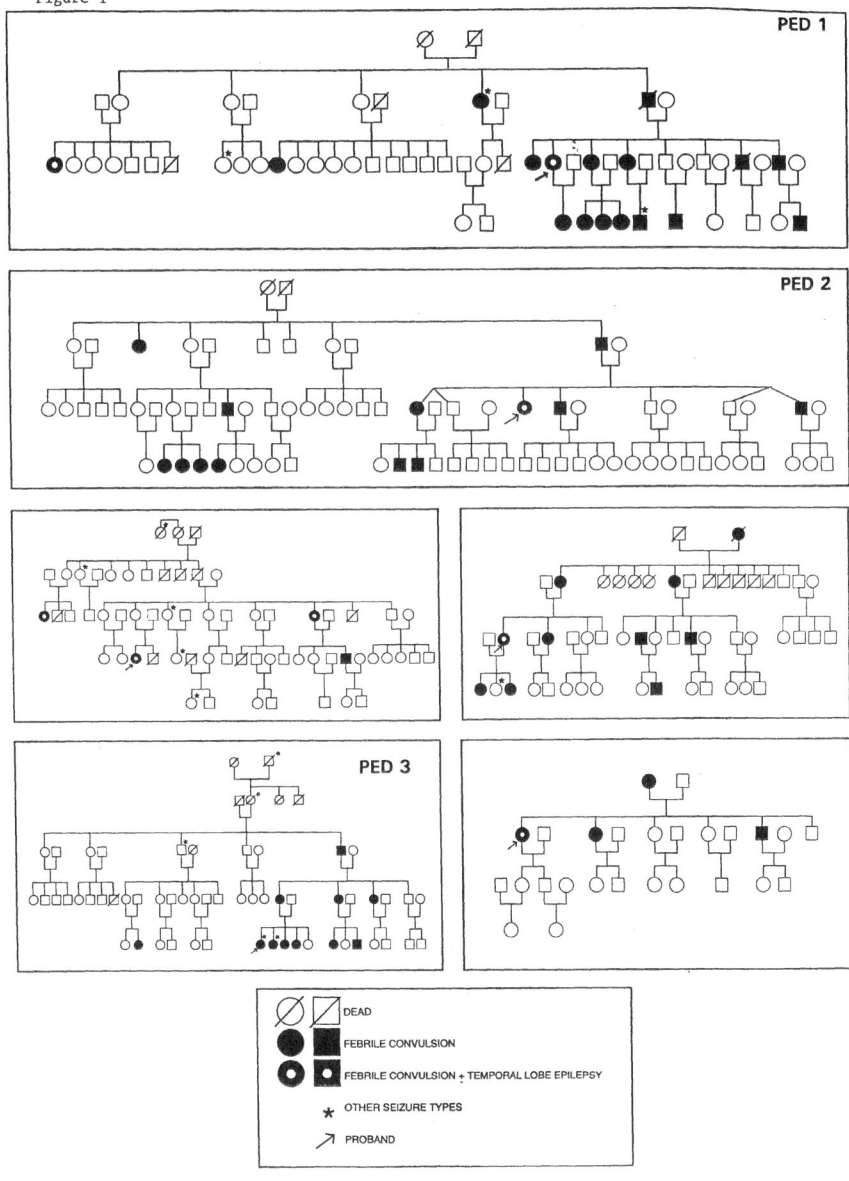

Fig. 1. Six multiplex families with inherited febrile convulsions.

is consistent with previous clinical and experimental evidence suggesting that status epilepticus may cause mesial temporal sclerosis (Pringle et al., 1993).

Genetics of febrile convulsions

Although fever is a necessary precipitant of febrile convulsions, a familial predisposition to this disorder has long been recognized. A positive family history is often obtained when a child presents with a febrile convulsion and similar seizures are at least two to three times more frequent in family members than in the general population with risks to first degree relatives in the range of 10–20 per cent (Frantzen et al., 1970; Nelson & Ellenberg, 1976; Tsuboi & Endo, 1977). Tsuboi & Endo (1977) reported that of 615 children with febrile convulsions, more than half (52 per cent) had a relative similarly affected and in the study by Frantzen et al. (1970), 40 per cent had a positive family history.

Twin studies also support a genetic contribution to the development of febrile convulsions, with concordance rates in monozygotic twins as high as 70 per cent and in dizygotic twins of up to 20 per cent having been reported (Lennox-Buchthal, 1971; Schiotz-Christensen, 1972; Tsuboi, 1982; Corey et al., 1990). There is also evidence of high risk of febrile convulsions in selected ethnic populations, particularly the Japanese who have a rate of 7 per cent (Tsuboi, 1977) and in Guam where up to 14 per cent of Chamarro Indians are affected (Stanhope et al., 1972).

Although a role of hereditary factors in febrile convulsions is not disputed, there is less agreement and conflicting evidence on the type of inheritance. Several genetic models have been proposed including autosomal dominant (Frantzen et al., 1970; Lennox-Buchthal, 1973; Rich et al., 1987; Maher & McLachlan, 1997), autosomal recessive (Schuman & Miller, 1966; Tsuboi, 1982) and polygenic or multifactorial (Tsuboi, 1976; Fukuyama et al., 1979; Rich et al., 1987). Our assessment of eight selected large multigenerational families with a striking aggregation of febrile convulsions supported an autosomal dominant mode of inheritance in these particular families (Maher & McLachlan, 1997). Seventy-five of 333 family members (23 per cent) had febrile convulsions. In addition, 43 per cent of children of probands, 51 per cent of their siblings and 46 per cent of their first degree relatives were similarly affected (Table 2). Concordance with the probands fell from 46 per cent in first degree relatives (parents, siblings, children of probands) to 24 per cent in second degree relatives (grandparents, uncles, aunts and children of siblings of probands) to 9 per cent in third degree relatives (great-grandparents, siblings of grandparents, children of uncles and aunts). The findings support an autosomal dominant inheritance pattern in these families since approximately 50 per cent of children, siblings and first degree relatives of probands had the disorder. Other factors supporting this view include male to male transmission, vertical transmission through multiple generations, and exclusive unilateral grouping of febrile convulsions in families (either maternal or paternal relatives of the proband were affected).

Table 2. Transmission of febrile convulsions.

1	Multiple generations affected	Yes
2	Male to male transmission	Yes
3	Affected children of probands	43%
	Affected siblings of probands	51%
	Affected first-degree relatives of probands	46%
4	Unilateral grouping of secondary cases	Yes
5	Males and females equally affected	No
6	Consanguinity	No

Systematically obtained febrile seizure pedigrees were collected and analysed by Johnson and collaborators (1996). They determined that febrile seizures within these kindreds was probably inherited as an autosomal dominant disorder, however, polygenic inheritance could not be excluded. Under the assumption that febrile seizures was an autosomal dominant disorder, they calculated a penetrance of 0.64 for their families which is in close agreement with the estimated penetrance of 0.60 determined for our families (Fig. 1). Rich et al. (1987) used complex segregation analysis of 467 families with febrile convulsions to suggest a single major locus model with dominant seizure susceptibility if the proband had multiple febrile convulsions but a multifactorial mode of inheritance if only a single uncomplicated febrile convulsion occurred. There was evidence in our families that febrile convulsions were more severe in the probands, thus supporting the findings of Rich et al. (1987).

Table 3. Combined two-point lod scores between proposed febrile seizure genes and markers on chromosome 8 and 19

Locus	Lod Score at θ						
	0.00	0.01	0.05	0.10	0.20	0.30	0.40
D8S260	−4.98	−3.96	−2.47	−1.55	−0.64	−0.24	−0.05
Ped 1*	−4.31	−3.46	−2.13	−1.31	−0.48	−0.10	0.03
Ped 2*	−0.56	−0.50	−0.43	−0.23	−0.16	−0.14	−0.08
D8S533	−3.47	−3.28	−2.45	−1.73	−0.95	−0.49	−0.18
Ped 1	−2.44	−2.32	−1.70	1.14−	−0.52	−0.21	−0.05
Ped 2	−1.03	−0.96	−0.75	−0.59	−0.42	−0.28	−0.13
D8S553	−3.58	−3.22	−2.17	−1.38	−0.54	−0.15	0.01
Ped 1	−2.16	−1.95	−1.34	−0.88	−0.40	−0.17	−0.06
Ped 2	−1.42	−1.27	−0.84	−0.51	−0.14	−0.02	0.06
D8S543	−4.42	−4.25	−3.52	−2.67	−1.47	−0.74	−0.29
Ped 1	−2.22	−2.15	−1.84	−1.41	−0.77	−0.40	−0.17
Ped 2	−2.20	−2.10	−1.68	−1.26	−0.70	−0.34	−0.12
D8S530	−4.99	−4.08	−2.65	−1.73	−0.77	−0.28	−0.04
Ped 1	−1.97	−1.29	−0.60	−0.28	−0.02	0.06	0.05
Ped 2	−3.02	−2.79	−2.05	−1.45	−0.75	−0.34	−0.10
D8S279	−5.85	−5.44	−4.61	−3.84	−2.46	−1.28	−0.47
Ped 1	−2.70	−2.38	−1.93	−1.73	−1.33	−0.78	−0.33
Ped 2	−3.15	−3.06	−2.68	−2.11	−1.13	−0.49	−0.14
D19S216	−10.84	−7.30	−5.04	−3.20	−1.23	−0.33	−0.03
Ped 1	−4.14	−3.36	−2.56	−1.84	−0.91	−0.42	−0.14
Ped 2	−6.70	−3.94	−2.48	−1.36	−0.32	0.09	0.17
D19S427	−9.59	−6.37	−4.09	−2.90	−1.71	−0.72	−0.15
Ped 1	−2.84	−2.84	−2.46	−2.12	−1.65	−0.91	−0.35
Ped 2	−6.75	−3.53	−1.63	−0.78	−0.06	0.19	0.20
D19S177	−8.13	−5.04	−3.23	−2.26	−0.95	−0.29	−0.00
Ped 1	−1.35	−1.36	−1.40	−1.24	−0.63	−0.26	−0.06
Ped 2	−6.78	−3.68	−1.83	1.02−	−0.32	−0.03	0.06

*Lod scores for the two individual families are presented as Ped 1 and Ped 2.

Although the possibility of multifactorial inheritance cannot be excluded in our families, we attempted to prove or disprove the hypothesis that our findings were accounted for on the basis of a single autosomal dominant gene by undertaking linkage analysis of the genome in three of the families. We initially focused on two candidate regions where suggestive evidence of linkage to markers on chromosome 8 (Wallace et al., 1996) and chromosome 19 (Dubovsky et al., 1996) have been described. Wallace et al. (1996), presented suggestive evidence of linkage of a major FC locus to a region on chromosome 8q13–21. The locus spanned approximately 8 cM and was flanked by D8S533 and D8S279. We evaluated two multiplex kindreds (Ped 1 and Ped 2; Fig. 1) for linkage to this region on chromosome 8. Two-point linkage analysis was performed using the computer program MLINK from the LINKAGE package (Lathrop & Lalouel, 1984). Our pedigrees were analysed for linkage using the original parameters of Wallace et al. (1996), which were a penetrance rate of 0.60, a 3 per cent phenocopy rate and a disease allele frequency of 0.0001. As part of a genome screening effort, we also analysed the data using a penetrance of 0.70 and a disease allele frequency of 0.001. Overall, we were able to exclude this region of chromosome 8 as containing an FC gene in our two kindreds. Formal exclusion is based on a calculated lod score < -2.00.

We also evaluated the region of chromosome 19p which was recently reported to be linked to a febrile seizure locus (Dubovsky et al., 1996). Lod scores were calculated using a penetrance of 0.70 and a disease allele frequency of 0.001. In particular, we concentrated on the markers D19S216, D19S427 and D19S177. We were able to exclude this region in three kindreds (Ped's 1, 2 & 3; Fig. 1). The linkage data are presented in Table 3. The combined lod scores from each family effectively excluded the locus identified by Dubovsky (1996). These results are consistent with the hypothesis that febrile seizures is a genetically heterogeneous disorder. Given that febrile seizures is a very common disorder with approximately one in twenty people having had a febrile seizure, the allele frequency of a number of independent disease genes may be quite large. Under these circumstances there is a possibility that multiplex pedigrees may segregate more than one disease allele or even disease gene. If this were the case, it could become extremely difficult to pinpoint a locus using large pedigrees and two-point linkage analysis. In order to minimize this possibility, we have initiated a genome-wide search with DNA from affected sibling pairs and their parents. While such an approach does not guarantee that each family will be genetically homogeneous, it dramatically reduces the possibility in any one kindred. In fact, the affected sib pair approach is robust enough to handle the effects of a small number of siblings, whose febrile seizures were due to mutations in different genes.

Genetics of temporal lobe epilepsy

In the same way that generalized epilepsy has been equated with idiopathic epilepsy of genetic or hereditary origin, partial (focal) epilepsy has become synonymous with symptomatic epilepsy of acquired or lesional origin. As has been pointed out previously (Andermann, 1991) and as discussed throughout this book, there is considerable evidence that the latter concept is not entirely correct. In fact, the first suggestion that genetic factors might play a role in the development of partial epilepsy was made over 30 years ago when several studies found an increased prevalence of seizures and epileptiform abnormalities in the EEGs of relatives of patients with partial epilepsy. Rodin & Whalen (1960) reported a familial occurrence of focal temporal abnormalities in the EEG, consistent with autosomal dominant inheritance and in a later study (Rodin & Gonzalez, 1966) found 'abnormal' EEGs in 30 per cent of families of 20 patients with temporal lobe epilepsy. Remarkably, they also indicated that 50 per cent of families had a history of seizures and 27 per cent of epilepsy. This compares to 2–3 per cent of families with a history of seizures documented in other studies (see Ottman, 1989). Bray & Weiser (1964) assessed 754 EEGs carried out on family members of forty patients with 'temporal lobe' (their quotation marks) epilepsy and found epileptiform abnormalities in 30 per cent of families compared to only 5 per cent in control families without a history of focal epilepsy. However, several of the EEGs illustrated clearly show what we now recognize are typical spikes of benign rolandic epilepsy, a quite separate and distinctive disorder. Other reports from around this time may have suffered from the same problem of misdiagnosis. Several other studies have found a prevalence rate of seizures of 2–7 per cent in relatives of patients with partial seizures (see Ottman, 1989 for references) which is somewhat higher than in the general population.

In an interesting study, Rimoin & Metrakos (1961) assessed seizures and epileptiform EEG abnormalities in relatives of 158 individuals with infantile hemiplegia and 270 normal controls. Table 4 shows the results in relatives of hemiplegic patients with seizures, those without seizures and in the normal controls. More frequent seizures and EEG abnormalities occurred in relatives of those with infantile hemiplegia and seizures than in both controls and those with infantile hemiplegia without seizures supporting a hereditary contribution to the development of convulsions with this acquired focal brain disorder. An intriguing aspect of the study was the finding that lower rates of seizures and EEG abnormalities were found in infantile hemiplegia without seizures than in the normal controls suggesting that genetic factors may regulate susceptibility to seizures, not only by enhancing vulnerability to epileptiform activity in some individuals, but by a protective effect in others.

Table 4. Familial predisposition to seizures after infantile hemiplegia

	Relatives with	
	Seizures	Abnormal EEGs
Hemiplegia + seizures	2.0%	23%
Controls	1.7%	13%
Hemiplegia	1.0%	9%

Figure 2, adapted from Lindsay (1971), illustrates several mechanisms by which genetic factors could influence the development of temporal lobe epilepsy. Firstly, since virtually all children sustain fevers at some time or other which are high enough or appear rapidly enough to trigger a seizure, it is clear from the evidence presented earlier regarding heritability of febrile convulsions, that genetic factors directly determine whether such a convulsion will occur or not under the appropriate environmental circumstances. Secondly, there is a likely genetic influence on whether a febrile convulsion, if it occurs, is brief or prolonged. Since seizures longer than 30 min are more likely to lead to temporal lobe epilepsy later in life, this will indirectly affect the outcome. Thirdly, even prolonged febrile convulsions do not always lead to temporal lobe epilepsy, and thus there could be a role for genetic factors in the development of mesial temporal sclerosis at this stage as well. Finally, and most straight

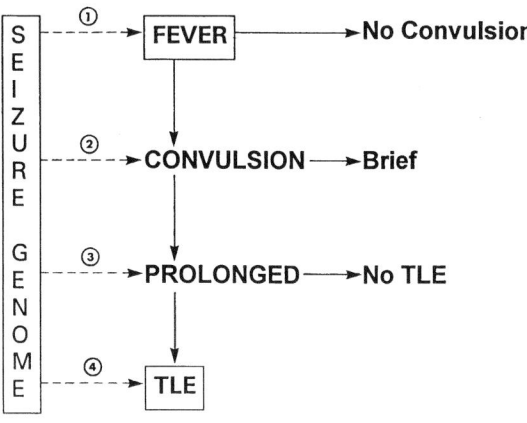

Fig. 2. Influence of seizure genome on development of temporal lobe epilepsy (TLE).

forward, is a direct phenotypic expression of a gene (or genes) as suggested by the autosomal dominant familial temporal lobe epilepsy described by Berkovic *et al.* (1996) and the family with partial epilepsy linked to chromosome 10q reported by Ottman *et al.* (1995).

Considering the number of children who have febrile convulsions, even those complicated by status epilepticus, pediatricians and pediatric neurologists who follow these cases over time are struck by how few progress to temporal lobe epilepsy. On the other hand, those who treat patients with intractable partial seizures at epilepsy surgery centres are impressed by how often febrile convulsions are a prologue to mesial temporal sclerosis. The resolution to this debate lies in unravelling the elements of the genetic code which predispose certain individuals to focal epilepsy following an acquired condition such as fever and which change a usually innocuous insult into one with permanent structural and functional brain sequelae.

References

Abou-Khalil, B., Andermann, E., Andermann, F., Olivier, A. & Quesney, L.F. (1993): Temporal lobe epilepsy after prolonged febrile convulsions: excellent outcome after surgical treatment. *Epilepsia* **34**, 878–883.

Andermann, E. (1991): Genetic studies of epilepsy in Montreal. In: *Genetic strategies in epilepsy research*, Anderson, V.E., Hauser, W.A., Leppik, I.E., Noebels, J.L. & Rich, S.S. (eds), pp. 129–137. Amsterdam: Elsevier.

Annegers, J.F., Hauser, W.A., Elveback, L.R. & Kurland, L.T. (1979): The risk of epilepsy following febrile convulsions. *Neurology* **29**, 297–303.

Annegers, J.F., Hauser, W.A., Shirts, S.B. & Kurland, L.T. (1987): Factors prognostic of unprovoked seizures after febrile convulsions. *N. Engl. J. Med.* **316**, 493–498.

Berg, A.T. (1992): Febrile seizures and epilepsy: The contributions of epidemiology. *Pediatr. Perinat. Epidemiol.* **6**, 145–152.

Berg, A.T. & Shinnar, S. (1996): Unprovoked seizures in children with febrile seizures: short-term outcome. *Neurology* **47**, 562–568.

Berkovic, S.F., McIntosh, A., Howell, R.A., Mitchell, A., Sheffield, L.J. & Hopper, J.L. (1996): Familial temporal lobe epilepsy: A common disorder identified in twins. *Ann. Neurol.* **40**, 227–235.

Blume, W.T., Desai, H.B., Girvin, J.P., McLachlan, R.S. & Lemieux, J.F. (1994): Effectiveness of temporal lobectomy measured by yearly follow-up and multivariate analysis. *J. Epilepsy* **7**, 203–214.

Bray, P.F. & Wiser, W.C. (1964): Evidence of a genetic etiology of temporal-central abnormalities in focal epilepsy. *N. Engl. J. Med.* **271**, 926–933.

Camfield, P., Camfield, C., Gordon, K. & Dooley, J. (1994): What types of epilepsy are preceded by febrile seizures? A population-based study of children. *Dev. Med. Child Neurol.* **36**, 887–892.

Corey, L., Berg, K., Pellock, J., Nance, W.E. & DeLorenzo, R. (1990): Seizure syndromes in Virginia and Norwegian twin kindreds. *Epilepsia* **31**, 814.

Dubovsky, J., Weber, J.L., Orr, H.T., Rich, S.S., Gil-Nagel, A., Anderson, V.E., Leppik, I.E. & Johnson, E.W. (1996): A second gene for familial febrile convulsions maps on chromosome 19p. *Am. J. Hum. Genet.* **59**, A223.

Falconer, M.A. (1971): Genetic and related aetiological factors in temporal lobe epilepsy: a review. *Epilepsia* **12**, 13–31.

Frantzen, E., Lennox-Buchthal, M., Nygaard, A. & Stene, J. (1970): A genetic study of febrile convulsions. *Neurology* **20**, 909–917.

French, J.A., Williamson, P.D., Thadani, V.M., Darcey, T.M., Mattson, R.H., Spencer, S.S. & Spencer, D.D. (1993). Characteristics of medial temporal lobe epilepsy: I. Results of history and physical examination. *Ann. Neurol.* **34**, 774–780.

Fukuyama, Y., Kagawa, K. & Tanaka, K. (1979): A genetic study of febrile convulsions. *Eur. Neurol.* **18**, 166–182.

Hauser, W.A. (1981): The natural history of febrile seizures. In: *Febrile seizures*, Nelson, K.B. & Ellenberg, J.H. (eds), pp. 5–17. New York: Raven Press.

Hauser, W.A. & Kurland, L.T. (1975): The epidemiology of epilepsy in Rochester, Minnesota 1935–67. *Epilepsia* **16**, 1–66.

Jensen, I. (1976): Temporal lobe epilepsy. Etiological factors and surgical results. *Acta Neurol. Scand.* **53**, 103–118.

Johnson, W.G., Kugler, S.L., Stenroos, E.S., Meulener, M.C., Rangwalla, I., Johnson, T.W. & Mandelbaum, D.E. (1996): Pedigree analysis in families with febrile seizures. *Am. J. Med. Genet.* **61,** 345–352.

Kanemoto, K., Takeuchi, J., Kawasaki, J. & Kawai, I. (1996): Characteristics of temporal lobe epilepsy with mesial temporal sclerosis, with special reference to psychotic episodes. *Neurology* **47,** 1199–1203.

Kuks, J.B., Cook, M.J., Fish, D.R., Stevens, J.M. & Shorvon, S.D. (1993): Hippocampal sclerosis in epilepsy and childhood febrile convulsions seizures. *Lancet* **342,** 1391–1394.

Lathrop, G.M. & Lalouel, J.M. (1984): Easy calculations of lod scores and genetic risks on small computers. *Am. J. Hum. Genet.* **36,** 460–465.

Lee, K., Diaz, M & Melchior, J.C. (1981): Temporal lobe epilepsy – not a consequence of childhood febrile convulsions in Denmark. *Acta Neurol. Scand.* **63,** 231–236.

Lennox-Buchthal, M. (1971): Febrile and nocturnal convulsions in monozygotic twins. *Epilepsia* **12,** 147–156.

Lennox-Buchthal, M. (1973): Febrile convulsions. A reappraisal. *Electroencephalogr. Clin. Neurophysiol.* **32,** 1–138.

Lindsay, J.M.M. (1971): Genetics and Epilepsy: A model from critical path analysis. *Epilepsia* **12,** 47–54.

Lindsay, J., Ounsted, C. & Richards, P. (1980): Long-term outcome in children with temporal lobe seizures. IV: Genetic factors, febrile convulsions and the remission of seizures. *Dev. Med. Child Neurol.* **22,** 429–439.

Maher, J. & McLachlan, R.S. (1995): Febrile convulsions: Is seizure duration the most important predictor of temporal lobe epilepsy? *Brain* **118,** 1521–1528.

Maher, J. & McLachlan, R.S. (1997): Febrile convulsions in selected large families: a single major locus mode of inheritance? *Dev. Med. Child Neurol.* **39,** 79–84.

Nelson, K.B. & Ellenberg, J.H. (1976): Predictors of epilepsy in children who have experienced febrile seizures. *N. Engl. J. Med.* **295,** 1029–1033.

Nelson, K.B. & Ellenberg, J.H. (1978): Prognosis in children with febrile seizures. *Pediatrics* **61,** 720–772.

Ottman, R. (1989): Genetics of the partial epilepsies: A review. *Epilepsia* **30,** 107–111.

Ottman, R., Risch, N., Hauser, W.A. *et al.* (1995): Localization of a gene for partial epilepsy to chromosome 10q. *Nat. Genet.* **10,** 56–60.

Ounsted, C., Lindsay, J. & Norman, R. (1966): *Biological factors in temporal lobe epilepsy. Clinics in Developmental Medicine, No. 22.* p. 135. London: Heinemann.

Pringle, C.E., Blume, W.T., Munoz, D.G. & Leung, S.L. (1993): Pathogenesis of mesial temporal sclerosis. *Can. J. Neurol. Sci.* **20,** 184–193.

Rich, S.S., Annegers, J.F., Hauser, W.A. & Anderson, V.E. Complex segregation analysis of febrile convulsions. (1987): *Am. J. Hum. Genet.* **41,** 249–257.

Rimoin, D.L. & Metrakos, J.D. (1961): The genetics of convulsive disorders in the families of hemiplegics. *Proc. 2nd Intern. Congr. Hum. Genet.* **3,** 1655–1658.

Rocca, W.A., Sharbrough, F.W., Hauser, W.A., Annegers, J.F. & Schoenberg, B.S. (1987): Risk factors for complex partial seizures: a population-based case-control study. *Ann. Neurol.* **21,** 22–31.

Rodin, E.A. & Whelan, J.L. (1960): Familial occurrence of focal temporal electroencephalographic abnormalities. *Neurology* **10,** 542–545.

Rodin, E.A. & Gonzalez, S. (1966): Hereditary components in epileptic patients. *JAMA* **198,** 221–225.

Schiottz-Christensen, E. (1972): Genetic factors in febrile convulsions. *Acta Neurol. Scand.* **48,** 538–546.

Schuman, S.H. & Miller, L.J. (1966): Febrile convulsions in families: Findings in an epidemiologic survey. *Clin. Pediatr.* **5,** 604–608.

Sofijanov, N., Sadikario, A., Dukovski, M. & Kutures, M. (1983): Febrile convulsions and later development of epilepsy. *Am. J. Dis. Child* **137,** 123–126.

Stanhope, J.M., Brody, J.A., Brink, E. & Morris, C.E. (1972): Convulsions among the Chamarro people of Guam, Mariana Islands. Part II. Febrile convulsions. *Am. J. Epidemiol.* **95,** 299–304.

Tsuboi, T. (1976): Polygenic inheritance of epilepsy and febrile convulsions. Analysis based on a computational model. *Br. J. Psychiat.* **129,** 239–242.

Tsuboi, T. (1977): Genetic aspects of febrile convulsions. *Hum. Genet.* **38,** 169–173.

Tsuboi, T. (1982): Febrile Convulsions. In: *Genetic basis of the epilepsies*, Anderson, V.E., Hauser, W.A., Penry, J.K., King, C.F. (eds), pp. 123–124. New York: Raven Press.

Tsuboi, T. & Endo, S.H. (1977): Febrile convulsions followed by nonfebrile convulsions. A clinical, electroencephalographic and follow-up study. *Neuropediatrics* **8,** 209–223.

VandenBerg, B.J. & Yerushalmy, J. (1969): Studies on convulsive disorders in young children. I. Incidence of febrile and nonfebrile convulsions by age and other factors. *Pediatr. Res.* **3,** 298–304.

Verity, C.M., Butler, N.R. & Golding, J. (1985): Febrile convulsions in a national cohort followed up from birth. I. Prevalence and recurrence in the first five years of life. *Br. Med. J.* **290,** 1307–1310.

Wallace, R.H., Berkovic, S.F., Howell, R.A., Sutherland, G.R. & Mulley, J.C. (1996): Suggestion of a major gene for familial febrile convulsions mapping to 8q13–21. *J. Med. Genet.* **33,** 308–312.

Chapter 17

Reading epilepsy: clinical and genetic background

Thomas Mayer and Peter Wolf

Epilepsie-Zentrum Bethel, Klinik Mara I, Maraweg 21, D-33617 Bielefeld, Germany

Bickford *et al.* (1956) was the first who described seizures precipitated by reading. He distinguished two types: a 'primary' form in which reading is the only mode of precipitation and a 'secondary' form, in which seizures occur also in other conditions. Discussions about this division made Bickford change the terms into specific (instead of primary) and non-specific (instead of secondary).

We know only little about the epidemiology of reading epilepsy (RE). There are about 120 cases published until now so that RE seems to be a rare syndrome. The vast majority of cases belong to the specific or primary form. Whereas RE is a well-defined epileptic syndrome, and the only example where a specific mode of seizure precipitation was recognized as the presenting and name-giving feature, the 'secondary' cases show much individual variability and are not today considered as a syndrome or an 'epilepsy'. RE is classified as one of the idiopathic localization-related epilepsies because of the typical partial seizures with relation to an anatomical region of the brain. Criticism regarding this classification has been made, for example by Radhakrishan *et al.* (1995). They were impressed by four of 18 own cases with RE and juvenile myoclonic epilepsy (JME), which is an unusual cluster. This 'co-occurrence' was never described before and the authors proposed considering RE a generalized epilepsy with seizures precipitated by specific modes of activation. There are indeed some hints of a relationship to the idiopathic generalized epilepsies, e.g. the benign course, good response to valproic acid (VPA), age of onset, seizures with myoclonias in clear consciousness and progression to generalized tonic–clonic seizures (GTCS). But RE and JME are not the same syndromes, because first, the small number of observations with both syndromes does not allow such conclusion and second, the myoclonic jerks of the upper limb typical for JME were not precipitated by reading but occurred spontaneously in the patients with both syndromes.

There are clear indications of a genetic background in RE with a hereditary predisposition in 40–45 per cent of the patients, but no large multiplex family with this syndrome has yet been found.

In the last 6 years we discovered 12 new cases with RE in our centre, which point out more details of this syndrome. We believe that the prevalence of the syndrome is higher than was thought. With more patients there will be a better chance to elucidate the genetic background of the RE syndrome as we wish to show in this paper.

Clinical features

RE is a syndrome with a male preponderance (men : women = 1.8 : 1). The age of onset is not in early school age when reading is learned but in the adolescence and young adult age (mean: 17.7 years). In a meta-analysis of Wolf (1992) only three patients were at onset younger than 12 years and only five older than 25 years.

One of the most impressive features of the syndrome is its clinical uniformity. According to the International Classification of Epilepsies and Epileptic Syndromes, 'all or almost all seizures in this syndrome are precipitated by reading (especially aloud) and are independent of the content of the text. They are simple focal motor – involving masticatory muscles, or visual, and if the stimulus is not interrupted, GTCS may occur'.

The most constant symptoms are abnormal sensations or movements in the musculature which is involved in reading and talking: tongue, throat, jaw, lips, face. Patients decribing their seizure symptoms use expressions for the seizures such as numbness, stiffness, tightness, clicking sensation or stammering.

The reading induced epileptic movements can easily be overlooked by observers. They are mostly myoclonic and only rarely tonic. The myoclonic jerks may occur isolatedly, sometimes repetitive with the possibility of progression to a secondarily GTCS, but in most patients GTCS occur rarely. In the view of the patients the GTCS typically marks the beginning of the epilepsy. Only in a few patients are partial seizures the only seizure type.

The clinical features mostly are bilateral but sometimes asymmetric or unilateral. A few patients also describe some kind of visual or ocular manifestation as the only or additional symptom to the motor seizure, e.g. reading precipitated epileptic nystagmus shortly before a GTCS (Meyer & Wolf, 1973) or ictal dyslexia. Modes of precipitation are not only reading but in more than a quarter talking, in 11 per cent writing, seldom reading figures, Braille or music. If reading of music is provocative, the arms playing the instrument jerk.

In cases where writing is provocative the myoclonic jerks involve the writing arm. Loud reading is more provocative than silent reading, the more difficult a text is (unusual text, nonsense text, text in an unknown language) the more it becomes provocative.

Table 1. Clinical features of reading epilepsy

Seizures induced by reading, speaking and writing
Seizures: (myo)clonic, seldom tonic, tonic–clonic
Abnormal sensations or movements in: tongue, throat, jaw, lips, face
Sensations: stiffness, numbness, tightness, clicking sensations, stammering
Consciousness: clear in (myo)clonic or tonic seizures

EEG

There is no characteristic EEG pattern in patients with RE. Wolf investigated the EEG of published and own patients with RE in a meta-analysis (1992). He found that the interictal EEG showed in 84/106 cases no pathological signs, in 11/106 patients bilateral spike wave activity, and in five patients paroxysmal temporal discharges.

In six out of 65 investigated cases (9 per cent) there was a photoparoxysmal reaction. Intermittent photic stimulation with the other 59 patients (91 per cent) remained negative, which shows that RE is not a variant of photosensitivity.

The ictal EEG showed in 73 cases paroxysmal activity which was, in 23 cases bilateral symmetric, in

28 cases bilateral asymmetric, and in 22 cases focal. The typical discharge is a single or very short volley of steep or sharp waves, spikes or spike and wave complexes.

75 per cent of the cases with focal ictal EEG findings had temporo-parietal foci, occasionally extended to central or occipital, with 25 per cent frontal, sometimes extended to central or anterior temporal. In the majority (78 per cent) of the cases with lateralizing EEGs, lateralization to the language dominant hemisphere was found.

Genetic aspects

In a meta-analysis of Wolf (1992) regarding all published patients with RE there was information on the family in 75 out of 111 cases belonging to 69 families. Thirty-four of these 75 patients (belonging to 28 families) had affected relatives: 20 of them had affected first degree relatives, eight patients had 13 second or third degree relatives.

A total of 47 relatives of patients with RE have had seizures. There was more information about seizures and epilepsies about 20 of these 47 relatives and all of these were first degree relatives (Table 2).

Table 2. Genetic aspects of reading epilpesy

Total cases	111
Information on family	75/111 (68%)
Affected relatives	34 in 28 families
Patients with affected 1st degree relatives	20 with 34 affected relatives
Patients with other affected relatives	8 with 13 affected relatives

The majority (11/20) of the affected relatives with syndrome diagnosis suffered also from RE. One of these relatives with RE is an identical twin. Another set of monozygotic twins was found by Berkovic (personal information). Furthermore, there were three relatives with idiopathic generalized epilepsy, two with febrile convulsions, one with GTCS since the age of three, two with seizures not precipitated by reading, and one with a symptomatic epilepsy (Table 3). It seems to be a tendency of relatives, unless they suffer from the same syndrome, to have either *Gelegenheitsanfälle* (occasional seizures) or idiopathic generalized epilepsies, just as in other idiopathic localization-related epilepsies.

Table 3. Relatives of patients with reading epilepsy (meta-analysis of Wolf, 1992)

Kind of epilepsy	Number of relatives
Unclear	27
Reading epilepsy	11
Idiopathic generalized	3
Febrile seizures	2
GTCS since age 3	1
Seizures unprovoked by reading	2
Symptomatic focal epilepsy	1

Case reports

In the last 6 years we have observed three patients with a co-occurrence of RE and JME, and one patient with RE and GTCS on awakening. The following case reports detail the relationship of the two idiopathic syndromes in these patients. Such concomitant occurences of two inherited syndromes allow insights into the genetics of RE.

Case report 1

The 45 year old patient (H.R.) suffered since the age of 17 from myoclonic jerks in the arms and legs especially in the morning, sometimes with a fall. He has been photosensitive since that time and he realized he got more jerks, when sitting in front of his computer. Twice he had a GTCS after sleep deprivation. After the second GTCS treatment with VPA began and he became seizure-free regarding GTCS and myoclonic jerks for several years. Since the age of 30 he noticed high frequency short myoclonic jerks in the mouth and jaw when reading or speaking aloud. He noticed more of those jerks if a text was difficult or when he had to talk about difficult subjects. He never got a GTCS precipitated by reading. There were no affected members in his family. The neurological examination and the CT scan were normal. In former EEG recordings, 3 Hz spike and poly-spike-wave activity was described. A routine EEG including intermittent light stimulation was now without pathological signs recorded at the age of 45. Provocation by reading showed left temporal spikes in spite of antiepileptic therapy with 1000 mg VPA per day and blood levels of VPA at 90.8 µg/ml.

Case report 2

A 24 year old woman (S.N.) had her first seizures at the age of three (GTCS ?). There was no more information about these seizures and she was treated with VPA until age 13. Then VPA medication was stopped and she remained seizure-free until age 16. From that time she noticed myoclonic jerks in the hand and arms in the morning, which she interpretated as a kind of clumsiness but not as minor epileptic seizures. At the age of 22 she had a GTCS after sleep deprivation and a lot of alcohol. She did not accept any treatment because she believed that this was the first epileptic seizure in her adult life. After that seizure she only occasionally had myoclonic jerks in the arms early in the morning, but at the age of 23 she became seizure-free without any therapy. At the age of 24 she suddenly became aware of myoclonic jerks on the right side of the face provoked by reading and speaking. She noticed these jerks especially when reading a difficult text, speaking about personal problems or when she felt angry or depressed and tried to read. After 1 year she had her second GTCS after sleep deprivation in the evening. This seizure happened in a store when she was looking for a special kind of meal. After several trials she tried to read a food description written in very small letters and with difficult expressions. After some short myoclonic jerks at her mouth she had the second GTCS of her adult life.

In her family there is a female cousin of the patient's mother who has epilepsy, but no details were available. The neurological status was normal. The ictal and interictal EEG showed left temporal sharp waves. She also was photosensitive with intermittent photic stimulation of 12 and 18 Hz. Magnetic resonance imaging showed the temporal horn of the lateral ventricle was larger on the left side, but no focal lesion was found. The patient is a law student with unusual hobbies such as diving and parachuting. With a treatment of phenobarbitone she had no more GTCS for 1 year, but reading induced myoclonic jerks. Now she takes 1200 mg VPA per day and only she is aware of short myoclonic jerks in the face only in very difficult or exciting conversations.

Case report 3

Patient J.S. is a 47-year-old female laboratory technician without familial antecedents who has had two GTC seizures in her life time. The first was at age of 17 during an operation on a nasal septum which had to be interrupted. The second occurred at age 29 shortly after another surgical procedure. Since the first GTCS, she occasionally had bilaterally myoclonias of the arms, 'as if a bird beat its wings', in full consciousness. These occurred more readily after increased alcohol intake or with prolonged TV watching. These myoclonias were treated intermittently with benzodiazepines which she took if feelings of unrest or tension of the neck indicated to her an increased probability of having jerks. After her second GTCS an EEG was taken and phenytoin (PHT) was prescribed which she took for several years.

In that period she first noticed that often with continuous reading she would develop jaw jerking. She found out, however, that more difficult texts, reading English or reading aloud were more provocative. With loud reading, she was unable to go on not only because of the jerks but because she could not read any longer what she saw. These symptoms occurred more readily when she felt exhausted or if she had not had enough sleep. If jaw jerking occurred, she paused, and the jerking would immediately stop.

Over the years, these symptoms had slowly increased, and jaw jerking could now also occur in emotional discussions, especially when she was angry. Occasionally, when writing a long letter, she could get jerks in her right arm, sometimes together with jaw jerks. These jerks during writing she found clearly different from the above mentioned bilateral myoclonias. Her past history was otherwise normal, and her physical examination unrevealing. A CT scan at age 32 had been described as showing slight cortical atrophy. A routine EEG was taken with a medication of 300 mg PHT and showed rare subclinical irregular rapid spike waves at rest and with hyperventilation which increased with photic stimulation, where they could be precipitated by eye closure. They appeared either on the left or bilaterally with left preponderance, mainly in the frontal, central and anterior temporal areas. She now reads quite easily. Unfortunately we could not record her ictal EEG. VPA was prescribed in a dose of 900 mg per day and she has indeed never since had any provoked or unprovoked myoclonias.

Case report 4

Patient U.N. is a 28-year-old woman with epilepsy since the age of 12. Her first GTCS was in the early morning at 4 a.m. She awoke with an unusual feeling in the head and in the whole body. She tried to go to the bed-room of her parents when she suddenly lost control of both legs. She dropped down losing consciousness and had a tonic–clonic seizure. After this first seizure she had three more GTCS on awakening, mostly after sleep deprivation. She remained seizure-free with a treatment of an unknown dose of phenobarbitone (PB) from the age of 15. There is no information about EEG recordings taken at that time. At the age of 25 she cautiously reduced medication of PB over a period of one year. Half a year after stopping PB medication she became aware of short myoclonic jerks while talking. Her husband thought that she had a kind of hiccup and neither of them were concerned about these symptoms. One evening while reading a book to her little daughter she felt tired and suddenly noticed a cluster of myoclonic jerks in the mouth, though she never got a GTCS any more. Medical treatment was started because she was afraid of the myoclonic jerks and she remembered the GTCS of childhood. There was no response to carbamazepine in the treatment of the myoclonic jerks, but with 100 mg of PB she only had jerks precipitated by talking or reading when she felt angry or tired. Her physical examination was normal and no focal lesions were found in the MRT.

In her family there is a female cousin suffered from a post-traumatic epilepsy. The interictal EEG-recording at the age of 28 was normal, the ictal EEG showed left temporal steep transients. With a treatment of 1000 mg VPA she has now remained seizure-free for two years.

Discussion

It is quite obvious that RE is a syndrome with a genetic background. There seems to be a tendency in affected relatives of patients with RE to have either idiopathic generalized epilepsies or single seizures (*Gelegenheitsanfälle*). Several affected relatives had RE, and a report on one monozygotic twin pair was published (Forster & Daly, 1973). There are no morphological lesions in MRI or CT scans in most of the cases. The neurological status is normal, and the clinical features are typical and uniform.

The age at onset is specific, the course is benign and VPA (Vanderzant *et al.*, 1982) is the most effective antiepileptic drug with clonazepam as the second most effective drug (Hall & Marshall, 1980). Association with photosensitivity (Blumenthal & Dunn, 1961; Maricardi *et al.*, 1991) was described in 9 per cent of cases (Wolf, 1982) but not more frequently in those cases with a positive family history. Until now we have no clear idea about the mode of inheritance and about the localization of the gene of RE.

In the classification of the ILAE, RE is a idiopathic localization-related epilepsy. There is no transition between this syndrome and the perirolandic epilepsy, the most frequently found localization-related epilepsy. The co-occurence with JME in some cases raises the question of whether RE could be a idiopathic generalized epilepsy syndrome. Arguments for that point of view are, for example, the age of onset, good response to VPA, clear consciousness during the myoclonic jerks, progression to GTCS (Radhakrishan *et al.*, 1995). In a case report Matricardi *et al.* (1991) described a 14-year-old girl with reading induced seizures, absences, television-induced seizures and pattern sensitivity. In this case reading could induce generalized spike-wave activity with simple absences. This patient, however, did not have the specific (primary) type of RE.

Typical cases of RE have also occasionally been described in association with symptomatic focal epilepsies without any generalized traits. Ritaccio *et al.* (1992) described a 24-year-old man with RE after removal of a left frontal arteriovenous malformation. They suggested that RE may be a reflex or action myoclonus localized to Brodmann's area 6. Miyamoto *et al.* (1995) showed focal hyperperfusion in ictal HMPAO-single photon emission computed tomography (SPECT) of the frontal lobes bilaterally and of the left temporal area. Positron emission tomography (PET)-studies (Posner *et al.*, 1988; Koepp *et al.*, 1995) have demonstrated bilateral activitation of the striate cortex and visual association cortex during reading. These facts indicate that RE is a localization-related epilepsy which asymmetrically involves those regions of both hemispheres which are functionally involved in the processes of reading. The precipitated seizures are partial seizures which involve sometimes both sides of the face due to the bilateral innervation of the affected musculature.

As in other idiopathic epilepsies inheritance may be polygenic. Until now there has been no multiplex family with RE. The association with another idiopathic syndrome could be helpful to find the gene of RE. The syndrome of JME seems to be genetically heterogeneous (Sander *et al.*, 1996; Greenberg *et al.*, 1996). Linkage and association studies provide strong evidence that a gene locus on chromosome 6 is involved in the expression of JME in some families and also in the expression in the idiopathic generalized epilepsy with grand mal on awakening (Greenberg *et al.*, 1996). Serratosa *et al.* (1996) suggested that a special pattern in EEG-recording (3.5–6 Hz polyspike wave or spike wave pattern) with this syndrome is responsible for gene localization of JME on chromosome 6 p.

The relatively frequent co-occurrence of RE with JME could indicate that RE is a polygenic disorder sharing one gene with JME. This would be consistent with the observation that, in the affected first degree relatives, idiopathic generalized epilepsies are the second largest group after RE. On the other hand, no affected relatives with JME have yet been reported.

There are now seven cases with RE plus JME, three in our epilepsy centre, and four of Radhakrishan *et al.* (1995). The characteristics of these cases are shown in Table 4.

Interestingly, there is an interval in the age of onset of JME and RE in our patients. In these cases RE had replaced JME as the clinical pattern. In the cases of Radhakrihan *et al.* (1995) there is no information about a different age of onset in RE and JME. The types of seizure in both syndromes are short myoclonic jerks but with different localization and without precipitation in JME. In both epilepsy syndromes, people are aware of their myoclonias, although these myoclonic jerks are associated with generalized epileptic discharges in EEG recordings in JME and sometimes in RE. GTCS could occur but these seizures are not very frequent in either syndrome. All of the patients with RE plus JME showed myoclonic jerks in the face during talking, not only during reading. It seems possible that the cases in which talking also precipitates myoclonic jerks are a separate group, related to those patients with praxis-induced seizures (Inoue *et al.*, 1994), since in three of the four cases of Radhakrishan *et al.* (1995) with RE and JME, calculating and playing chess could induce seizures. Alternatively, they could be a subgroup of the core patients with pure RE. To test this hypothesis, more patients with the co-occurrence of RE and JME must be studied.

Table 4. *Characteristics of seven cases with RE and JME (cases from Mayo Clinic, Rochester (1–4) and epilepsy centre*

Case	Sex	Age at onset JME/RTE	Trigger (other than reading)	Associated symptoms	Seizures
1	F	46	Calculating, listening to conversation	Unable to concentrate	Myocl.
2	F	14	Nil	Nil	Myocl., GTCS
3	M	16	Chess playing, calculating	Interuption of breathing absences	Myocl., GTCS, Abs.
4	F	17	Calculating, speaking, writing	Stuttering	Myocl., GTCS
5	F	16/29	Speaking, TV-watching	Unable to word the text	Myocl., GTCS
6	M	17/30	Speaking	Stuttering with high frequency of seizures	Myocl.
7	F	16/24	Speaking	Nil	Myocl., GTCS

If the EEG pattern of the patients is compared with RE and JME as may be seen in Table 5, five of seven patients with the association of both syndromes have both generalized ictal and interictal EEG patterns. But in the two cases where the interictal EEG is normal, the ictal epileptic discharges are focal.

Table 5. *Characteristics of seven cases with RE and JME*

Case	EEG interictal	EEG ictal	Photosensivity	Therapy
1	Generalized SW-activity	Generalized SW-activity	Negative	DPH/PRM: partial control
2	Generalized atypical SW-activity	Generalized SW-activity	Negative	DPH/PRM: partial control
3	Generalized spikes and polyspikes	Generalized spikes and polyspikes	Negative	VPA: exc. control
4	Generalized spikes and polyspikes	Generalized spikes and polyspikes	Negative	VPA: exc. control
5	Generalized spikes	Generalized spikes	Positive	VPA: exc. control
6	Normal	Spikes left temporal	Positive (?)	VPA: good control
7	Normal	Steep transient left temporal	Positive (?)	VPA: ?

Conclusion

In Table 6 the syndromes of RE and JME are compared with each other to show differences and similarities. In general it seems obvious that these are two different idiopathic syndromes.

Table 6. Comparison between RE and JME

	RE	JME
Genetic background	Yes, unclassified mode	Yes, unclassified mode
Interictal EEG	Usually negative	Usually positive
Ictal EEG	Very brief SW	Generalized PSW
Specific focal seizures	Yes	No
Specific generalized seizures	No	Yes
Relation to anatomical region	Yes, complex	Probable, but unidentified
Exogenous pathogenetic factors	Unusual	Unusual
Specific age of onset	15–25	12–18
Benign spontaneous course	Typical	Possible
Precipitation	Specific	Non-specific (sleep deprivation), sometimes specific: photosensitive; praxis

Interestingly there is no close relationship to any other kind of idiopathic localization-related epilepsy. Rolandic epilepsy differs with respect to age at onset, seizure types, therapy stategies and precipitation (negative in Rolandic epilepsy). So it seems to be obvious that RE and rolandic epilepsy are genetically different syndromes with different gene loci.

The next steps will be to investigate the families of patients with RE and JME to look for affected but unidentified relatives, any photosensitivity, and to perform detailed genetic analysis with all affected family members when a multiplex family is found. There may be a chance for this, thanks to the many new cases with RE identified over the past few years.

References

Baxter, D.W. & Bailey, A.A. (1961): Primary reading epilepsy. *Neurology* **11**, 445–449.

Bickford, R.G. (1973): Discussion, *Trans. Am. Neurol. Ass.* **98**, 187–188.

Bickford, R.G., Whelan, J.L., Klass, D.W. & Corbin, K.B. (1956): Reading epilepsy: clinical and electroencephalographic studies of a new syndrome. *Trans. Am. Neurol. Ass.* **81**, 100–102.

Bingel, A. (1957): Reading epilepsy. *Neurology* **7**, 752–756.

Blumenthal, I.J. & Dunn, A. (1962): Reading epilepsy: case report. *Electroencephalogr. Clin. Neurophysiol.* **14**, 270–273.

Blumenthal, I.J. & Dunn., A. (1967): Reading epilepsy combined with intermittent photic stimulation. Case report. *Excerpta Med. Int. Congr.* **134**, 85–89.

Brooks, J.E. & Jirauch, P.M. (1971): Primary reading epilepsy. A misnomer. *Arch. Neurol.* **25**, 97–104.

Ch'ien, L.T. & Little, S.C. (1971): Reading epilepsy. *Ala. J. Sci.* **8**, 227–231.

Christie, S., Guberman, A., Tansley, B.W. & Couture, M. (1988): Primary reading epilepsy: investigation of critical seizure-provoking-stimuli. *Epilepsia* **26**, 288–293.

Cirignotta, F., Zucconi, M., Mondini, S. & Lugaresi, E. (1986): Writing epilepsy. *Clin. Electroencephalogr.* **17**, 21–23.

Cohn, R., Allison, M.E. & De Bolt, W.L. (1961): Reading epilepsy. *Electroencephalogr. Clin. Neurophysiol.* **13**, 315.

Commission on Classification and Terminology of the International League against Epilepsy (1989): Proposal for revised classification of epilepsies and epileptic syndromes. *Epilepsia* **30**, 389–399.

Chritchley, M., Cobb, W. & Sears, T.A. (1959): On reading epilepsy. *Epilepsia* **1**, 403–417.

Daly, R.F. & Forster, F.M. (1975): Inheritance of reading epilepsy. *Neurology* **25**, 1051–1054.

Forster, F.M. & Daly, R.F. (1973): Reading epilepsy in identical twins. *Trans. Am. Neurol. Ass.* **98**, 186–188.

Forstner, G., Ferguson, R. & Jones, D.P. (1961): Reading epilepsy. *Can. Med. Assoc. J.* **85**, 608–609.

Greenberg, D.A., Durner, M., Resor, S., Rosenbaum & D. Shinnar, S. (1995): The genetics of idiopathic generalized epilepsies of adolescent onset. *Neurology* **45**, 942–946.

Hall, J.H. & Marshall, P.C. (1980): Clonazepam therapy in reading epilepsy. *Neurology* **30**, 550–551.

Inoue, Y., Seino, M., Kubato, H., Yamakaku, K., Tanaka, M. & Yagi, K. (1994): Epilepsy with praxis-induced seizures. In: *Epileptic seizures and syndromes*, P.Wolf (ed.), pp 81–91. London: John Libbey.

Kartsounis, L.D. (1988): Comprehension as the effective trigger in a case of primary reading epilepsy. *J. Neurol. Neurosurg. Psychiatr.* **51**, 128–130.

Koepp, M.J., Richardson, M.P., Brooks, D.J., Poline, J.B., Friston, K.J. & Duncan, J.S. (1995): [11C]-Diprenorphine activation study in patients with reading epilepsy. *Epilepsia* **36**, Suppl..3 , 138.

Lasater, G.M. (1962): Reading epilepsy. *Arch. Neurol.* **6**, 492–495.

Lee, S.J., Sutherling, W.W., Persing, J.A. & Butler, A.B. (1980): Language-induced seizure. A case of cortical origin. *Arch. Neurol.* **37**, 433–436.

Matricardi, M., Brinciotti, M. & Paciello, F. (1991): Reading epilepsy with absences, television-induced seizures, and pattern sensitivity. *Epilepsy Res.* **9**, 145–147.

Matthews, W.B. & Wright, F.K. (1967): Hereditary primary reading epilepsy. *Neurology* **17**, 919–921.

Mesri, J.C. & Pagano, M.A. (1987): Reading epilepsy. *Epilepsia* **28**, 301–304.

Meyer, J.G. & Wolf, P. (1973): Über primäre Leseepilepsie. *Mit einem kasuistischen Beitrag. Nervenarzt* **44**, 155–160.

Miyamoto, A., Takahashi, S., Tokumitsu, A. & Oki, J. (1995): Ictal HMPAO-single photon emission computed tomography findings in reading epilepsy in a Japanese boy. *Epilepsia* **36**, 1161–1163.

Newmann, P.K. & Longly, B.P. (1984): Reading epilepsy. *Arch. Neurol.* **41**, 13–14.

Posner, M.I., Petersen, S.E., Fox, P.T. & Raichle, M.E.(1988): Localization of cognitive operations in the human brain. *Science* **240**, 1627–1631.

Radhakrishan, K., Silbert, P.L. & Klass, D.W. (1995): Reading epilepsy. An appraisal of 20 patients diagnosed at the Mayo Clinic, Rochester, Minnesota, between 1949 and 1989, and delineation of the epileptic syndrome. *Brain* **118**, 75–89.

Ramani, V. (1983): Primary reading epilepsy. *Arch. Neurol.* **40**, 39–41.

Ried, S., Behl, I. & Schmidt, D. (1991): Leseepilepsie: eine Variante des Impulsiv-Petit mal? In: *Epilepsie 90*, Scheffner, D. (ed.), pp. 168–173. Reinbeck: Einhorn-Presse.

Ritaccio, A.L., Hickling, E.J. & Ramani, V. (1992): The Role of Dominant Premotor Cortex and Grapheme to Phoneme Transformation in reading epilepsy. *Arch. Neurol.* **49**, 933–939.

Rowan, A.J., Heathfield, K.G.W. & Scott, D.F. (1970): Is reading epilepsy inherited? *J. Neurol. Neurosurg. Psychiatry* **33**, 476–478.

Saenz-Lope, E., Herranz-Tanarro, F.J. & Masdeu, J.C. (1985): Primary reading epilepsy. *Epilepsia* **26**, 649–656.

Sander, T, Hildmann, T., Janz, D., Bianchi, A., Bauer, G., Scaramelli, A. & Beck-Mannagetta, G. (1996): Lack of linkage between idiopathic generalized epilepsies and the gene encoding the neural cell adhesion molecule. *Epilepsy Res.* **25**, 139–145.

Serratosa, J.M., Delgado-Escueta, A.V., Medina, M.T., Zhang, Q., Iranmanesh, R. & Sparkes, R.S. (1996): Clinical and genetic analysis of a large pedigree with JME. *Ann. Neurol.* **39**, 187–195.

Vanderzant, Ch., Fitz, R., Holmes, G., Greeberg, H.S. & Sackellares, J. Ch. (1982): Treatment of primary reading epilepsy with valproic acid. *Arch. Neurol.* **39**, 452–453.

Wolf, P. (1978): Reading epilepsy: evidence for a cognitive factor in seizure precipitation. In: *Advances in epileptology*, Meinradi, H. & Rowan, A.J. (eds), pp. 85–90. Amsterdam, Lisse: Swets Zeitlinger.

Wolf, P. (1989): Reflex epilepsies and syndrome classification. An argument for considering primary reading epilepsy as an idiopathic localization-related epilepsy. In: *Reflex seizures and reflex epilepsies*, Beaumanoir, A., Gastaut, H. & Naquet, R. (eds), pp. 283–286. Genève: Médecine et Hygène.

Wolf, P. & Goosses, R. (1986): Relation of photosensitivity to epileptic syndromes. *J. Neurol. Neurosurg. Psychiatry* **49,** 1386–1391.

Wolf, P. (1992): Reading epilepsy. In: *Epileptic syndromes in infancy, childhood and adolescence* (2nd. edition), Roger, J., Dravet, Ch., Bureau, M., Dreifuss, F.E., Perret, A. & Wolf, P. (eds), pp. 281–298. London: John Libbey.

Chapter 18

Pathophysiology and genetics of hot-water epilepsy

P. Satishchandra[1], Gautam R. Ulla[3], Anindya Sinha[4], S.K. Shankar[2]

Department of Neurology[1] and Neuropathology[2], National Institute of Mental Health & Neurosciences (NIMHANS), Bangalore, India; [3]Department of Physiology, M.S.Ramaiah Medical College, ME-RL, Bangalore, India; [4]National Institute of Advanced Studies, Indian Institute of Science, Bangalore, India

The convulsions precipitated by a sensory stimulus are described as reflex or sensory epilepsy (Gastuat 1973). As the seizure-inducing mechanism rather than the aetiology constitutes the common factor in these seizures, the term 'sensory precipitation of seizures' proposed by Penfield (1941) is probably more appropriate. Epilepsy precipitated by the stimulus of bathing with hot water pouring over the head is known as 'hot-water epilepsy (HWE) (Mani *et al.*, 1968, 1975; Subramanyam, 1972; Szymonowicz & Meloff, 1978; Satishchandra *et al.*, 1988) or 'water-immersion epilepsy' (Mofenson *et al.*, 1965) or 'bathing epilepsy' (Shaw *et al.*, 1988; Lenoir *et al.*, 1989).

Allen (1945) from New Zealand described the first case of seizures precipitated by contact with hot water. Following this, there were isolated case reports from Australia (Keipert, 1969), United States (Stensman & Ursing, 1971), Canada (Szymonowicz & Meloff, 1978), United Kingdom (Parasonage *et al.*, 1976) and Japan (Kurata, 1979; Miyao *et al.*, 1982; Morimoto *et al.*, 1985). However, large numbers of patients with HWE have been reported from India (Mani *et al.*, 1975; Subramanyam, 1972; Satishchandra *et al.*, 1985, 1988; Gururaj & Satishchandra, 1992). A large series consisting of 279 cases of HWE seen over 4 years in a tertiary institution (1980–83) has been published from Bangalore, South India (Satishchandra *et al.*, 1988). A recently concluded house-to-house survey (Bangalore urban-rural Neuroepidemiological survey) in South India, found that HWE accounts for 6.9 per cent of all epilepsies in this community giving a prevalence of 60 per 100,000 (Satishchandra *et al.*, unpublished data).

Clinical features

Seizures in HWE are precipitated by a hot water bath or immersion in a hot water tub. In Southern India it is customary to bathe everyday, however washing of the head is done generally once every 3–15 days. People pour mugfuls of hot water from a bucket in quick succession directly over the body or head. The temperature of the hot water used ranges between 40–50 °C (ambient room temperature is 25–30 °C). This type of HWE has been reported in people having a hot shower or tub bath from all over the world (Table 1). Children are more frequently affected, although it has been reported in adults from South India (Mani *et al.*, 1968; Subramanyam, 1972; Satishchandra *et al.*, 1985, 1988). Males are affected more frequently in the ratio of 2–2.5 times that of females. The frequency of these seizures depends upon the frequency of head bathing. At a later stage in the natural history, 5–10 per cent of these patients have seizures even during a 'body bath', when water is not poured over head.

The seizures are of complex partial type with or without secondary generalization. Symptoms at onset included a dazed look, a sense of fear, irrelevant speech, and visual and auditory hallucinations with complex automatisms. One third of all reported cases have generalized tonic–clonic seizures (Table 1). These seizures have been witnessed in the laboratory and have been documented on video in few cases (Stensman & Ursing, 1971; Kurata, 1979; Szymonowicz & Meloff, 1978; Satishchandra et al., 1988). About 10 per cent of subjects expressed intense pleasure and continued to pour hot water over the head until they lost consciousness. These seizures last 1–3 min and could occur either at the beginning or at the end of the bath. A positive history of epilepsy among the family members has been reported in 7–23 per cent of cases. Spontaneous non-reflex epilepsy was reported a few years later in 16–38 per cent of patients (Mani et al., 1975; Subramanyam, 1972; Satishchandra et al., 1988). Neurological examination is normal.

Table 1. Published literature of hot water epilepsy

Authors (date)	No. of cases	Sex	Age at onset	Type of seizures	Temperature of water (in °C)	Development of non-reflex epilepsy
Allen (1945)	1	M	10 y	CPS	?	No
Mofenson et al.(1965)	1	M	7 m	Gen	37–48	No
Mani et al. (1968, 1975)	108	72 M 28 F	6–15 y	CPS Gen	40–50	16 %
Keipert (1969)	1	M	5 m	CPS	?	No
Stensman & Ursing (1971)	1	M	7 m	CPS	37.5	No
Onuma et al. (1972)	1	F	2 y	CPS	> 39	No
Subramanyam (1972)	26	58 M 42 F	2 m – 35 y	CPS Gen	40–55	38 %
Parsonage et al. (1976)	3	2 M 1 F	5–21 y	CPS	?	No
Szymonowicz & Meloff (1978)	1	M	18 m	CPS	37–38	100 %
Itoh et al. (1979)	1	M	5.5 y	Gen	39	No
Kurata (1979)	12	33 M 67 F	5 m – 9 y	Gen Atonic	40–43	100 %
Miyao et al. (1982)	3	2 M 1 F	3 y	Gen	?	100 %
Satishchandra et al. (1988)	279	72 M 28 F	2 m – 58 y	CPS Gen	40–50	25.4 %
Roos (1988)	1	M	8 m	CPS	40	?
Shaw et al. (1988)	1	M	5 m	CPS	37	No
Lenoir et al. (1989)	2	1 M 1 F	12 m	CPS	37	50 %
Gururaj & Satishchandra (1992)	78	61 M 17 F	6 m – 58 y	CPS Gen	40–50	12.8 %

CPS: Complex partial seizures; Gen: Generalized seizures;
Y: Year, M – Month; ?: Not reported; M: Male; F: Females.

Interictal scalp electroencephalography is usually normal or shows diffuse abnormalities in 15–20 per cent of cases (Subramanyam, 1972; Mani et al., 1975; Satishchandra et al., 1988). Lateralized or localized spike discharges have been reported in a few isolated cases (Onuma et al., 1972; Szymonowicz & Meloff, 1978; Morimoto, 1985). Ictal EEG recording has technical limitations. However, seven reports in the literature have ictal recordings during provocation in water immersion epilepsy. They have demonstrated left temporal rhythmic delta activity (Stensman & Ursing, 1971), sharp and slow waves in the left hemisphere (Parsonage et al., 1976), bilateral spikes (Morimoto et al., 1985) and temporal spikes (Shaw et al., 1988). Roos et al. (1987) had simultaneous split-screen video EEG recording in one patient of 'bathing epilepsy' and demonstrated delta waves starting from the right hemisphere with rapid secondary generalization.

Pathophysiology

Stensman & Ursing (1971) suggested that this type of epilepsy is precipitated by complex tactile and temperature dependent stimuli. Though it was possible to provoke the seizure in the laboratory by pouring hot water over the heads of these patients, hot water towels, sauna or blowing hot air on the head failed to induce seizures. This suggests that the triggering stimulus is complex and would involve a combination of factors such as contact of scalp with hot water, temperature of the water and specific cortical areas of stimulation etc. As complex partial seizures are the commonest variety of seizure, and ictal EEG demonstrates focal activity in the temporal or frontal lobe, Syzmonowicz & Meloff (1976) suggested that there could be structural lesions in the temporal lobe. However, available information from CT/MRI in such patients have not shown the presence of any focal structural lesions. Even if such lesions were present, it is still not clear whether the mechanism of seizure depends upon locally increased neuronal excitability in the lesions or pathological involvement of lower centres such as the hypothalamus, or both (Parsonage et al., 1976). Shankar & Satishchandra (1994) published pathological findings in four of their hot water epilepsy patients. All had spontaneous non-reflex epilepsy subsequent to the onset of HWE. Two succumbed during status epilepticus and one due to incidental vertebrobasilar insufficiency. Another developed symptoms of raised intracranial tension 15 years after the onset of HWE and had a diffuse low grade astrocytoma in the thalamus. Pathological examination of these brains demonstrated a variable degree of hippocampal sclerosis (Table 2). The neuronal loss and gliosis seen in the anterior hippocampus of these brains were similar to that described with chronic temporal lobe epilepsy (Rasmussen, 1983). Associated anoxic changes prevented any critical quantitative assessment of the hippocampal or parahippocampal pathology.

Published literature from India reports that 11–27 per cent HWE patients had febrile convulsions prior to the development of this reflex epilepsy (Mani et al., 1975; Satishchandra et al., 1988; Subramanyam 1972). This association has not been noted from other parts of the world for other types of focal epilepsy. Febrile convulsions were found to be associated with complex partial seizures as an important risk factor in 20 per cent of the population (Rocca et al., 1987) in a case-control study from Rochester Minnesota. Hence association of febrile convulsions and HWE is not higher than that one would expect. The clinical behaviour of HWE patients during incidental febrile episodes with respect to susceptibility to seizures is under investigation.

Experimental seizures can be induced in mature rats by repeated exposure of the head to hot water (45 °C), which is comparable to the phenomenon of 'kindling' by repeated stimulation using subthreshold electrical currents. Klauenberg & Sparber (1984) called this 'hyperthermic kindling'. Satishchandra et al. (1988) postulated 'hyperthermic kindling' might be responsible for the development of HWE in humans. To further understand the pathophysiological and pharmacological mechanisms underlying HWE, an experimental animal model mimicking human HWE in its entirety – precipitating stimulus, the ictal events and EEG – has been developed (Satishchandra et al., 1993; Ullal et al., 1996).

Table 2. Pathological features in HWE epilepsy*

Case no.	Age (yr) and sex	Duration of epilepsy (yr)	Type of seizures	Pathology	Cause of death
1	23 M	15	GTCS	Right thalamic glioma spreading to Rt.temporal lobe and surface meninges	Hypothalamic failure during postoperative period
2	65 M	53	CPS	Cerebral atrophy with mild neuronal loss and hippocampal sclerosis on both sides	VBI
3	12 M	1	CPS	Neuronal loss, moderate degree of gliosis in dentate, gyrus of hippocampus right more than left	Status epilepticus
4	1.5 M	1	SPS	Ischaemic changes in left frontal and parietal with laminar necrosis	Status epilepticus
			CPS	Ischaemic changes with sclerosis in hippocampus and reticular nuclei of brainstem	

*All had non-reflex spontaneous epilepsy following hot water epilepsy.
GTCS: Primary generalized epilepsy, CPS: complex partial seizures, SPS: Simple partial seizures, VBI: Vertebrobasilar insufficiency.

The rapid rise in rectal temperature following thermal stimulus in seizure-susceptible rats in comparison to the seizure-resistant ones indicate the possible role of the thermoregulatory centre in initiating the seizure discharge (Ullal et al., 1996a). There could be certain constitutional genetic traits among the Wistar rats which makes some animals seizure-resistant and others seizure prone (Ullal et al., 1995). Stimulating seizure sensitive rats at predetermined frequency for seven times in 96 h followed by delayed 8th and 9th stimulation on 15th and 30 days after the 7th stimulus, a progressive increase in seizure duration and severity and decrease in rectal and hippocampal temperature threshold was noted. This feature persisted subsequently, even after 30 days, suggesting a phenomenon of 'hyperthermic kindling' in these animals. Such hyperthermic seizures in animals could easily be blocked by using antiepileptic drugs such as phenobarbital and benzodiazepine, but phenytoin and calcium channel blocker nifedipine were ineffective (Ullal et al., 1996b).

Recording the body temperature through a thermistor kept inside the auditory canal in the susceptible humans with HWE, during hot water head bathing has demonstrated a 'rapid spurt' in the temperature of 2–3 °F within the short span of 2 min. Further it takes 10–12 min for this temperature to return to the baseline, once the bath is completed, which is in comparison to the rise of 0.5 to 0.6 °F noted in the normal healthy volunteers, which return to baseline immediately at the end of the bath. This suggests that this special form of induced hyperthermia could be responsible for causing HWE in these susceptible individuals (Satishchandra et al., 1995). We postulate that HWE patients probably have an aberrant thermoregulatory system and hence are extremely sensitive to the rapid rise in temperature occurring during hot water head bathing which precipitates seizures. This aberrant thermoregulation seems to be genetically determined and further work to elucidate this hypothesis is currently under investigation. The rat model described simulates human HWE and gives new evidence that human HWE is not a true reflex epilepsy but a 'hyperthermic' seizure (Ullal et al., 1996a).

Genetics of hot water epilepsy

A family history of hot water epilepsy has been reported in 7–15 per cent of Indian probands (Satishchandra et al., 1988; Mani et al., 1975). Ito et al. (1979) from Japan reported HWE in

Chapter 18 Pathophysiology and genetics of hot-water epilepsy

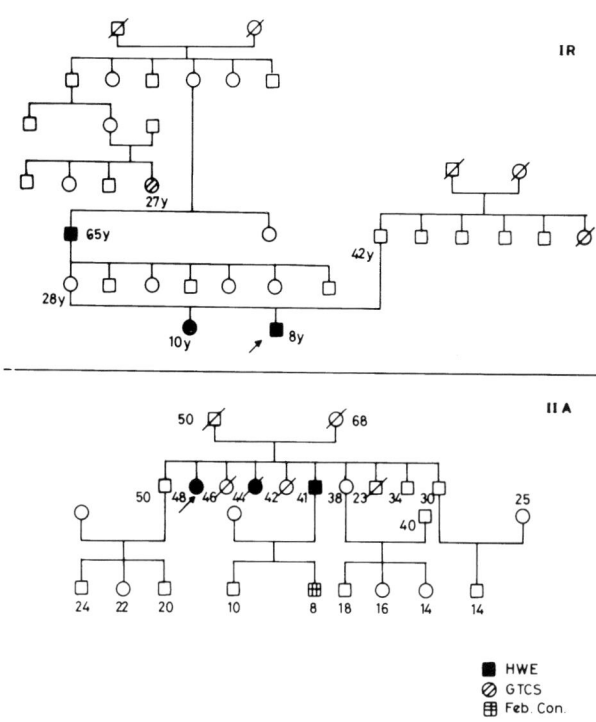

Fig. 1. Pedigree charts of familial hot-water epilepsy.

monozygotic twins. Among 279 patients of HWE reported from South India, there were three dizygotic twins each with one member affected (Satishchandra et al., 1988). HWE was familial in 18 per cent of cases in an epidemiological study conducted in rural Bangalore, South India. This included one family with all the seven members having HWE for more than 24 months (Gururaj & Satishchandra, 1992).

Following the observation of induced hyperthermia and postulation of aberrant thermoregulation in the susceptible population, recently Satishchandra et al. (1995) reviewed their cases for familial HWE and found five families with two or three members manifesting the disease (Figs. 1, 2 and 3).

The classical example of a hyperthermic seizure is the febrile convulsion. Febrile convulsions affect 2–5 per cent of all children under the age of 5 years. They have a variety of causes, but a genetic component has been recognized for a long time. Its mode of inheritance is still not known. Earlier published reports have suggested a polygenic mode of inheritance (Tsuboi, 1982; Maher & McLachian, 1995), an autosomal dominant inheritance with reduced penetrance (Frantzen et al., 1970) or an autosomal recessive inheritance (Schuman & Miller, 1966). Recently a large family has been described from Australia in which febrile convulsion appeared to result from autosomal dominant inheritance at a single major locus. Previously mapped epilepsy genes were excluded and a genome-wide search, using microsatellite markers, suggested that a locus on chromosome 8q13–21 may be involved (Wallace et al., 1996).

The genetic mechanism underlying the expression of hot water epilepsy in humans is still not known. We studied five pedigrees; two of these families also exhibited primary generalized epilepsy among siblings and offspring of individuals affected by HWE. A single-locus model was invoked to explain the inheritance pattern of HWE in these families (Strickberger, 1976). Dominant inheritance, either autosomal or sex-linked, was unlikely since quite a few generations in these pedigrees showed absolutely no evidence of being afflicted. An X-linked recessive trait was also an unlikely mechanism since (i) the parental generation in all three families with groups of severely affected siblings were completely asymptomatic (families IR, IIA and VN); and (ii) in that event, none of the daughters of the normal males and the asymptomatic (but necessarily) carrier females in these families should have been affected by HWE.

An autosomal recessive mutation leading to HWE in the homozygous condition is, however, a distinct possibility and can explain the specific appearance of the disease phenotype and its observed distribution among offspring of both sexes in all the five lineages. This would also require, of course,

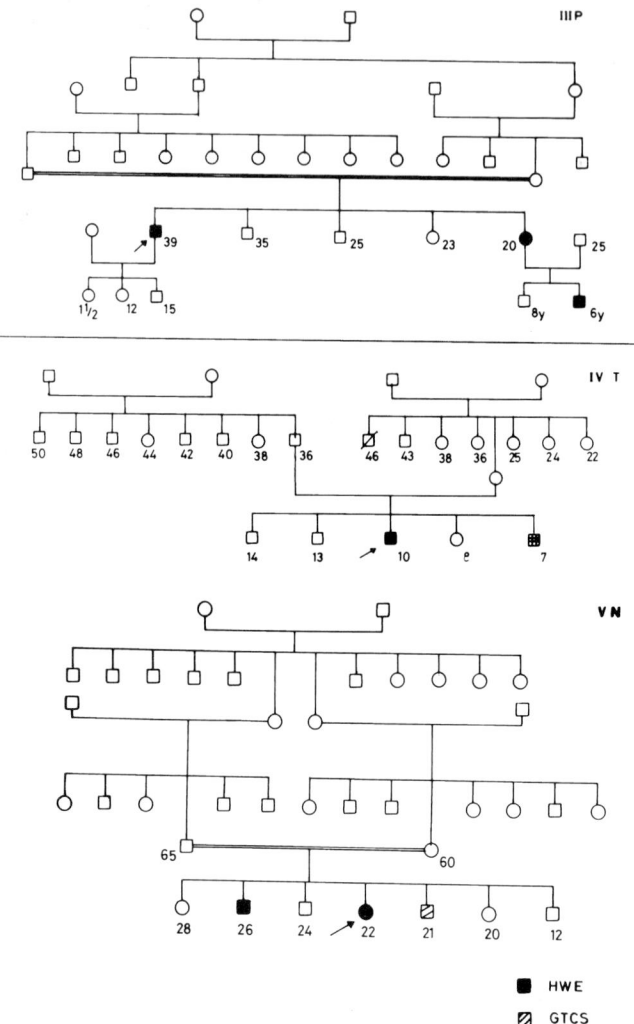

Figs. 2 & 3. Pedigree charts of familial hot-water epilepsy.

that both be asymptomatic carriers of the trait. We speculate that although the frequency of such a mutation in a particular population would be fairly low, the traditionally high incidence of consanguineous marriages in many South Indian families (Ramadevi et al., 1982) could lead to a marked increase in the appearance of HWE in these populations. This is exemplified rather strikingly by two of the five observed lineages IIIP and VN where marriages between first cousins have yielded a number of HWE-afflicted children.

There does not appear to be any strong evidence of a genetic link between HWE and primary generalized epilepsy although, in a single family (VN) the latter did affect a sibling of two individuals with full-blown HWE. Febrile convulsions, on the other hand, occurred in close relatives (both siblings and offspring) of HWE-afflicted individuals in two of the five lineages (IIA and IVT respectively).

The single-locus model is, however, insufficient to explain any genetic linkage between these conditions; the influence of a modifier locus (or loci) or of environmental factors may need to be invoked to account for their co-occurrence.

We are currently exploring more complex multigenic models for the possible genetic link between HWE and febrile convulsions; these would, however, require substantiation through detailed genetic analysis of a much larger number of lineages given the paucity of detailed family records. We are also developing a mouse model system to conduct classical and molecular genetic studies on HWE. In addition, such a model system could effectively contribute to our further understanding of the pathophysiology and biochemistry of this disease.

Acknowledgement : We thank Mr. M.V. Srinivasan for secretarial assistance.

References

Allen, I.M. (1945): Observation on cases of reflex epilepsy. *N.Z. Med. J.* **44**, 135–142.

Frantzen, E., Lennox-Buchthal, M., Nygaard, A. & Stene, J. (1970): A genetic study of febrile convulsions. *Neurology* **20**, 909–917.

Gastuat, H. (1973): *Dictionary of Epilepsy Part I*. Geneva: World Health Organization.

Gururaj, G. & Satishchandra, P. (1992): Correlates of hot water epilepsy in rural South India: A descriptive study. *Neuroepidemiology* **11**, 173–179.

Itoh, N., Kurita, I. & Konno, K. (1979): A case of hot-water epilepsy in the monozygotic co-twin. *Folia Psychiat. Neurol. (Japan)* **33**, 329–330.

Keipert, J.A. (1969): Epilepsy precipitated by bathing: water-immersion epilepsy. *Aust. Paediatr. J.* **5**, 244–247.

Klauenberg, B.J. & Sparber, S.B. (1984): A kindling like effect inducted by repeated exposure to heated water in rats. *Epilepsia* **25**, 292–301.

Kurata, S. (1979): Epilepsy precipitated by bathing – A follow up study. *Brain Dev.* (Domestic ed). **11**, 400–405.

Lenoir, P., Ranet, J. & Demeirleir, L. (1989): Bathing induced seizures. *Pediatr. Neurol.* **5**, 124–125

Mani, K.S., Gopalakrishnan, P.N., Vyas, J.N. & Pillai, M.S. (1968): Hot-water epilepsy – A peculiar type of reflex epilepsy, a preliminary report. *Neurology (India)* **16**, 107–110.

Mani, K.S., Mani, A.J. & Ramesh, C.K. (1975): Hot water epilepsy, A peculiar type of reflex epilepsy. Clinical and electroencephalographic features in 108 cases. *Trans. Am. Neurol. Assoc.* **99**, 224–226.

Maher, J. & McLachlan, R.S. (1995): Febrile convulsions. Is seizure duration the most important predictor of temporal lobe epilepsy? *Brain* **118**, 1521–1528.

Merlis, J.K. (1974): Reflex epilepsy. In: *Handbook of Clinical Neurology* (Vol 15), Vinken, P.J. & Bruyn, G.W. (eds), pp. 440–456. Amsterdam: North Holland Publishing.

Miyao, M., Tezuka, M., Kuwajima, K. & Kamoshita, S. (1982): Epilepsy induced by hot water immersion. *Brain Dev.* **4**, 158.

Mofenson, H.C., Weymuller, C.A. & Greensher, J. (1965): Epilepsy due to water immersion – An unusual case of reflex sensory epilepsy, *JAMA* **191**, 600–601.

Morimoto, T., Hayakawa, T., Sugie, H., Awaya, Y. & Fukuyama, Y. (1985): Epileptic seizures precipitated by constant light, movement in daily life and hot water immersion. *Epilepsia* **26**, 237–242.

Onuma, T., Fukushima, Y., Takeda, T., Osawa, T. & Sato, T. (1972): A case of epilepsy precipitated by hot-water immersion. *Clin. Neurol. (Tokyo)* **12**, 386–393.

Parsonage, M.J., Moran, J.H. & Exley, K.A. (1976): So called water immersion epilepsy. *Epileptology Proc 7th Internat Symp. on Epilepsy*, pp. 50–60. Stuttgart: Thieme.

Rasmussen, T.B. (1983): Surgical treatment of complex partial seizures – results, lesions and problems. *Epilepsia* **24** (Suppl.), 565–576.

Ramadevi, A.R., Rao, N.A. & Bittles, A.H. (1982): Inbreeding in the State of Karnataka, South India. *Hum. Herid.* **32**, 8–10.

Rocca, W.A., Sharbrough, F.W., Hauser, W.A., Annegers, J.F. & Schoenberg, B.S. (1987): Risk factors for complex partial seizures: a population based case-control study. *Ann. Neurol.* **21,** 22–31.

Roos, R.A.C. & Van Diyk, J.E. (1988): Reflex epilepsy induced by immersion in hot water. *Eur. Neurol.* **28,** 6–10.

Satishchandra, P., Shivaramakrishna, A. & Kaliaperumal, V.G. (1985): Hot water epilepsy – A variant of reflex epilepsy in parts of South India. *J. Neurol.* **232** (Suppl.), 212.

Satishchandra, P., Shivaramakrishna, A., Kaliaperumal, V.G. & Schoenberg, B.S. (1988): Hot water epilepsy – A variant of reflex epilepsy in Southern India. *Epilepsia* **29,** 52–56.

Satishchandra, P., Ullal, G.R. & Shankar, S.K. (1993): Experimental animal model for hot water epilepsy. *Epilepsia* **34** Suppl (2), 101

Satishchandra, P., Ullal, G.R. & Shankar, S.K. (1995): Newer insight into the complexity of hot-water epilepsy. *Epilepsia* **36**(Suppl. 3), 206–207.

Satishchandra, P., Ullal, G.R. & Shankar, S.K. (1996): Genetics of Hot-Water Epilepsy. Presented at Workshop in 'Genetics of focal epilepsies: experimental and clinical correlates at Avignon, France, Sept. 1996.

Schuman, S.H. & Miller, L.J. (1966): Febrile convulsions in families: findings in an epidemiological survey. *Clin. Pediatr. (Phil.)* **5,** 604–608.

Shankar, S.K. & Satishchandra, P. (1994): Autopsy study of brains in hot water epilepsy. *Neurology (India)* **42,** 56–57.

Shaw, N.J., Livingston, J.H., Minns, R.A. & Clarke, M. (1988): Epilepsy precipitated by bathing. *Dev. Med. Child Neurol.* **30,** 108–111.

Stensman, R. & Ursing, B. (1971): Epilepsy precipitated by hot water immersion. *Neurology* **21,** 559–562.

Strickberger, M.W. (1976): *Genetics* (2nd ed). New York: McMillan Publishing Company.

Subrahmanayam, H.S. (1972): Hot water epilepsy. *Neurology (India)* **20**(Suppl. II): 241–243.

Szymonowicz, W. & Meloff, K.L. (1978): Hot water epilepsy. *Can. J. Neurol. Sci.* **5,** 247–251.

Tsuboi, T. (1982): Febrile convulsions. In: *Genetic basis of the epilepsies*, Anderson, V.E., Hauser, W.A., Penry, J.K. & Sing, C.F. (eds), pp.123–134. New York: Raven Press.

Ullal, G.R., Satishchandra, P. & Shankar, S.K. (1995): Seizure patterns, hippocampal and rectal temperature threshold with hyperthermic kindling in rats on hot-water stimulation. *Epilepsia* **36** (Suppl. 3) 552.

Ullal, G.R., Satishchandra, P. & Shankar, S.K. (1996a): Hyperthermic seizures: an animal model for hot-water epilepsy. *Seizure* 221–228.

Ullal, G.R., Satishchandra, P. & Shankar, S.K. (1996b): Effect of antiepileptic drugs and calcium channel blocker on hyperthermic seizures in Rats: animal model for hot-water epilepsy. *Indian J. Physiol. Pharmacol.* **40,** 303–308.

Velmurugendran, C.U. (1985): Reflex epilepsy. *J. Neurol.* **232**(Suppl.), 212.

Wallace, R.H., Berkovic, S.F., Howell, R.A., Sutherland, G.R. & Mulley, J.C. (1996): Suggestion of a major gene for familial febrile convulsions mapping to 8q 13–21. *J. Med. Genet.* **33,** 308–312.

Part VI
Molecular biology

Chapter 19

Molecular biology in autosomal dominant nocturnal frontal lobe epilepsy

Ortrud K. Steinlein

Institute for Human Genetics, University of Bonn, Germany

Although it has long been recognized that genetic factors play a major role in the aetiology of idiopathic epilepsies, the molecular mechanisms are largely unknown. Familial clustering of common generalized idiopathic epilepsy subtypes suggests a multiplicative contribution of several loci. In contrast to the common idiopathic epilepsies, like childhood absence epilepsy, juvenile absence epilepsy, or juvenile myoclonic epilepsy, some rare focal and generalized forms are inherited as autosomal dominant traits. Genes for two monogenic traits, benign familial neonatal convulsions and autosomal dominant nocturnal frontal lobe epilepsy, have been assigned to the same candidate region on chromosome 20q13.2-q13.3. The region was physically mapped and partially subcloned into cosmids. Expression analysis identified the gene coding for the neuronal nicotinic acetylcholine receptor inside the candidate region. Screening for mutations revealed a missense mutation (Ser248Phe) in the second transmembrane domain of the gene as the molecular defect underlying nocturnal frontal lobe epilepsy in a large Australian pedigree. The mutation lead to hypoactivity of the receptor via accelerated desensitization, thus possibly disturbing the balance between inhibitory and excitatory synaptic transmission.

Autosomal dominant nocturnal frontal lobe epilepsy

Autosomal dominant nocturnal frontal lobe epilepsy (ADNFLE) was linked to the chromosomal region 20q13.2-q13.3 in one large Australian pedigree (Phillips *et al.*, 1995). This autosomal dominant partial epilepsy is characterized by clusters of brief nocturnal motor seizures, which are often misdiagnosed as night terrors, nightmares, hysteria, or paroxysmal nocturnal dystonia. Seizures start in childhood or early adulthood and usually persist through adult life. Most of the seizures occur shortly after the patients fall asleep or in the early hours of the morning. Some patients also experience seizures during daytime naps. Loss of consciousness due to secondary generalization is reported by several patients at some time. In most cases the seizures can be controlled by carbamazepine, while sodium valproate is generally not effective (Scheffer *et al.*, 1995; see Chapter 9, this volume). ADNFLE was the first human partial epilepsy syndrome shown to follow an autosomal dominant mode of inheritance. Interestingly, two other genetic loci have been previously assigned to the chromosomal region around the polymorphic markers CMM6 (D20S19) and RMR6 (D20S20) on chromosome 20q13.2-q13.3 (Fig. 1): benign familial neonatal convulsions (gene symbol *EBN1*;

Leppert et al., 1989) and the low voltage electroencephalogram (gene symbol *EEGV1*; Steinlein et al., 1992a).

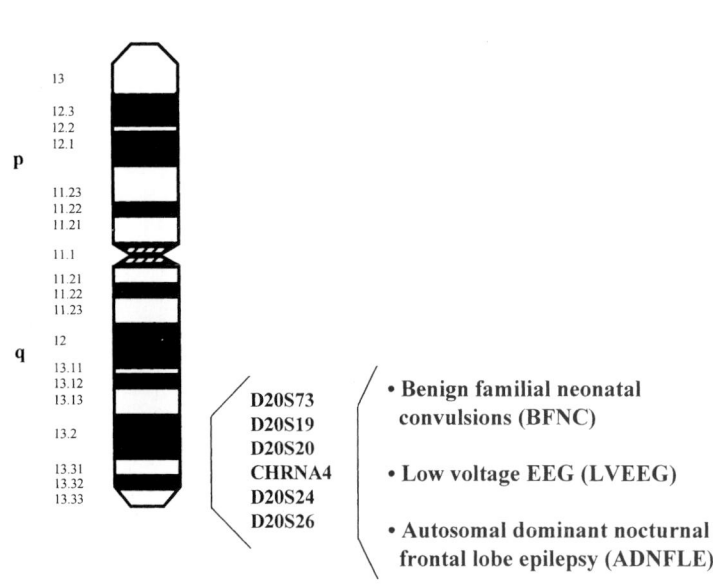

Fig. 1. *Chromosome 20. The exact physical order of the polymorphic markers is not known. CHRNA4 is located in the 160 kb interval between D20S20 and D20S24.*

Benign familial neonatal convulsions

Benign familial neonatal convulsions (BFNC) are an example of a rare autosomal dominant epilepsy first described by Rett & Teubel (1964). Unprovoked partial or generalized clonic convulsions, which occur during wakefulness and sleep, typically start around day three after birth and in most cases disappear spontaneously after several weeks or months. Seizure duration varies between seconds and several minutes, with a seizure frequency between three and six per day. The interictal electroencephalogram and subsequent intellectual development are usually normal. BFNC, in most cases, has a favourable outcome, but about 12 per cent of the patients will have epileptic seizures again later in their life. Most of these later seizures are generalized, tonic, or tonic–clonic. Interestingly, some of the patients have only nocturnal seizures (Ronen et al., 1993). Locus heterogeneity has been shown, and in the meantime evidence was found for the localization of a second BFNC gene on chromosome 8 (gene symbol *EBN2*; Lewis et al., 1993; Steinlein et al., 1994).

Low voltage EEG

Despite the fact that the normal human electroencephalogram (EEG) shows a high degree of inter-individual variability, the resting EEG pattern of healthy adults maintains its individual characteristics, which is largely genetically determined, over many years (Vogel, 1986). Some variants of the EEG have been shown to be monogenetically inherited. The low voltage EEG (LVEEG) is a common variant of the normal human EEG (prevalence 4–5 per cent) with an autosomal dominant mode of inheritance. It is characterized by the absence or reduction of alpha activity in the resting

EEG. The only exceptions are short segments of alpha rhythm appearing immediately after the closure of the eyes (Anokhin *et al.*, 1992). Several mechanisms generating alpha waves have been proposed, but they are still poorly understood and little is known about their site of origin. A thalamic pacemaker involved in the synchronization of the EEG and an intracortical surface parallel network of neurons are possible explanations. In any case, the mechanisms leading to the synchronization of the electrophysiological brain activity are complex. But as shown by the autosomal dominant mode of inheritance of the LVEEG, the variation of one single gene is sufficient to change or suppress the pattern of synchronization. Thirty per cent of the studied families with LVEEG have been linked to D20S19 (Steinlein *et al.*, 1992a).

Genetic studies

Despite the co-localization of the genes, BFNC and ADNFLE are clinically distinct epileptic disorders. Frontal lobe seizures have never been described in BFNC patients and vice versa. Furthermore, no family members with LVEEG have been described in families with BFNC or ADNFLE so far. However, due to the high frequency of LVEEG in the adult population and the unknown effect of epilepsy, or a predisposition to epilepsy, on this EEG variant, an association between this phenotype and BFNC or ADNFLE might be difficult to prove. However, with respect to the localization in the same candidate region, it can not be ruled out that at least some of these phenotypes are due to different mutations in the same gene, and are therefore allelic.

The candidate region for the three phenotypes on chromosome 20q13.2-q13.3 (Fig. 1) has been studied using the methods of positional cloning, including genetic and physical mapping as well as cosmid- and P1 cloning (Steinlein *et al.*, 1992b). The polymorphic markers in this region, like D20S20, D20S19, D20S73 (MS217), and D20S24 (IP20K09), are closely linked on the physical map. Unfortunately, due to the lack of recombination events observed in sufficiently large families, the distal and proximal boundaries, and therefore the exact size of the candidate region are not known. Probably the region spans not more than 500–1000 kb. Several so-called CpG-islands were found inside the region. CpG-islands are short stretches of unmethylated CpG nucleotides, which are often located close to expressed sequences. They provide a landmarks in the genome, and are useful for the optimization of cloning strategies. With respect to the short physical intervals a combined cosmid- and P1-cloning method was chosen. The 420 kb of genomic DNA cloned from the candidate region were screened for expressed sequences. Several cDNA's belonging to different genes have been identified in the region. As predicted from the homology between parts of mouse chromosome 2 and human chromosome 20 (Pilz *et al.*, 1992), the gene coding for the $\alpha 4$ subunit of the neuronal nicotinic acetylcholine receptor (CHRNA4) was found to be located in the candidate region (Steinlein *et al.*, 1994). CHRNA4 has been mapped between the polymorphic markers D20S20 and D20S24 (IP20K09).

Neuronal nicotinic acetylcholine receptors

Two different types of receptors respond to acetylcholine: muscarinic and nicotinic receptors. The nicotinic acetylcholine receptors can be further subdivided into the muscle and the neuronal type. Together with glycine-, $GABA_A$- and $5-HT_3$-receptors the neuronal nicotinic acetylcholine receptors (nAChRs) belong to a supergene family of ligand gated receptors. While only two different subtypes of the muscle receptor exist (foetal and adult type, differing by one subunit), the nAChRs are highly diverse. The large number of possible neuronal subtypes is due to the observation that at least 11 subunits might be expressed in the brain (Le Novere, 1995). The pentameric receptors are formed through varying combinations of subunits arranged around a central channel (Fig. 2). Several subunits have been identified. They are classified as α subunits ($\alpha 2$-$\alpha 9$), if they share, as part of the acetylcholine binding site, a pair of cysteines with the $\alpha 1$ subunit of the muscle-type AChR. Subunits without these cysteine residues are called non-α or β subunits ($\beta 2$-$\beta 4$). The major nAChR subtype in chicken and rat brain was found to be composed of the ACh-binding subunit $\alpha 4$ and the structural

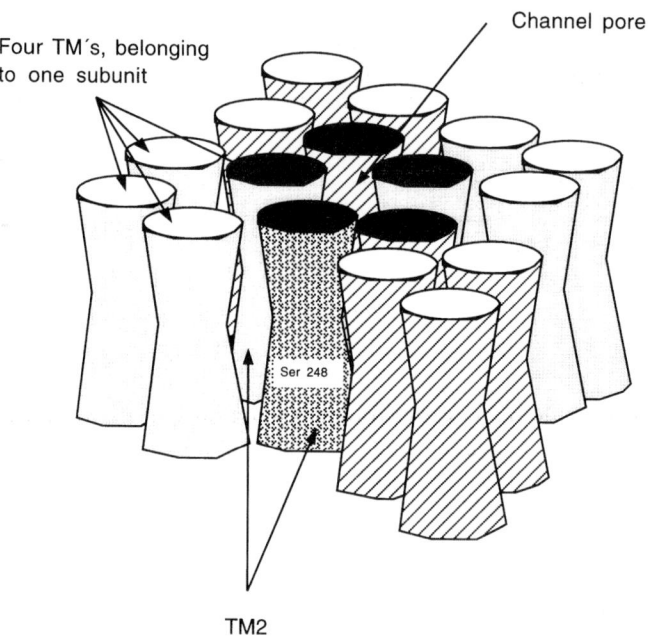

Fig. 2. Model of the neuronal nicotinic acetylcholine receptor. The second transmembrane domains (TM2) of five subunits contribute to the walls of the ion channel. The position of Ser248 is indicated. Transmembrane domains 1 and 3–4 are only shown for four subunits.

subunit β2. It is unknown if this is also true for the human brain. Despite the high number of possible distinct receptor subtypes which can be formed by varying combinations of the different subunit types, not much information has been obtained about the biological role of nAChRs in the mammalian brain. Preliminary results suggest that they may play an important role in the presynaptic enhancement of fast excitatory synaptic transmission (McGehee et al., 1995; Buisson et al., this volume).

α4-Subunit gene (CHRNA4)

The CHRNA4 gene consists of six exons (Fig. 3). Comparison with other members of the neuronal nicotinic AChR subunit family confirmed the conservation of the size of the exons previously described for other species. The open reading frame consists of 627 amino acid residues, with the main part of the coding region distributed in exon 5. The ATG start codon is included in exon 1, the termination signal in exon 6 is followed by at least 637 bp of the 3′ untranslated region. All of the exon-intron splice sites are consistent with the AG/GT rule. Four hydrophobic domains coding for the potential membrane spanning regions (transmembrane domains) are found in characteristic positions (Steinlein et al., 1996). The lumen of the ion channel has shown to be lined by residues from the second membrane spanning region (Hucho et al., 1986; Imoto et al., 1988). The first transmembrane domain probably also contributes to the channel lining (DiPaola et al., 1990). Intron lengths varied between 1.6 and 5.5 kb. A microsatellite marker was found to be located in the first intron of the gene (Weiland & Steinlein, 1996). The complete coding region of the CHRNA4 gene is estimated to be contained within approximately 17 kb of genomic DNA (Steinlein et al., 1996).

Primer pairs covering the entire coding region, including the exon-intron boundaries, of the CHRNA4 gene have been designed and PCR (polymerase chain reaction) amplifications from DNA of affected pedigree members from the chromosome 20q linked Australian ADNFLE family (Phillips et al.,

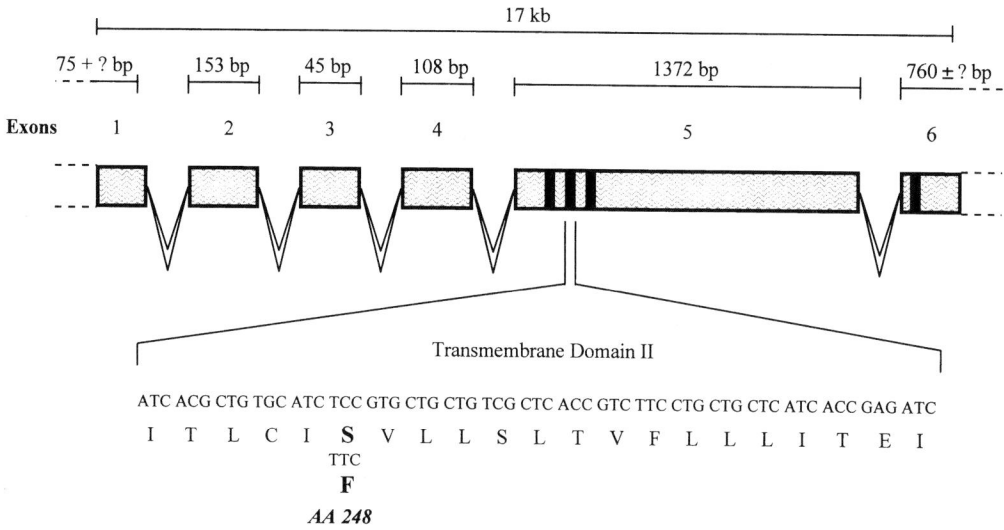

Fig. 3. The exon structure of the CHRNA4 gene is shown together with parts of the nucleotide and deduced amino acid sequence of the wildtype and Ser248Phe-mutant gene (S, serine; F, phenylalanine). The position of the introns is only indicated and they are not drawn to size. Transmembrane domains 1–3, which are located in exon 5, and transmembrane domain 4 (exon 6) are indicated by filled squares. bp, base pairs; AA, amino acid residues.

1995), BFNC patients and probands with LVEEG were carried out. The PCR fragments were analysed by single strand confirmation analysis (SSCA). So far, no mutations could be identified, neither in BFNC patients nor in probands with LVEEG. However, the number of examined individuals is too small to exclude CHRNA4 as a candidate gene for both phenotypes. Mutations might have been overlooked if they did not produce band shifts in SSCA. Furthermore, the promoter region remains to be cloned and analysed. Even the possibility of intronic mutations has to be considered.

The Ser248Phe mutation

However, positive results have been obtained by SSCA with the Australian ADNFLE family. Altered mobility in single strand confirmation analysis was detected for two overlapping fragments. The fragments were subcloned and sequenced after amplification with vector specific primers. Furthermore, direct sequencing of PCR fragments from genomic DNA was performed. The clones carrying the aberrant allele showed a C to T transition (Fig. 4). The missense mutation replaced the neutral serine by a complex aromatic phenylalanine in the sixth amino acid position (homologous to Ser248 of the Torpedo α-subunit) of the transmembrane domain 2 (Steinlein et al., 1995). Data base analysis showed that serine is conserved in this position in most of the other subunits of the human neuronal nicotinic acetylcholine receptor (nAChR). Serine is replaced by another amino acid residue only in subunits α7 and α8; these subunits diverged very early in the history of the multigene family of nAChR subunits and have distinct structural and pharmacological properties. Furthermore, Ser248 is found in species evolutionarily as diverse as for example the goldfish *Carassius auratus* and the locust *Schistocerca gregaria*.

The Ser284Phe mutation was shown to be present in all affected family members, as well as in the four individuals available for testing who were obligate carriers, one individual who was below the

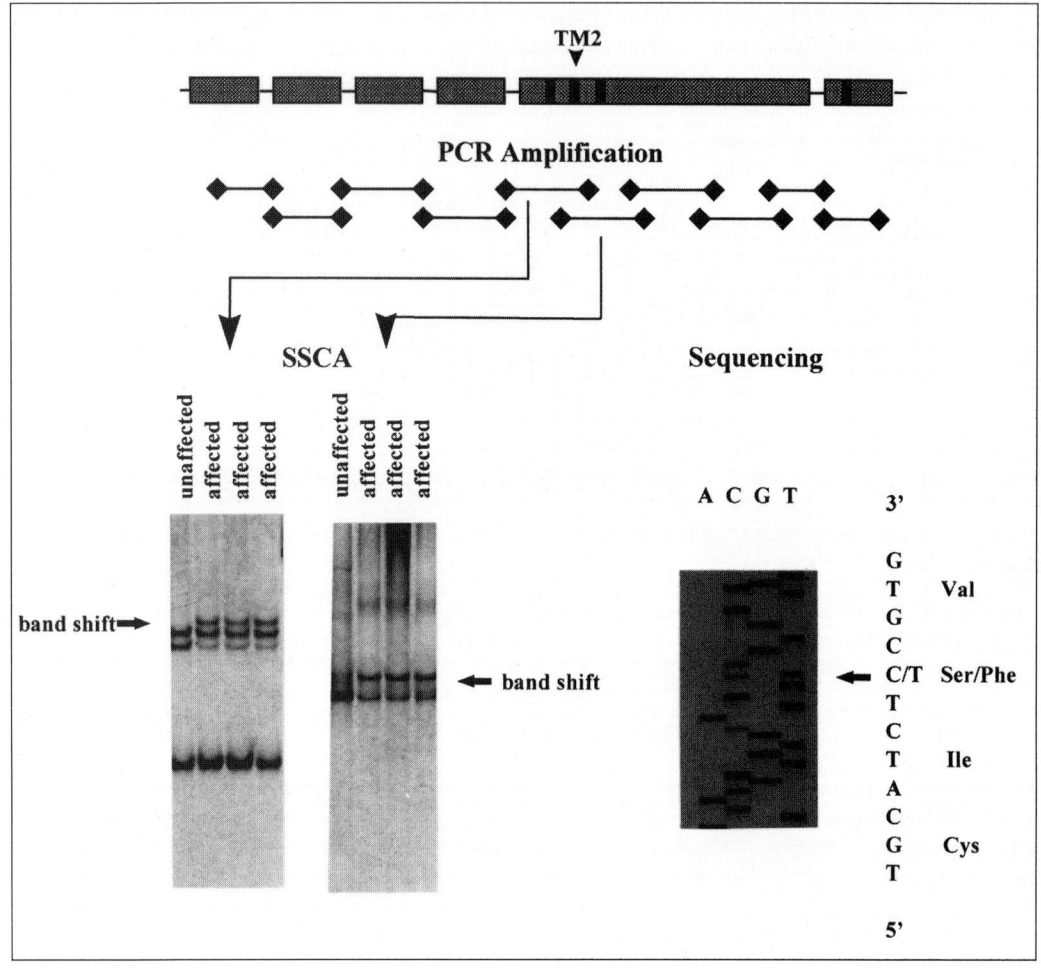

Fig. 4. Top: Schematic representation of the PCR amplification of the CHRNA4 gene;
Left lower side: Single strand confirmation analysis (SSCA)-pattern of the Ser248Phe mutation in two overlapping PCR fragments, shown for three ADNFLE patients and one unaffected pedigree member.
Right lower side: Sequencing of the Ser248Phe mutation in an ADNFLE patient. Fragments were amplified out of the DNA from a patient with one 5′biotinylated (5′-biotin-GGCGAGTGGGTCATCGTGG–3′) and one non-biotinylated primer (5′-GCTCGGGCCAGAAGCGCGG –3′). The primers bind to parts of exon 5 of the CHRNA4 gene. After the amplification the fragment was sequenced by an internal primer (5′-GGGCATGGTGTGCGTGCGTG–3′) using the Sequenase Version 2.0 kit (Amersham). The mutation, a C to T nucleotide exchange leading to the replacement of serine in amino acid position 248 by phenylalanine, is indicated by an arrow.

mean age of manifestation and two additional unaffected individuals. The latter finding can be explained by incomplete penetrance. Due to as yet unknown reasons, only about 80 per cent of the gene carriers actually develop epilepsy. In some cases the patients might be only mildly affected, and not diagnosed as having epilepsy. The mutation was not found in 333 independent control individuals. Thus it is unlikely that it is a rare but benign polymorphism of the coding sequence. Furthermore, mutagenesis experiments showed that the Ser248Phe mutation changes the pharmacological and functional properties of the receptor. The rate of desensitization seems to depend on the hydrophobicity profile of the amino acids residues lining the ion channel. The coexpression of the mutated α4-subunit and the wild type β2-subunit in Xenopus oocytes gave rise to a receptor which, if compared with the wild type α4β2 receptor, showed a ≥10 fold acceleration of the desensitization rate. Furthermore, the time the receptor needed to recover from to a conducting state was significantly prolonged (Weiland *et al.*, 1996). Thus the substitution of a strongly hydrophobic phenylalanine for a hydrophilic serine lead to marked hypoactivity of the affected receptor.

Recently, a second CHRNA4 mutation (776ins3) has been described in a Norwegian ADNFLE family (Steinlein *et al.*, 1997): the insertion of three nucleotide codes for an additional leucine residue at the extracellular end of the second transmembrane domain. Electrophysiological studies investigating the mutate nAChR in Xenopus oocytes have shown that the 776ins3 mutation gives rise to a profound modification of the receptor function.

Due to the fact that not much is known about the role of nAChRs in the central nervous system, one can only speculate about functional consequences of the mutation. If nAChRs are indeed presynaptically located (McGehee *et al.*, 1995), they may be involved in the regulation of other neurotransmitter systems, like GABA or glutamate and thus influencing the excitability level of neurons. It has been hypothesized that the predominant role of nAChR in the brain could be that of a modifier of neuronal excitability. Maybe the balance between inhibitory and exhibitory synaptic input is disturbed by the Ser248Phe mutation and 776ins3 mutations, thus leading to the decrease of the seizure threshold. However, a lot of basic research needs to be done before we can sufficiently explain the mechanisms leading from a mutation in the second transmembrane domain of an acetylcholine receptor to a partial epilepsy syndrome with nocturnal seizures.

Addendum

Two novel voltage-dependent potassium channel genes, KCNQ2 and KCNQ3, have now been described to be mutated in BFNC families linked either to chromosome 20q13.3 or 8q24 (Biervert *et al.*, 1998; Charlier *et al.*, 1998; Singh *et al.*, 1998). The KCNQ2 gene on chromosome 20q13.3 is separated by approximately 30 kb from CHRNA4. Electrophysiological studies showed that the truncation of the KCNQ2 gene caused by a 5bp deletion in an Australian BFNC family affects channel function (Biervert *et al.*, 1998).

References

Anokhin, A., Steinlein, O., Fischer, C., Mao, Y., Vogt, P., Schalt, E. & Vogel, F. (1992): A genetic study of the human low-voltage electroencephalogram. *Hum. Genet.* **90**, 99-112.

Biervert, C., Schroeder, B.C., Kubisch, C., Berkovic, S.F., Propping, P., Jentsch, T.J. & Steinlein, O.K. (1998): A potassium channel mutation in neonatal human epilepsy. *Science* **279**, 403–406.

Buisson, B., Curtis, L., Bertrand, D. (1997): Neuronal nicotinic acetylcholine receptor and epilepsy. This volume.

Charlier, C., Singh, N.A., Ryan, S.G., Lewis, T.B., Reus, B.E., Leach, R.J. & Leppert, M. (1998): A pore mutation in a novel KQT-like potassium channel gene in an idioipathic epilepsy family. *Nat. Genet.* **18**, 53–55.

DiPaola, M., Kao, P. & Karlin, A. (1990): Mapping the alpha subunit site photolabeled by the noncompetitive inhibitor (3H)-quinacrine azide in the active state of the nicotinic acetylcholine receptor. *J. Biol. Chem.* **265**, 11017-11029.

Hucho, F., Oberthur, W. & Lottspeich, F. (1986): The ion channel of the nicotinic acetylcholine receptor is formed by the homologous helices MII of the receptor subunits. *FEBS Lett.* **205**, 137-142.

Imoto, K., Busch, C., Sakmann, B., Mishina, M., Konno, T., Nakai, J., Bujo, H., Mori, Y., Fukuda, K. & Numa, S. (1988): Rings of negatively charged amino acids determine the acetylcholine receptor channel conductance. *Nature* **355**, 645-648.

Leppert, M., Anderson, V.E., Quattlebaum, T., Stauffer, D., O'Conell, P., Lathrop, M., Lalouel, J.M. & White, R. (1989): Benign familial neonatal convulsions linked to genetic markers on chromosome 20. *Nature* **337**, 647-648.

Lewis, T.B., Leach, R.J., Ward, K., O'Connell, P. & Ryan, S.G. (1993): Genetic heterogeneity in benign familial neonatal convulsions: identification of a new locus on chromosome 8q. *Am. J. Hum. Genet.* **53**, 670-675.

Le Novere, N. & Changeux, J.P. (1995): Molecular evolution of the nicotinic acetylcholine receptor: an example of multigene family in excitable cells. *J. Mol. Evol.* **40**, 155-172.

McGehee, D.S., Heath, M.J.S., Gelber, S., Devay, P. & Role, L.W. (1995): Nicotine Enhancement of fast excitatory synaptic transmission in CNS by presynaptic receptors. *Science* **269**, 1692-1696.

Phillips, H.A., Scheffer, I.E., Berkovic, S.F., Hollway, G.E., Sutherland, G.R., Mulley, J.C. (1995): Localisation of a gene for autosomal dominant nocturnal frontal lobe epilepsy to 20q13.2. *Nat. Genet.* **10**, 117-118.

Pilz, A.J., Willer, E., Povey, S., & Abbott, C.M. (1992): The genes coding for phosphoenolpyruvate carboxykinase-1 (PCK1) and neuronal nicotinic acetylcholine receptor a4 subunit (CHRNA4) map to human chromosome 20, extending the known region of homology with mouse chromosome 2. *Ann. Hum. Genet.* **56**, 289-293.

Rett, A. & Teubel, R. (1964): Neugeborenenkrämpfe im Rahmen einer epileptisch belasteten Familie. *Wiener Klin. Wochenschr.* **76**, 609-613.

Ronen, G.M., Rosales, T.O., Connolly, M., Anderson, V.E. & Leppert, M. (1993): Seizure characteristics in chromosome 20 benign familial neonatal convulsions. *Neurology* **43**, 1355–1360.

Scheffer, I.E., Bhatia, K.P., Lopes-Cendes, I., Fish, D.R., Marsden, D., Andermann, E., Andermann, F., Desbiens, R., Keene, D., Cendes, F., Manson, J.I., Constantinou, J.E.C., McIntosh, A. & Berkovic, S.F. (1995): Autosomal dominant nocturnal frontal lobe epilepsy: A distinctive clinical disorder. *Brain* **118**, 61–73.

Singh, N.A., Charlier, C., Stauffer, D., DuPont, B.R., Leach, R.J., Melis, R., Ronen, G.B., Bjerre, I., Quattlebaum, T., Murphy, J.V., McHarg, M.L., Gagnon, D., Rosales, T.O., Peiffer, A., Anderson, V.E. & Leppert, M. (1998): A novel potassium channel gene, KCNQ2, is mutated in an inherited epilepsy of newborns. *Nat. Genet.* **18**, 25–29.

Steinlein, O., Anokhin, A., Mao, Y., Schalt, E. & Vogel, F. (1992a): Localization of a gene for the human low voltage EEG on 20q and genetic heterogeneity. *Genomics* 12, 69–73.

Steinlein, O., Fischer, C., Keil, R., Smigrodzki, R. & Vogel, F. (1992b): D20S19, linked to Low voltage EEG, benign neonatal convulsions, and Fanconi anaemia, maps to a region of enhanced recombination and is localized between CpG islands. *Hum. Mol. Genet.* **1**, 325–329.

Steinlein, O., Smigrodzki, R., Lindstrom, J., Anand, R., Köhler, M., Tocharoentanaphol, C. & Vogel, F. (1994): Refinement of the localization of the gene for neuronal acetylcholine receptor α4 subunit (CHRNA4) to human chromosome 20q13.2-q13.3. *Genomics* **22**, 493–495.

Steinlein, O., Schuster, V., Fischer, C. & Häussler, M. (1995a): Benign familial neonatal convulsions: confirmation of genetic heterogeneity and further evidence for a second locus on chromosome 8q. *Hum. Genet.* **95**, 411–415.

Steinlein, O., Mulley, J., Propping, P., Wallace, R., Phillips, H., Sutherland, G., Scheffer, I. & Berkovic, S. (1995b): A missense mutation in the neuronal nicotinic acetylcholine receptor α4 subunit is associated with autosomal dominant nocturnal frontal lobe epilepsy. *Nat. Genet.* **11**, 201–203.

Steinlein, O., Weiland, S., Stoodt, J. & Propping, P. (1996): Exon-Intron Structure of the Human Neuronal Nicotinic Acetylcholine Receptor a4 Subunit (CHRNA4). *Genomics* **32**, 289–294.

Vogel F (1986): Grundlagen und Bedeutung genetisch bedingter Variabilität des normalen menschlichen EEG. *Z. EEG-EMG* **17**, 173–188.

Weiland, S. & Steinlein, O. (1996): Dinucleotide polymorphism in the first intron of the human neuronal nicotinic acetylcholine receptor α4 subunit gene (CHRNA4). *Clinical Genetics* **50**, 433–434.

Weiland, S., Witzemann, V., Villarroel, A., Propping, P. & Steinlein, O. (1996): An amino acid exchange in the second transmembrane segment of a neuronal nicotinic receptor causes partial epilepsy by altering its desensitization kinetics. *FEBS Letters* **398**, 91–96.

Chapter 20

Neuronal nicotinic acetylcholine receptor and epilepsy

B. Buisson, L. Curtis and D. Bertrand

Department of Physiology, CMU, 1 rue Michel Servet, 1211 Geneva 4, Switzerland

The brain is specialized in the processing of information originating from inside and outside of the body. It is believed that vegetative and/or emotional information is processed by the most primitive structures of the brain whereas 'cognitive tasks' result from activity of the neocortex. Integration and control of multiple simultaneous 'inputs' is performed by specialized neuronal circuits which are localized in restricted brain areas. However, complex tasks involve multiple interactions between different neuronal networks (Damasio, 1994). At the molecular level numerous peptides and proteins have been identified in the regulation of neuronal growth, survival and communication (Jessell & Kandel, 1993; Katz & Shatz, 1996; Lewin & Barde, 1996; Tessier-Lavigne & Goodman, 1996; Thoenen, 1995). Alteration of any of these molecular players could lead to pathological profiles. One of these pathologies, also known under the term of epilepsy, is characterized by recurrent 'crises' and affects at least 1 per cent of the population.

Epilepsy is a disorder characterized by recurring seizures, which are hypersynchronous discharges originating in one brain region and which in some cases propagate to a broader zone. According to their aetiology, epilepsies can be classified as *symptomatic* or *idiopathic*. Acquired anatomical lesions such as tumours, brain infarcts, or other pathological affections can provoke dysfunction of neuronal tissues, leading to *symptomatic* epileptic seizures. In contrast, the *idiopathic* epilepsies occur in the absence of any evident macroscopic anomalies, and are thought to be caused by exogenous or endogenous molecular insults. An abnormal synchronization of neuronal firing which often involves recurrent activities in the neocortex and/or the hippocampus is observed during seizure. The apparent clinical manifestation of seizure is determined by three factors: (a) the neuronal population in which the abnormal synchronous firing originates, (b) the areas to which this electrical activity spreads, and (c) the time-course of the spread and recovery. This simple analysis underlines the key role of the neuronal architecture in the genesis and the spread of synchronous neuronal discharges.

Brain neurons are organized in structural networks which are genetically determined and developmentally regulated (Katz & Shatz, 1996; Tessier-Lavigne & Goodman, 1996). Their architecture as well as their plasticity strongly depend upon inter-neuronal exchanges. Thus, neuronal membranes express a very large panel of proteins which are specialized in cell-to-cell recognition, cell guidance and cell communication processes (Jessell & Kandel, 1993; Katz & Shatz, 1996; Tessier-Lavigne & Goodman, 1996). One class of these specialized molecules are the voltage-gated channels (Hille, 1992). Voltage-gated channels are proteins which are selectively permeable to one type of ion (cations: Na^+, K^+, Ca^{2+}, or anions: Cl^-) and are at the origin of each neuron's endogenous electrophysiological properties. Given the characteristics of their voltage-gated channels, some neurons can display spontaneous oscillations of their membrane potential, which occurs at a determined frequency (Stériade & Llinàs, 1988). The electrical activity of a neuron propagates from its cell body to its axon termini in a regenerative fashion. Chemical or electrical synapses (Jessell & Kandel, 1993) are specialized structures allowing the coupling between two cells. Electrical synapses are restricted to a very small number of neurons and constitute a physical coupling between two cells. The large majority of synapses are so called chemical synapses and involve the release of small molecules: the neurotransmitters and/or neuropeptides (Jessell & Kandel, 1993; Südhof, 1995). A chemical synapse can be further subdivided into three compartments with: (a) the presynaptic bouton where small vesicles are docked close to the plasmatic membrane (Südhof, 1995), (b) the synaptic cleft which separates pre- and postsynaptic membranes (no wider than 100 nm) and (c) the postsynaptic membrane where a large quantity of receptors are embedded.

Today, more than twenty neurotransmitters and a large quantity of neuropeptides have been found to participate in the transmission of information at chemical synapses (reviewed in Hökfelt, 1991). Invasion of the synaptic bouton by the action potential causes a brief release (in the ms scale) of a high concentration (up to mM) of neurotransmitter. After a short diffusion through the synaptic cleft (less than 0.2 ms), the neurotransmitter activates ionotropic receptors (ligand-gated channels; Galzi & Changeux, 1995) and/or metabotropic receptors (Bockaert, 1995). Activation of anionic selective ligand-gated channels, such as those formed by $GABA_A$ or glycine receptors induces an hyperpolarization of the postsynaptic membrane and the transmission is called 'inhibitory' (Betz, 1990; Betz, 1992). In contrast, opening of cationic selective ligand-gated channels such as those of the AMPA/NMDA glutamate (Bettler & Mulle, 1995; McBain & Mayer, 1994; Sucher et al., 1996), nicotinic (Bertrand & Changeux, 1995), purinergic (Gibb & Halliday, 1996; North, 1996) or serotoninergic (5-HT_3 receptors; (Maricq et al., 1991; Yang et al., 1992)) causes a depolarization of the postsynaptic membrane and the transmission is defined as 'excitatory'. Interestingly, some nicotinic receptors have been identified at presynaptic or preterminal sites where they are able to enhance the efficacy of both inhibitory (Léna & Changeux, 1997; Léna et al., 1993; McMahon et al., 1994) and excitatory synaptic transmission (Gray et al., 1996; McGehee et al., 1995; Vidal & Changeux, 1993).

Neuropeptides, which are released mainly under repetitive action potentials, are thought to activate only metabotropic receptors. Binding of the neurotransmitter and/or neuropeptides to postsynaptic metabotropic receptors leads to the activation of second messenger pathways. Those signaling pathways can induce a modification of the ligand-gated channels' properties (through phosphorylation/dephosphorylation mechanisms) and as a correlate can modulate the efficacy of synaptic transmission (Gurantz et al., 1994; Margiotta & Pardi, 1995; McBain & Mayer, 1994; Pin & Bockaert, 1995; Tong et al., 1995; Vijayaraghavan et al., 1990).

Moreover, postsynaptic cells have the ability to modify the activity of their surrounding cells through the intermediary of retrograde messengers such as arachidonic acid (AA) or nitric oxide (NO). Both molecules are released subsequently to a transient increase of the intracellular calcium in the postsynaptic cell which closely follows an excitatory transmission. They have been identified to be potent allosteric modulators of NMDA- (AA and NO; Manzoni et al., 1992; Miller et al., 1992) and nicotinic receptors (AA: Vijayaraghavan et al., 1995).

Finally, it is of value to recall that postsynaptic cells often control the survival of presynaptic neurons through the release of very small quantities of neurotrophins (Lewin & Barde, 1996; Thoenen, 1995) which are able to stabilize neuronal connections (Lo, 1995) as well as to enhance synaptic transmission (Kang & Schuman, 1995). In some cases, the release of neurotrophins is controlled by the 'firing' of the presynaptic cells (Ernfors et al., 1991; Isackson et al., 1991).

In a single neuron, spatial and temporal summation of the synaptic signals will lead to the firing of an action potential, if the integration of the neurotransmitter-induced anionic and cationic currents drives the membrane potential to its threshold value. In the case of neurons which present a spontaneous electrical activity, the excitatory and inhibitory inputs modulate the neuron's firing rate. The balance between excitation and inhibition depends upon three factors: (a) the basal electrophysiological properties of the neuron (essentially determined by voltage-gated channels), (b) the particular synapses activated at a precise time and (c) the cellular distribution of ligand-gated channels (post- and pre-synaptic).

According to the previous considerations, any modification of the neuronal network morphogenesis or of the synaptic transmission can lead to the anarchical synchronous discharges observed during epileptic seizures. The aim of this work is to examine in the light of the most recent findings the correlation existing between one type of known ligand-gated channels, the neuronal nicotinic acetylcholine receptors (nAChRs), and some forms of genetically transmissible epilepsies (Scheffer et al., 1995; Steinlein et al., 1995).

Structure and function of the neuronal nAChRs

Our knowledge about the structure of the neuronal nAChRs mainly derives from biochemical and electron microscopic studies made on the muscle receptors and more specifically those obtained in large quantity from the electric fish *Torpedo*. The extreme density of the receptors in the electric organ of *Torpedo*, which leads to a pseudo crystalline arrangement, allowed first electron micrographic studies with negative staining to be done (reviewed in Changeux, 1990) and then high-resolution electron microscopy (Unwin, 1996). In parallel, the identification and cloning of the genes coding for five subunits of *Torpedo* nAChRs allowed the deduction of the amino acid sequences of the corresponding proteins as well as their pattern of hydrophobicity (reviewed in Devillers-Thiéry et al., 1993). The general features of the nAChR subunits were soon identified and it was deduced that these proteins possess four transmembrane segments each arranged with both their N-terminal and C-terminal ends facing the extracellular domain. From these and other data it was proposed that a single muscle nAChR result, from the assembly of five subunits arranged around an axis of pseudosymmetry in the following stoichiometry: 2α, β, γ, δ, with the γ subunit being replaced by the ε subunit in the adult form of the receptor (reviewed in Changeux, 1990). When examined from above, the receptor displays a donut-like shape whereas a clear asymmetry is observed on side views with a prominent portion of the protein sticking outside the membrane in the synaptic cleft. Low stringency screenings of neuronal cDNA libraries with muscle oligonucleotides soon led to the identification and cloning of several genes coding for putative neuronal nAChRs. Up to now, eight α ($\alpha 2$-$\alpha 9$) and three β ($\beta 2$-$\beta 4$) subunits have been identified in the chick and mammals. The corresponding human forms of nAChRs were identified in recent studies and these subunits share up to 77 per cent homology of the gene sequences with those of the rat or chick (Lindstrom, 1996; Monteggia et al., 1995; Peng et al., 1994). Subdivision in α and β is based upon their homology with the muscle subunits. Several evidences have shown that the α subunits, which are readily identifiable by the presence of two adjacent cysteins in their extracellular domain (position 192–193 in the muscle), constitute the major component of the acetylcholine (ACh) binding site. In contrast, the neuronal non-α subunits most resemble the muscle β subunits and are also called structural subunits. Reconstitution in host systems (Bertrand et al., 1991a; Boulter et al., 1987; Buisson et al., 1996; Gopalakrishnan et al., 1996) have shown that functional neuronal nAChRs can be obtained by the co-expression of an α and a β subunit. An exception to this rule is, however, observed with the $\alpha 7$ subunits that can reconstitute functional nAChRs when expressed alone (Couturier et al., 1990; Gopalakrishnan et al., 1995) suggesting that they might assemble in homo-oligomers. It is thought that, as in the muscle receptor, neuronal nAChRs result from the assembly of five subunits in a stoichiometry of two α and three β for the heteromeric receptors whereas homomeric receptors would contain five identical subunits (Lindstrom, 1996; Palma et al., 1996). An important characteristic of all ligand-gated channels is their capacity to form both the ligand-binding site and the ionic pore. In the case of the neuronal nAChRs the ligand binding domain is thought to be at the interface between two neighbouring subunits (one α and its adjacent

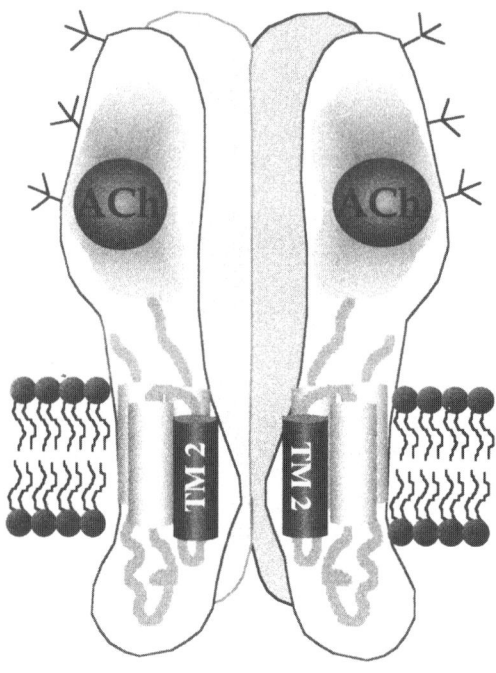

Fig. 1. Side view of a neuronal nAChR embedded in the cellular membrane.

subunit) while the aqueous pore lies in the centre of the subunit assembly (reviewed in Bertrand & Changeux, 1995; Galzi & Changeux, 1995). The structural organization of a neuronal nAChR is schematized in Fig. 1.

Significant progress in the understanding of the function of the ligand-gated channels has been made possible by the combination of molecular biological and electrophysiological experiments. Namely, by examination of the effects caused by point mutations on the functional properties of a given ligand-gated channel it became possible to approach its structure function relationship at the amino-acid level. Mutagenesis done in the putative ACh-binding domain, previously identified using photoaffinity labelling (Galzi et al., 1990), demonstrated that substitution of a single residue could reduce the apparent affinity of the receptor (EC_{50}) by as much as a hundred fold without affecting the time course of the response (Galzi et al., 1991). Other investigations subsequently confirmed the contribution of both the α and its adjacent subunits in the formation of the ACh binding site (Corringer et al., 1995). Finally, construction of chimeras between the α7 neuronal nAChR and the serotoninergic 5-HT$_3$ receptor illustrated that ligand-gated channels contain domains that can be exchanged between receptor species while preserving the functionality of the receptor (Eiselé et al., 1993).

In other studies, the properties of the aqueous pore and its determinant were examined. In agreement with previous observations it was confirmed that the second transmembrane segments (TM-2) form the walls of the ionic pore. Furthermore, it was found that mutation of a single residue in TM-2 in the homomeric α7 neuronal nAChR can suppress the calcium permeability of this channel (Bertrand et al., 1993a), whereas the additional insertion of an extra amino acid at the channel inner mouth could switch its ionic selectivity from cationic to anionic (Galzi et al., 1992, reviewed in Bertrand et al., 1993b). Surprisingly, however, substitution of an uncharged leucine residue by a threonine could induce profound effects both in the apparent affinity of the receptor, its time course of response, as well as its pharmacology (Bertrand et al., 1992; Revah et al., 1991).

From all these experiments it was concluded that functional properties of a given ligand-gated channel are defined by the ensemble of its structural elements but that mutation of a single residue in some critical points such as the ligand binding domain or the ionic pore can induce profound alteration of the whole receptors' characteristics. As a conclusion, and given the present state of our knowledge, it is not yet possible to predict the effect induced by a point mutation requiring its effects to be assessed by functional studies.

Neuronal nAChRs in the human brain

Numerous investigations performed with selective ligands and specific oligonucleotides have revealed a wide distribution of nAChRs in chick and rodent brains. In humans, autoradiographic studies also suggest the presence of nAChRs in many areas. High-affinity binding sites for (-)-nicotine have been detected in the thalamus, the hippocampus, the basal ganglia and the cortex (Adem et al., 1988; Court & Clementi, 1995; Court et al., 1992; Perry et al., 1992; Sugaya et al., 1990). By analogy with experiments performed with rodents (Clarke et al., 1985; Deutch et al., 1987; Flores et al., 1992; Marks et al., 1992; Picciotto et al., 1995; Swanson et al., 1983), it could be proposed that nAChRs of the α4β2 subtype constitute most, if not all, of the high-affinity nicotine binding sites in the human brain. Moreover, binding and functional studies indicate that reconstituted human α4β2 nAChRs display a high affinity for (-)-nicotine (Buisson et al., 1996; Gopalakrishnan et al., 1996). Binding of iodinated α-bungarotoxin (^{125}I-αBgt) has been detected in the hippocampus (dentate gyrus, CA1, CA2 and CA3), the presubiculum, and the subiculum (Rubboli et al., 1994a) and suggests together with in situ hybridizations (see below) the presence of α7-containing nAChRs in those areas. Cloning of the human cDNAs encoding for the different nAChRs subunits started only a few years ago (for a review see Lindstrom, 1996). Thus, in situ hybridization studies performed in the human brain are just at the beginning. As presented in Fig. 2, mRNAs encoding for α3, α4 and α7 have been detected in the cortex (Brodman areas 4 and 10; Schröder et al., 1995; Schröder et al., 1996; Wevers et al., 1995).

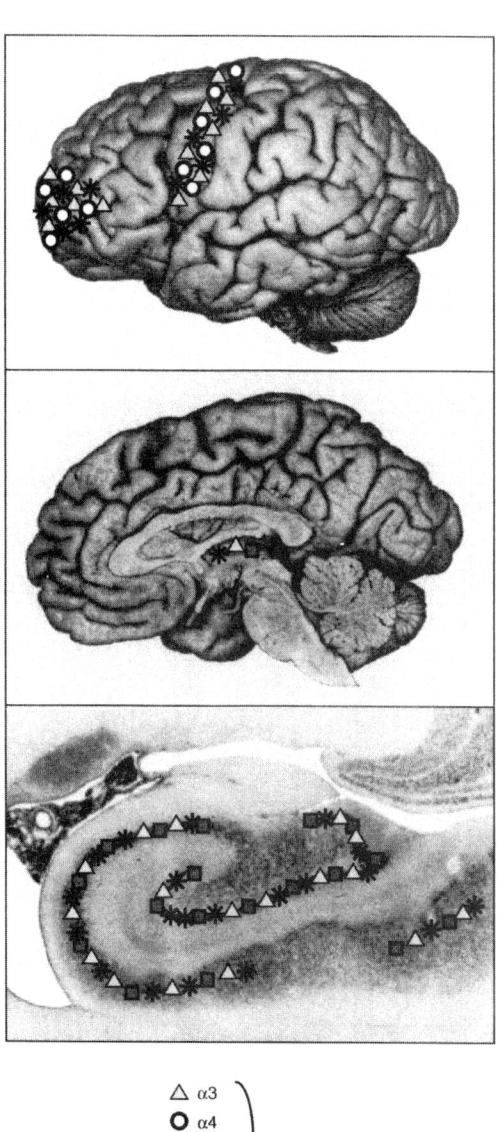

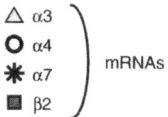

Fig. 2. Localization of mRNAs encoding for the α3, α4 and α7 subunits in the human brain. Top panel illustrates mRNA presence in Brodman areas 4 and 10. Middle panel, the thalamus is clearly identified in the sagittal section. Bottom illustrates the distribution of the nAChRs subunits in the hippocampus.

Transcripts for α3, α7 and β2 have been localized in the thalamus and the hippocampus (dentate granular layer, CA1 and CA2 pyramidal neurons; Rubboli et al., 1994a; Rubboli et al., 1994b). To date, in situ hybridization for the α4 subunit has not been performed in the thalamus. Nevertheless, PET imaging indicates a very high and selective labelling of the baboon thalamus by the α4β2 selective ligand epibatidine (Ding et al., 1996) thereby providing indirect evidence for the presence of this nAChR type in the thalamus. Thus, it seems highly probable that the human thalamus also expresses high levels of α4β2 nAChRs. As observed in other studies, care should be taken with *in situ* investigations: the presence of a given mRNA does not guarantee the expression of the corresponding protein nor provide information on its level of expression. As an illustration, mRNAs and proteins of α4 and α7 nAChR subunits have been probed in the cortex of control and Alzheimer's patients (Wevers *et al.*, 1997): although no significant difference is observed between Alzheimer's patients and age-matched controls in the distribution pattern and in the number of neurons expressing α7 and/or α4 mRNAs, there is a marked reduction in the intensity and number of immunopositive neurons (for both α4 and α7) in all cortical layers in the brain of Alzheimer patients (Wevers *et al.*, 1997). Thus, immunolabelling experiments reveal a strong impairment of α4 and α7 nAChR proteins expression in Alzheimer disease and highlight the necessity of immunocytochemical studies for control and pathological brains. The use of subunit specific monoclonal antibodies (Lindstrom, 1996) allows a precise localization of brain nAChRs as recently illustrated by the confocal microscopy images obtained for the labelling of nAChRs of chick pretectum and ciliary ganglion (Horch & Sargent, 1995; Ullian & Sargent, 1995). Finally, it is of value to recall that the nAChRs' expression in human brain decreases markedly with age even in the absence of any identified neurological pathology (Court & Clementi, 1995; Schröder *et al.*, 1996).

Mutation S248F: a loss of function

Since different forms of epilepsy appear to be inherited, many investigators have hypothesized a possible genetic link (Noebels, 1996). Studies performed in different laboratories have identified a specific form of epilepsy that is genetically transmissible: autosomal dominant nocturnal frontal lobe epilepsy (ADNFLE; Scheffer *et al.*, 1995). More specifically, ADNFLE was found to be associated with a gene of chromosome 20 at location q13.2-q13.3 (Phillips *et al.*, 1995) and was soon correlated with a missense mutation in the gene coding for the α4 subunit of neuronal nAChRs (Steinlein *et al.*, 1995; Steinlein, this volume). This mutation corresponds to a substitution of a serine residue by a phenylalanine in the TM-2 segment which, as described above, forms the channel wall.

In order to examine the effects caused by this missense mutation the equivalent substitution of the amino-acid was done on the well characterized chick α4 subunit (Bertrand *et al.*, 1990). Intranuclear co-injection, in *Xenopus* oocytes, of the mutated cDNA with the one coding for the wild type β2 subunit led to the reconstitution of functional nAChRs whose properties were examined using the two electrode voltage clamp recording technique (Bertrand *et al.*, 1991a). Comparison of the ACh-evoked currents obtained in the same batches of oocytes for the wild type α4β2 nAChR or the mutated receptor revealed marked differences (Fig. 3).

The maximal amplitude of the ACh-evoked current in the mutant never exceeded one tenth of the current detected for the wild type receptors for equivalent quantities of cDNAs injected. Assuming that the mutation does not alter the amount of protein synthetized by the oocytes this observation suggests either that mutated receptors assembled less efficiently or that it affected the channel conductance or mean open time. Another observation was made from the measurement of the ACh dose-response curve. In these experiments the sensitivity of the receptor is assessed by applying short pulses of ACh in growing order of concentrations. Plots of the peak current as a function of agonist concentration yield a typical dose-response curve and allow the determination of the receptors' apparent affinity or EC_{50}. Measurements done in wild type and mutated nAChRs showed a consistent difference in the ACh dose-response curve with the mutant being roughly ten times less sensitive to ACh than the wild type. In addition a faster decline, or desensitization, of the response of the mutated receptor was observed for sustained ACh-applications. Taken together, data collected with a chick receptor demonstrate that mutation of the residue S248F (numbered accordingly to the human subunit) in the α4 subunit produces a loss of function of the neuronal α4β2 nAChRs. Comparable observations have been recently performed with the human α4β2 nAChRs (Weiland *et al.*, 1996).

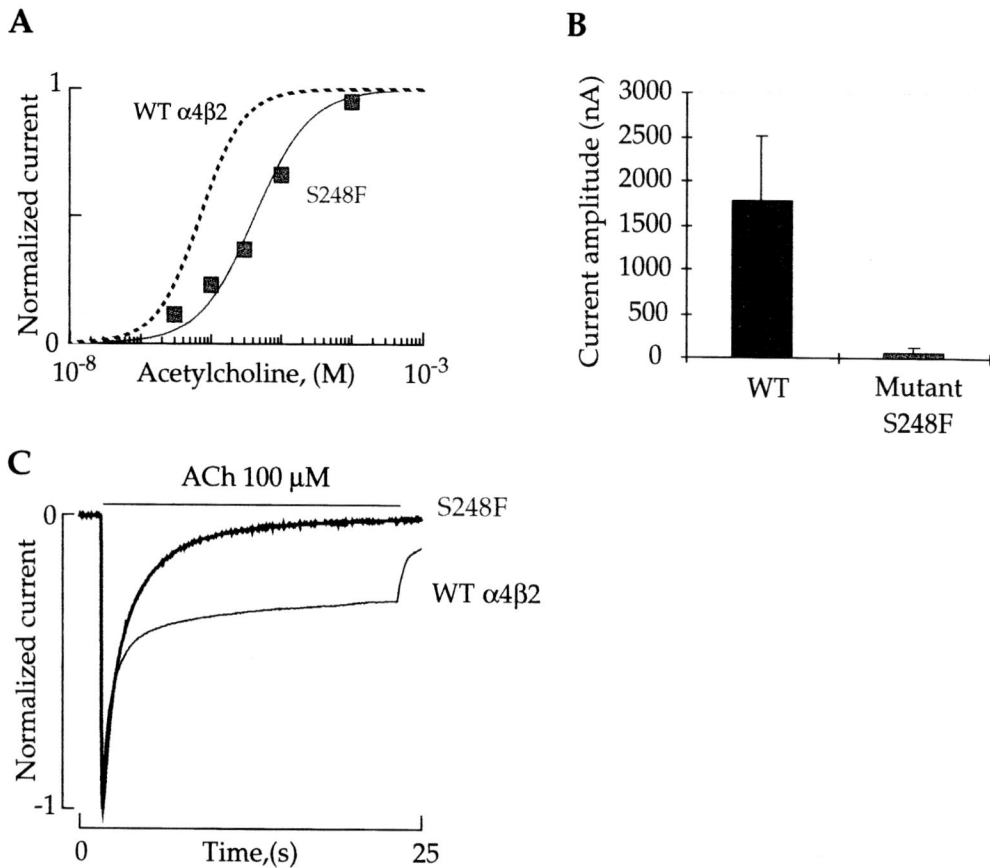

Fig. 3. Mutation of the amino acid S248F (numbered accordingly to the human gene) causes a loss of function. (A) ACh dose-response curves of the wild type and mutant nAChR are illustrated. (B) Oocytes expressing the mutant receptor display ACh-evoked currents of significantly lower amplitude than their siblings which express the wild type receptor. (C) Mutant nAChRs display a stronger desensitization in response to sustained ACh applications. All recordings were done in voltage clamp and cells were held at –100 mV.

Discussion

Fast synaptic transmission within the brain involves two kinds of synapses: excitatory and inhibitory. Glutamate, ACh and ATP activate cationic ligand-gated channels which lead to a membrane depolarization and a subsequent increase of the network excitability. In contrast, GABA (and glycine) activates anionic receptors which hyperpolarize the membrane and decrease the neuronal excitability. Since an imbalance between excitation and inhibition has been associated with the onset and spread of brain seizures: most of the investigations and therapies have focused their efforts on the GABA receptors (both ionotropic and metabotropic subtypes). Potentiation of the GABA effects indeed represents one way of decreasing the global brain excitability and of reducing the probability of seizure onsets.

Genetic investigations in human have associated a point mutation in the α4 nAChR subunit with one form of epilepsy (ADNFLE; Phillips *et al.*, 1995; Steinlein *et al.*, 1995; Steinlein, this volume). At first, it could seem surprising that an excitatory ligand-gated channel could be linked with one kind of epilepsy. Moreover, depending upon the structure considered nAChRs are localized either pre- and/or postsynaptically (Gray et al., 1996; Léna et al., 1993; McGehee et al., 1995; McMahon et al., 1994; Zhang et al., 1996). Thus, the main challenge is now to understand how such a mutated nAChR could determine an epileptic phenotype. Electrophysiological recordings suggest that the chick equivalent S248F mutation induces a global loss of function for the α4β2 nAChRs. Comparable findings have been recently described for the reconstituted human S248F-α4β2 nAChR (Weiland et al., 1996; Steinlein, this volume). If the S248F mutation of the human α4 nAChR subunit is associated with a loss of function of the corresponding nAChRs, the question that remains to be answered is: how can such a mutation lead to the phenotypical profile of ADNFLE? In the mouse, knock-out of the nAChR β2 subunit which prevents the formation of functional α4 containing nAChRs results only in subtle comportmental differences with respect to the wild type (Picciotto et al., 1995). In agreement, the high-affinity binding of (-)-nicotine is fully abolished in slices of these β2 deficient mice, demonstrating the loss of the α4β2 subtype of nAChRs. Interestingly, the $β2^-/β2^-$ mice have not been reported to show any seizures. Because β2 subunits can assemble potentially with at least four different α subunits (α2, α3, α4 and α5), the β2 knock-out probably induces more effects than the ones caused by the single S248F α4 mutation. When considering these observations and the neuro-anatomical differences between rodents and humans, it is difficult to make parallels between the β2 knock-out and the S248F mutation. A possible role of the α4 subunit could be its participation in neuronal development. The nAChR α4 mRNA is already detected in the foetus at day 11 and throughout adulthood in the rat nervous system (Zoli et al., 1995). Preliminary data indicate that the α4 mRNA can be detected in the human cortex as early as the 19th week of gestation and that its distribution at birth resembles that of the adult cerebral cortex (Schröder et al., 1996). These data are reinforced by the fact that (-)-nicotine binding sites are detected in the cortex (Court et al., 1992; Perry et al., 1992) and in the hippocampus (Court & Clementi, 1995) in the 22nd week of gestation. Moreover, since many in vitro experiments have demonstrated that nAChRs are involved either in the inhibition of neurite outgrowth (Owen & Bird, 1995; Small et al., 1995) or in the guidance of growth cones (Zheng et al., 1994), it is likely that identical mechanisms take place in the genesis of neuronal networks. Thus, and as suspected for the rat (Zoli et al., 1995), it seems possible that human nAChRs could play a morphogenetic role in brain ontogenesis, especially in the thalamus and in cortical areas. A fine disorganization of neuronal circuits (loss of inhibitory neurons and presumptive thalamocortical terminals) has been previously observed in the human epileptic neocortex (DeFelipe et al., 1993). At this level we can only speculate that the S248F α4 could induce some alterations of the neuronal connections which occurred during the last steps of the CNS ontogenesis.

Other comments can be suggested from the studies of clinical profile of ADNFLE. Because seizures associated with the S248F α4 mutation appear only when the patient is dozing (stage 2 of sleep), or shortly before awakening (Scheffer et al., 1995), it is likely that the set point of seizures is linked with a particular step of the sleep cycle and involves the activation of determined neuronal networks. The EEG oscillations that can be recorded during sleep and arousal are thought to result from neuronal activities of synaptically coupled thalamocortical neurons (Contreras et al., 1997; Krosig et al., 1993; Stériade & Contreras, 1995; Stériade et al., 1993). According to Steriade and collaborators (1993) 'The EEG spindles are the epitome of brain electrical synchronization at the onset of sleep, an electrographic landmark for the transition from waking to sleep that is associated with loss of perceptual awareness'. In vitro and in vivo recordings have demonstrated that such EEG signals are generated by the interactions of thalamocortical with cortical neurons as well as GABAergic neurons of the reticular thalamic nucleus (Stériade et al., 1993; see Fig. 4).

When considering this simple network and in accordance with the current literature it can reasonably be speculated that each of these neurons could express α4-containing nAChRs. Because α4 mRNAs have been identified in cortical pyramidal neurons, α4-containing nAChRs could be expressed in postsynaptic (cortex) and/or presynaptic (thalamus) compartments of these cells (Schröder et al.,

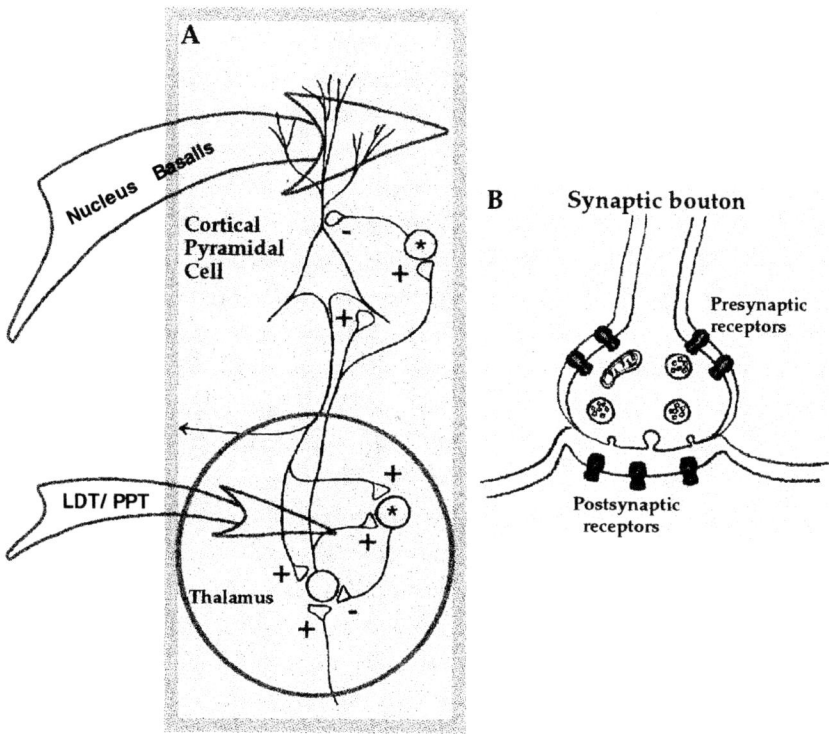

Fig. 4. Thalamo-cortical network. (A) Simplified representation of the neuronal pathways existing between the thalamus and cortex. Signs symbolize excitatory and/or inhibitory synapses. Stars label small GABAergic interneurons. Arrows indicate the cholinergic innervations coming from the Nucleus Basalis of Meynert and from the latero-dorsal tegmentum and pedunculopontine tegmentum (LDT, PPT). (B) Schematic drawing of a synaptic bouton with the pre- and postsynaptic ligand-gated channels. Activation of the presynaptic ligand-gated channels increases the intracellular calcium concentration and thereby the neurotransmitter release.

1996; Wevers et al., 1994). Nicotine binding in the rat cerebral cortex has been associated with thalamocortical afferents (Clarke, 1991) and suggests that thalamocortical neurons could express presynaptic nAChRs. Moreover, presynaptic enhancement of a non-NMDA glutamate transmission in the rat prefrontal cortex has been demonstrated by the work of Vidal & Changeux (1993). It is likely that the human thalamus expresses a high level of α4β2 nAChRs which could be located either presynaptically or postsynaptically on the membranes of thalamocortical and/or reticular thalamic neurons as illustrated by the strong epibatidine binding in the baboon thalamus (Ding et al., 1996). Thus, α4-containing nAChRs could be expressed by many types of neurons involved in the thalamo-cortical network. According to their cellular site of expression (presynaptic versus postsynaptic) S248F-α4 nAChRs could induce seizures by impairing the excitation/inhibition balance at any point of the network, leading to abnormal thalamic discharges that could spread to the frontal cortex. Local applications of nAChRs antagonists (which can simulate a loss of function) on brain slices could bring further insight on the origin of epileptic foci. Moreover, and as discussed above, the S248F α4 could induce abnormal connections in the thalamocortical network during the last steps of the brain ontogenesis. Finally, it is of value to mention that this thalamocortical network (Fig. 4) has been previously implicated in another type of epilepsy: the generalized absence seizures (Snead, 1995).

While thalamocortical and intrathalamic pathways are prime candidates for the regions implicated in ADNFLE, nicotinic transmission have been suggested to play a role in other brain areas (Clarke, 1993; Clarke, 1995). The ventral tegmental area contains nAChRs which are thought to modulate synaptic transmission (Blaha *et al.*, 1996; Brodie, 1991). The cholinergic pathways of the ventral tegmental area are part of the ascending reticular system, known to play a crucial role in the sleep-arousal transitions (Steriade *et al.*, 1993). The substantia nigra pars compacta, also part of the ascending reticular system and thought to contain functional nAChRs (Clarke *et al.*, 1985), has been shown to exert an inhibitory effect on certain forms of experimental seizures (Danober *et al.*, 1995).

Neuronal nAChRs are regulated by ligands such as calcium (Buisson *et al.*, 1996; Eiselé *et al.*, 1993; Galzi *et al.*, 1996; Léna & Changeux, 1993b; Mulle *et al.*, 1992; Vernino *et al.*, 1992) and steroids (Bertrand *et al.*, 1991b; Buisson & Bertrand, 1997; Valera *et al.*, 1992) which have been identified as allosteric effectors. Progesterone strongly inhibits the reconstituted human α4β2 nAChR with an IC_{50} in the μM range (reviewed in Buisson & Bertrand, 1997). Considering this remark, it is interesting to note that Scheffer *et al.* (1995) indicate that a number of women with ADNFLE have associated changes in seizure frequency (both increase and decrease) with menarche, pregnancy and menopause. It seems then very likely that, under certain physiological conditions, steroids could exacerbate the effects of the S248F α4 mutation. However, the steroid potentiation of the $GABA_A$ receptors (Barker, 1987; Majewska, 1986) must be taken into account at the same time and could add onto the modulation of the nAChRs. Finally, Scheffer *et al.* (1995) point out that seizures associated with ADNFLE decrease with ageing with a marked reduction after 40–50 years. This last observation should suggest that the 'negative' effect of the S248F α4 mutation could be weakened by a loss of nAChR expression. As an illustration, at the age of 50 years nicotine binding sites in the CA1 of the hippocampus have decreased by about 50 per cent compared to those of the infant (Court & Clementi, 1995; Schröder *et al.*, 1996).

In conclusion, S248F α4-containing nAChRs could provoke morphogenetic alterations that could lead to an abnormal neuronal network architecture and/or could impair the excitation/inhibition balance at some synapses. Thus, under certain physiological circumstances (spindle waves at sleep onset) these anomalies might trigger epileptic discharges. Furthermore, synaptic transmission cannot be viewed as a unique system; rather the entire architecture of the neuronal network should be taken in consideration. The present observation is that a loss of function of the nAChR can result in epileptic discharges that can be due either to a direct effect on synapses or indirectly through the modulation of another transmitter release (Léna & Changeux, 1997; Léna *et al.*, 1993; McMahon *et al.*, 1994). According to this hypothesis, compounds acting on a specific nAChR could be used as powerful enhancers of the GABA release and thereby widen the present antiepileptic pharmacopea.

Addendum

Following the final preparation of this chapter, three investigations of the role of nAChRs in ADNFLE appeared in the literature. Firstly, the group of Steinlein has identified an insertion mutation in the human α4 nAChR gene in another family with ADNFLE (Steinlein *et al.*, 1997). Secondly, this new α4 mutation, together with the S248F one, are characterized more extensively in two recent electrophysical studies using reconstituted receptors expressed in *Xenopus* oocytes (Bertrand *et al.*, 1997; Kuryatov *et al.*, 1997).

Acknowledgements: We would like to thank Mrs. S. Bertrand for her valuable collaboration and participation in the experiments, and to Prof. M. Stériade and Dr A. Wevers for communicating results in press. We are indebted to Dr. P.J. Corringer for providing the mutant cDNA. We thank Drs F. Picard, L. Danober and C. Marescaux for helpful suggestions. This work was supported by the Swiss National Science Foundation and the 'Office Fédéral de l'Education et des Sciences' to D.B.

References

Adem, A., Singh Jossan, S., D'Argy, R., Brandt, I., Winblad, B. & Nordberg, A. (1988): Distribution of nicotinic receptors in human thalamus as visualized by ^{3}H-nicotine and ^{3}H-acetylcholine receptor autoradiography. *J. Neural. Transm.* **73**, 77–83.

Barker, J.L., Harrison, N.L., Lange, G.D. & Owen, D.G. (1987): Potentiation of γ-amino-butyric-acid-activated chloride conductance by a steroid anaesthetic in cultured rat spinal neurones. *J. Physiol. (Lond.)* **386**, 485–501.

Bertrand, D., Ballivet, M. & Rungger, D. (1990): Activation and blocking of neuronal nicotinic acetylcholine receptor reconstituted in *Xenopus* oocytes. *Proc. Natl. Acad. Sci. (USA)* **87**, 1993–1997.

Bertrand, D. & Changeux, J.P. (1995): Nicotinic receptor: An allosteric protein specialized for intercellular communication. *Seminars in The Neurosciences* **7**, 75–90.

Bertrand, D., Cooper, E., Valera, S., Rungger, D. & Ballivet, M. (1991a): Electrophysiology of neuronal nicotinic acetylcholine receptors expressed in *Xenopus* oocytes following nuclear injection of genes or cDNA. In: *Methods in Neuroscience*, Conn, M. (ed.), pp. 174–193. New York: Academic Press.

Bertrand, D., Devillers, T.A., Revah, F., Galzi, J.L., Hussy, N., Mulle, C., Bertrand, S., Ballivet, M. & Changeux, J.P. (1992): Unconventional pharmacology of a neuronal nicotinic receptor mutated in the channel domain. *Proc. Natl. Acad. Sci. (USA)* **89**, 1261–1265.

Bertrand, D., Galzi, J.L., Devillers-Thiéry, A., Bertrand, S. & Changeux, J.P. (1993a): Mutations at two distinct sites within the channel domain M2 alter calcium permeability of neuronal α7 nicotinic receptor. *Proc. Natl. Acad. Sci. (USA)* **90**, 6971–6975.

Bertrand, D., Galzi, J.L., Devillers-Thiéry, A., Bertrand, S. & Changeux, J.P. (1993b): Stratification of the channel domain in neurotransmitter receptors. *Curr. Op. Neurobiol.* **5**, 688–693.

Bertrand, D., Valera, S., Bertrand, S., Ballivet, M. & Rungger, D. (1991b): Steroids inhibit nicotinic acetylcholine receptors. *Neuroreport* **2**, 277–280.

Bertrand, S., Weiland, S., Steinlein, O. & Bertrand, D. (1997): Physiological effects of mutations of the α4 neuronmal nicotinic receptor associated with epilepsy. *Soc. Neurosci. Abstr.* 156-4.

Bettler, B. & Mulle, C. (1995): Review: Neurotransmitter receptors II. AMPA and kainate receptors. *Neuropharmacology* **34**, 123–139.

Betz, H. (1990): Ligand-gated ion channels in the brain: the amino acid receptor superfamily. *Neuron* **5**, 383–392.

Betz, H. (1992): Structure and function of inhibitory glycine receptors. *Quart. Rev. Biophys.* **25**, 381–394.

Blaha, C.D., Allen, L.F., Das, S., Inglis, W.L., Latimer, M.P., Vincent, S.R. & Winn, P. (1996): Modulation of dopamine efflux in the nucleus accumbens after cholinergic stimulation of the ventral tegmental area in intact, pedunculopontine tegmental nucleus-lesioned, and laterodorsal tegmental nucleus-lesioned rats. *J. Neurosci.* **16**, 714–722.

Bockaert, J. (1995): Les récepteurs à sept domaines transmembranaires: physiologie et pathologie de la transduction. *Médecine-Science* **11**, 382–394.

Boulter, J., Connolly, J., Deneris, E., Goldman, D., Heinemann, S. & Patrick, J. (1987): Functional expression of two neuronal nicotinic acetylcholine receptors from cDNA clones identifies a gene family. *Proc. Natl. Acad. Sci. (USA)* **84**, 7763–7767.

Brodie, M.S. (1991): Low concentrations of nicotine increase the firing rate of neurons of the ventral tegmental area *in vitro*. In: *Effects of nicotine on biological systems*, Adlkofer, F. & Thureau, K. (eds), pp. 373–377. Basel: Birkhauser Verlag.

Buisson, B. & Bertrand, D. (1999): Steroid modulation of the nicotinic acetylcholine receptor. In: *Neurosteroids: a new regulatory function in the nervous system*, Baulieu, E.E., Robel, P. & Schumacher, M. (eds), in press. Totowa, NJ (USA): Humana Press Inc.

Buisson, B., Gopalakrishnan, M., Arneric, S.P., Sullivan, J.P. & Bertrand, D. (1996): Human α4β2 neuronal nicotinic acetylcholine receptor in HEK 293 cells: a patch-clamp study. *J. Neurosci.* **16**, 7880–7891.

Changeux, J.P. (1990): Functional architecture and dynamics of the nicotinic acetylcholine receptor: an allosteric ligand-gated ion channel, In: *Fidia Research Foundation Neuroscience Award Lectures*, Changeux, J.P., Llinàs, R.R., Purves, D. & Bloom, F.E. (eds), pp. 21–168. New York: Raven Press.

Clarke, P.B.S. (1993): Nicotine dependence-mechanisms and therapeutic strategies. *Biochem. Soc. Symp.* **59**, 83–95.

Clarke, P.B.S. (1991): Nicotinic receptors in rat cerebral cortex are associated with thalamocortical afferents. *Soc. Neurosci. Abstr.* **17**, 384.18.

Clarke, P.B.S. (1995): Nicotinic receptors and cholinergic neurotransmission in the central nervous system. *Ann. N.-Y. Acad. Sci.* **757**, 73–83.

Clarke, P.B.S., Schwartz, R.D., Paul, S.M., Pert, C.B. & Pert, A. (1985): Nicotinic binding in rat brain: autoradiographic comparison of [^{3}H]acetylcholine, [^{3}H]nicotine, and [^{125}I]-alpha-bungarotoxin. *J. Neurosci.* **5**, 1307–1315.

Contreras, D., Destexhe, A., Sejnowski, T.J. & Stériade, M. (1997): Spatiotemporal patterns of spindle oscillations in cortex and thalamus. *J. Neurosci.* **17**, in press.

Corringer, P.J., Galzi, J.L., Eiselé, J.L., Bertrand, S., Changeux, J.P. & Bertrand, D. (1995): Identification of a new component of the agonist binding site of the nicotinic alpha 7 homooligomeric receptor. *J. Biol. Chem.* **270**, 11749–11752.

Court, J. & Clementi, F. (1995): Distribution of nicotinic subtypes in human brain. *Alz. Disease Ass. Disorders* **9** Suppl. 2, 6–14.

Court, J.A., Piggott, M.A., Perry, E.K., Barlow, R.B. & Perry, R.H. (1992): Age associated decline in high affinity nicotinic binding in human brain frontal cortex does not correlate with changes in choline acetyltransferase activity. *Neurosci. Res. Com.* **10**, 125–133.

Couturier, S., Bertrand, D., Matter, J.M., Hernandez, M.C., Bertrand, S., Millar, N., Valera, S., Barkas, T. & Ballivet, M. (1990): A neuronal nicotinic acetylcholine receptor subunit (alpha 7) is developmentally regulated and forms a homo-oligomeric channel blocked by alpha-bungarotoxin. *Neuron* **5**, 845–856.

Damasio (1994): *Descartes' error. Emotion, reason and the human brain*, Grosset, A. (ed.). Putnam Books.

Danober, L., Depaulis, A., Vergnes, M. & Marescaux, C. (1995): Mesopontine cholinergic control over generalized non-convulsive seizures in a genetic model of absence epilepsy in the rat. *Neuroscience* **69**, 1183–1193.

DeFelipe, J., Garcia-Sola, R., Marco, P., del-Rosario-del-Río, M., Pulido, P. & Cajal, S.R.y. (1993): Selective changes in the microorganization of the human epileptogenic neocortex revealed by paravalbumin immunoreactivity. *Cerebral Cortex* **3**, 39–48.

Deutch, A.Y., Holliday, J., Roth, R.H., Chun, L.L.Y. & Hawrot, E. (1987): Immunohistochemical localization of a neuronal nicotinic acetylcholine receptor in mammalian brain. *Proc. Natl. Acad. Sci. (USA)* **84**, 8697–8701.

Devillers-Thiéry, A., Galzi, J.L., Eiselé, J.L., Bertrand, S., Bertrand, D. & Changeux, J.P. (1993): Functional architecture of the nicotinic acetylcholine receptor: a prototype of ligand-gated ion channels. *J. Membrane Bio.* **136**, 97–112.

Ding, Y.-S., Gatley, S.J., Fowler, J.S., Volkow, N.D., Aggarwal, D., Logan, J., Dewey, S.L., Liang, F., Carroll, F.I. & Kuhar, M.J. (1996): Mapping nicotinic acetylcholine receptors (nAChR) with PET. *Synapse* **24**, 403–407.

Eiselé, J.L., Bertrand, S., Galzi, J.L., Devillers-Thiéry, A., Changeux, J.P. & Bertrand, D. (1993): Chimaeric nicotinic-serotonergic receptor combines distinct ligand binding and channel specificities. *Nature* **366**, 479–483.

Ernfors, P., Bengzon, J., Kokaia, Z., Persson, H. & Lindvall, O. (1991): Increased levels of messenger RNAs for neurotrophic factors in the brain during kindling epileptogenesis. *Neuron* **7**, 165–76.

Flores, C.M., Rogers, S.W., Pabreza, L.A., Wolfe, B.B. & Kellar, K.J. (1992): A subtype of nicotinic cholinergic receptor in rat brain is composed of alpha 4 and beta 2 subunits and is up-regulated by chronic nicotine treatment. *Mol. Pharmacol.* **41**, 31–37.

Galzi, J.L., Bertrand, D., Devillers-Thiéry, A., Revah, F., Bertrand, S. & Changeux, J.P. (1991): Functional significance of aromatic amino acids from three peptide loops of the alpha 7 neuronal nicotinic receptor site investigated by site-directed mutagenesis. *FEBS Lett.* **294**, 198–202.

Galzi, J.L., Bertrand, S., Corringer, P.J., Changeux, J.P. & Bertrand, D. (1996): Identification of calcium binding sites that regulate potentiation of a neuronal nicotinic acetylcholine receptor. *EMBO J.* **15**, 5824–5832.

Galzi, J.L. & Changeux, J.P. (1995): Neuronal nicotinic receptors: Molecular organization and regulations. *Neuropharmacology* **34**, 563–582.

Galzi, J.L., Devillers-Thiéry, A., Hussy, N., Bertrand, S., Changeux, J.P. & Bertrand, D. (1992): Mutations in the ion channel domain of a neuronal nicotinic receptor convert ion selectivity from cationic to anionic. *Nature* **359**, 500–505.

Galzi, J.L., Revah, F., Black, D., Goeldner, M., Hirth, C. & Changeux, J.P. (1990): Identification of a novel amino acid α-Tyr 93 within the active site of the acetylcholine receptor by photoaffinity labeling: additional evidence for a three-loop model of the acetylcholine binding site. *J. Biol. Chem.* **265**, 10430–10437.

Gibb, A.J. & Halliday, F.C. (1996): Fast purinergic transmission in the central nervous system. *Seminars in the Neurosciences* **8**, 225–232.

Gopalakrishnan, M., Buisson, B., Touma, E., Giordano, T., Campbell, J.E., Hu, I.C., Donnelly-Roberts, D., Arneric, S.P., Bertrand, D. & Sullivan, J.P. (1995): Stable expression and pharmacological properties of the human α7 nicotinic acetylcholine receptor. *Eur. J. Pharmacol. Mol. Pharmacol. Sec.* **290**, 237–246.

Gopalakrishnan, M., Monteggia, L.M., Anderson, D.J., Molinari, E.J., Piattoni, K.M., Donnelly, R.D., Arneric, S.P. & Sullivan, J.P. (1996): Stable expression, pharmacologic properties and regulation of the human neuronal nicotinic acetylcholine alpha 4 beta 2 receptor. *J. Pharmacol. Exp. Ther.* **276**, 289–297.

Gray, R., Rajan, A.S., Radcliffe, K.A., Yakehiro, M. & Dani, J.A. (1996): Hippocampal synaptic transmission enhanced by low concentrations of nicotine. *Nature* **383**, 713–716.

Gurantz, D., Harootunian, A.T., Tsien, R.Y., Dionne, V.E. & Margiotta, J.F. (1994): VIP modulates neuronal nicotinic acetylcholine receptor function by a cyclic AMP-dependent mechanism. *J. Neurosci.* **14**, 3540–3547.

Hille, B. (1992): *Ionic channels of excitable membranes.* Sunderland, Massachusetts: Sinauer Associates Inc.

Hökfelt, T. (1991): Neuropeptides in perspective: the last ten years. *Neuron* **7**, 867–879.

Horch, H.L. & Sargent, P.B. (1995): Perisynaptic surface distribution of multiple classes of nicotinic acetylcholine receptors on neurons in the chicken ciliary ganglion. *J. Neurosci.* **15**, 7778–95.

Isackson, P.J., Huntsman, M.M., Murray, K.D. & Gall, C.M. (1991): BDNF mRNA expression is increased in adult rat forebrain after limbic seizures: temporal patterns of induction distinct from NGF. *Neuron* **6**, 937–948.

Jessell, T.M. & Kandel, E.R. (1993): Synaptic transmission: A bi-directional and self-modifiable form of cell-cell communication. *Neuron* **10**, 1–30.

Kang, H. & Schuman, E.M. (1995): Long-lasting neurotrophin-induced enhancement of synaptic transmission in the adult hippocampus. *Science* **267**, 1658–1662.

Katz, L.C. & Shatz, C.J. (1996): Synaptic activity and the construction of cortical circuits. *Science* **274**, 1133–1138.

Krosigk, M.V., Bal, T. & McCormick, D.A. (1993): Cellular mechanisms of a synchronized oscillation in the thalamus. *Science* **261**, 361–364.

Kuryatov, A., Gerzanich, V., Nelson, M., Olale, F. & Lindstrom, J. (1997): Mutation associated with autosomal dominant nocturnal frontal lobe epilepsy alters Ca^{++} permeability, conductance and gating of the human α4β2 nicotinic receptor. *Soc. Neurosci. Abstr.* 156-5.

Léna, C. & Changeux, J.P. (1993b): Allosteric modulations of the nicotinic acetylcholine receptor. *Trends Neurosci.* **16**, 181–186.

Léna, C. & Changeux, J.P. (1997): Role of Ca^{2+} ions in nicotinic facilitation of GABA release in mouse thalamus. *J. Neurosci.* **17**, 576–585.

Léna, C., Changeux, J.P. & Mulle, C. (1993): Preterminal nicotinic receptors on GABAergic axons: a study on thin slices and freshly isolated neurons in the rat interpeduncular nucleus. *J. Neurosci.* **13**, 2680–2688.

Lewin, G.R. & Barde, Y.-A. (1996): Physiology of the neurotrophins. *Ann. Rev. Neurosci.* **19**, 289–317.

Lindstrom, J. (1996): Neuronal nicotinic acetylcholine receptors. In: *Ion channels*, Narashi, T. (ed.), pp. 377–449. New York: Plenum Press.

Lo, D.C. (1995): Neurotrophic factors and synaptic plasticity. *Neuron* **15**, 979–981.

Majewska, M.D., Harrison, N.L., Schwartz, R.D., Barker, J.L. & Paul, S.M. (1986): Steroid hormone metabolites are barbiturate-like modulators of GABA receptor. *Science* **232**, 1004–1007.

Manzoni, O., Prezeau, L., Marin, P., Deshager, S., Bockaert, J. & Fagni, L. (1992): Nitric oxide-induced blockade of NMDA receptors. *Neuron* **8**, 653–662.

Margiotta, J.F. & Pardi, D. (1995): Pituitary adenylate cyclase-activating polypeptide type I receptors mediate cyclic AMP-dependent enhancement of neuronal acetylcholine sensitivity. *Mol. Pharmacol.* **48**, 63–71.

Maricq, A.V., Peterson, A.S., Brake, A.J., Myers, R.M. & Julius, D. (1991): Primary structure and functional expression of the $5HT_3$ receptor, a serotonin-gated channel. *Science* **254**, 432–437.

Marks, M.J., Pauly, J.R., Gross, S.D., Deneris, E.S., Hermans-Borgmeyer, I.H., Heinemann, S.F. & Collins, A.C. (1992): Nicotine binding and nicotinic receptor subunit RNA after chronic nicotine treatment. *J. Neurosci.* **12**, 2765–2784.

McBain, C.J. & Mayer, M.L. (1994): N-Methyl-D-Aspartic acid receptor structure and function. *Physiol. Rev.* **74**, 723–760.

McGehee, D.S., Heath, M.J.S., Gelber, S., Devay, P. & Role, L.W. (1995): Nicotine enhancement of fast excitatory synaptic transmission in CNS by presynaptic receptors. *Science* **269**, 1692–1696.

McMahon, L.L., Yoon, K.W. & Chiappinelli, V.A. (1994): Nicotinic receptor activation facilitates GABAergic neurotransmission in the avian lateral spiriform nucleus. *Neuroscience* **59**, 689–698.

Miller, B., Sarantis, M., Traynelis, S.F. & Attwell, D. (1992): Potentiation of NMDA receptor currents by arachidonic acid. *Nature* **355**, 722–725.

Monteggia, L.M., Gopalakrishnan, M., Touma, E., Idler, K.B., Nash, N., Arneric, S.P., Sullivan, J.P. & Giordano, T. (1995): Cloning and transient expression of genes encoding the human alpha 4 and beta 2 neuronal nicotinic acetylcholine receptor (nAChR) subunits. *Gene* **155**, 189–193.

Mulle, C., Léna, C. & Changeux, J.P. (1992): Potentiation of nicotinic receptor response by external calcium in rat central neurons. *Neuron* **8**, 937–945.

Noebels, J.F. (1996): Targeting epilepsy genes. *Neuron* **16**, 241–244.

North, R.A. (1996): P2X purinoceptors plethora. *Seminars in the Neurosciences* **8**, 187–194.

Owen, A. & Bird, M. (1995): Acetylcholine as a regulator of neurite outgrowth and motility in cultured embryonic mouse spinal cord. *Neuroreport* **6**, 2269–2272.

Palma, E., Bertrand, S., Binzoni, T. & Bertrand, D. (1996): Neuronal nicotinic α7 receptor expressed in *Xenopus* oocytes presents five putative binding sites for methyllycaconitine. *J. Physiol. (Lond.)* **491**, 151–161.

Peng, X., Katz, M., Gerzanich, V., Anand, R. & Lindstrom, J. (1994): Human alpha 7 acetylcholine receptor: cloning of the alpha 7 subunit from the SH-SY5Y cell line and determination of pharmacological properties of native receptors and functional alpha 7 homomers expressed in *Xenopus* oocytes. *Mol. Pharmacol.* **45**, 546–554.

Perry, E.K., Court, J.A., Johnson, M., Piggott, M.A. & Perry, R.H. (1992): Autoradiographic distribution of [^{3}H]nicotine binding in human cortex: relative abundance in subicular complex. *J. Chem. Neuroanat.* **5**, 399–405.

Phillips, H.A., Scheffer, I.E., Berkovic, S.F., Holloway, G.E., Sutherland, G.R. & Mulley, J.C. (1995): Localization of a gene for autosomal dominant nocturnal frontal lobe epilepsy to chromosome 20q13.2. *Nat. Genet.* **10**, 117–118.

Picciotto, M.R., Zoli, M., Léna, C., Bessis, A., Lallemand, Y., Le Novère, N., Vincent, P., Pich, E.M., Brulet, P. & Changeux, J.P. (1995): Abnormal avoidance learning in mice lacking functional high-affinity nicotine receptor in the brain. *Nature* **374**, 65–67.

Pin, J.P. & Bockaert, J. (1995): Get receptive to metatropic glutamate receptors. *Curr. Opin. Neurobiol.* **5**, 342–349.

Revah, F., Bertrand, D., Galzi, J.L., Devillers-Thiéry, A., Mulle, C., Hussy, N., Bertrand, S., Ballivet, M. & Changeux, J.P. (1991): Mutations in the channel domain alter desensitization of a neuronal nicotinic receptor. *Nature* **353**, 846–849.

Rubboli, F., Court, J.A., Sala, C., Morris, C., Chini, B., Perry, E. & Clementi, F. (1994a): Distribution of nicotinic receptors in the human hippocampus and thalamus. *Eur. J. Neurosci.* **6**, 1596–1604.

Rubboli, F., Court, J.A., Sala, C., Morris, C., Perry, E. & Clementi, F. (1994b): Distribution of neuronal nicotinic receptor in subunits in human brain. *Neurochem. Int.* **25**, 69–71.

Scheffer, I.E., Bhatia, K.P., Lopes, C.I., Fish, D.R., Marsden, C.D., Andermann, E., Andermann, F., Desbiens, R., Keene, D. & Cendes, F. (1995): Autosomal dominant nocturnal frontal lobe epilepsy. A distinctive clinical disorder. *Brain* **118**, 61–73.

Schröder, H., Giacobini, E., Wevers, A., Birtsch, A. & Schutz, U. (1995): Nicotinic receptors in Alzheimer's disease In: *Brain imaging of nicotine and tobacco smoking*, Domino, E.F. (ed.), pp. 73–93. Ann Arbor: NPP Books.

Schröder, H., Wevers, A., Happich, E., Schütz, U., Moser, N., de Vos, R.A.I., van Noort, G., Jansen, E.N.H., Giacobini, E. & Maelicke, A. (1996): Molecular histochemistry of nicotinic receptors in human brain. In: *Alzheimer disease: from molecular biology to therapy*, Becker, R. & Giacobini, E. (eds), pp. 269–273. Boston: Birkhäuser.

Small, D.H., Reed, G., Whitefield, B. & Nurcombe, V. (1995): Cholinergic regulation of neurite outgrowth from isolated chick sympathetic neurons in culture. *J. Neurosci.* **15**, 144–151.

Snead, O.C. (1995): Basic mechanisms of generalized absence seizures. *Ann. Neurol.* **37**, 146–157.

Steinlein, O.K., Mulley, J.C., Propping, P., Wallace, R.H., Phillips, H.A., Sutherland, G.R., Scheffer, I.E. & Berkovic, S.F. (1995): A missense mutation in the neuronal nicotinic acetylcholine receptor alpha 4 subunit is associated with autosomal dominant nocturnal frontal lobe epilepsy. *Nat. Genet.* **11**, 201–203.

Steinlein, O.K. (1999): Molecular biology in autosomal dominant nocturnal frontal lobe epilepsy (this volume).

Steinlein, O.K., Magnusson, A., Stood, J., Bertrand, S., Weiland, S., Berkovic, S.F., Nakken, K.O., Propping, P. & Bertrand, D. (1997): An insertion mutation of the CHRNA4 gene in a family with autosomal dominant nocturnal frontal lobe epilepsy. *Hum. Mol. Genet.* **6**, 943–947.

Stériade, M. & Contreras, D. (1995): Relations between cortical and thalamic cellular events during transition from sleep patterns to paroxysmal activity. *J. Neurosci.* **15,** 623–642.

Stériade, M. & Llinàs, R. (1988): The functional states of the thalamus and the associated neuronal interplay. *Physiol. Rev.* **68,** 649–742.

Stériade, M., McCormick, D.A. & Sejnowski, T.J. (1993): Thalamocortical oscillations in the sleeping and aroused brain. *Science* **262,** 679–685.

Sucher, N.J., Awobuluyi, M., Choi, Y.-B. & Lipton, S. (1996): NMDA receptors: from genes to channels. *Trends Pharmacol. Sci.* **17,** 348–355.

Südhof, T.C. (1995): The synaptic vesicle: a cascade of protein-protein interactions. *Nature* **375,** 645–653.

Sugaya, K., Giacobini, E. & Chiappinelli, V.A. (1990): Nicotinic acetylcholine receptor subtypes in human frontal cortex: changes in Alzheimer's disease. *J. Neurosci. Res.* **27,** 349–359.

Swanson, L.W., Lindstrom, J., Tzartos, S., Schmued, L.C., O'Leary, D.D.M. & Cowan, W.M. (1983): Immunohistochemical localization of monoclonal antibodies to the nicotinic acetylcholine receptor in chick midbrain. *Proc. Natl. Acad. Sci. (USA)* **80,** 4532–4536.

Tessier-Lavigne, M. & Goodman, C.S. (1996): The molecular biology of axon guidance. *Science* **274,** 1123–1132.

Thoenen, H. (1995): Neurotrophins and neuronal plasticity. *Science* **270,** 593–598.

Tong, G., Shepherd, D. & Jahr, C.E. (1995): Synaptic desensitization of NMDA receptors by calcineurin. *Science* **267,** 1510–1512.

Ullian, E.M. & Sargent, P.B. (1995): Pronounced cellular diversity and extrasynaptic location of nicotinic acetylcholine receptor subunit immunoreactivities in the chicken pretectum. *J. Neurosci.* **15,** 7012–7023.

Unwin, N. (1996): Projection structure of the nicotinic acetylcholine receptor: Distinct conformations of the alpha subunits. *J. Mol. Biol.* **257,** 586–596.

Valera, S., Ballivet, M. & Bertrand, D. (1992): Progesterone modulates a neuronal nicotinic acetylcholine receptor. *Proc. Natl. Acad. Sci. (USA)* **89,** 9949–9953.

Vernino, S., Amador, M., Luetje, C.W., Patrick, J. & Dani, J.A. (1992): Calcium modulation and high calcium permeability of neuronal nicotinic acetylcholine receptor. *Neuron* **8,** 127–134.

Vidal, C. & Changeux, J.P. (1993): Nicotinic and muscarinic modulations of excitatory synaptic transmission in the rat prefrontal cortex *in vitro*. *Neuroscience*, **56,** 23–32.

Vijayaraghavan, S., Huang, B., Blumenthal, E.M. & Berg, D.K. (1995): Arachidonic acid as a possible negative feedback inhibitor of nicotinic acetylcholine receptors on neurons. *J. Neurosci.* **15,** 3679–3687.

Vijayaraghavan, S., Schmid, H.A., Halvorsen, S.W. & Berg, D.K. (1990): Cyclic AMP-dependent phosphorylation of a neuronal acetylcholine receptor alpha-type subunit. *J. Neurosci.* **10,** 3 255–3262.

Weiland, S., Witzemann, V., Villarroel, A., Propping, P. & Steinlein, O. (1996): An amino acid exchange in the second transmembrane segment of a neuronal nicotinic receptor causes partial epilepsy by altering its desensitization kinetics. *FEBS Lett.* **398,** 91–96.

Wevers, A., Jeske, A., Lobron, C., Birtsch, C., Heinemann, S., Maelicke, A., Schroder, R. & Schroder, H. (1994): Cellular distribution of nicotinic acetylcholine receptor subunit mRNAs in the human cerebral cortex as revealed by non-isotopic *in situ* hybridization. *Brain Res. Mol. Brain Res.* **25,** 122–128.

Wevers, A., Monteggia, L., Nowacki, S., Bloch, W., Lindstrom, J., Maelicke, A., Arneric, S. & Schröder, H. (1997): Decreased densities of nicotinic receptor-subunit expressing neurons in the cortex of Morbus Alzheimer. *Ann. Anatomy* **92** (Suppl.), 179.

Wevers, A., Sullivan, J.P., Giordano, T., Birtsch, C., Monteggia, L.M., Nowacki, S., Arneric, S. & Schröder, H. (1995): Cellular distribution of the mRNA for the alpha 7 subunit of the nicotinic acetylcholine receptor in the human cerebral cortex. *Drug Develop. Res.* **36,** 103–110.

Yang, J., Mathie, A. & Hille, B. (1992): 5-HT3 receptor channels in dissociated rat superior cervical ganglion neurons. *J. Physiol. (Lond.)* **448,** 237–56.

Zhang, Z.-W., Coggan, J.S. & Berg, D. (1996): Synaptic currents generated by neuronal acetylcholine receptors sensitive to α-bungarotoxin. *Neuron* **17,** 1231–1240.

Zheng, J.Q., Felder, M., Connor, J.A. & Poo, M.M. (1994): Turning of nerve growth cones induced by neurotransmitters. *Nature* **368,** 140–144.

Zoli, M., N., L., Hill, J.A. & Changeux, J.P. (1995): Developmental regulation of nicotinic ACh receptor subunit mRNAs in the rat central and peripheral nervous systems. *J. Neurosci.* **15,** 1912–1939.

Chapter 21

Channelopathies: ion channels and paroxysmal disorders of the nervous system

Louis J. Ptáček

Howard Hughes Medical Institute, Department of Neurology; Department of Human Genetics; Human Molecular Biology and Genetics Program, University of Utah, SLC, UT; and Program in Neuroscience, University of Utah School of Medicine, Salt Lake City, Utah 84112, USA

Epilepsy represents a group of disorders in which recurrent seizures occur. The seizures are typically unprovoked and unpredictable. Epilepsy is estimated to affect 1–3 per cent of the population (Commission, 1989) and has strong genetic and environmental influences. The epilepsies are extremely heterogeneous, both clinically and genetically.

Many other disorders in humans occur intermittently in patients who are normal between attacks. In addition to the shared feature of episodic occurrence, these paroxysmal disorders share other features with the epilepsies including precipitating factors, therapeutic responses, and presumed pathophysiological bases. In this chapter, the similarities and differences among various episodic diseases will be examined, particularly those between epilepsy and the familial paroxysmal dyskinesias. Furthermore, an argument will be made that the growing knowledge of the role of ion channels in rare paroxysmal disorders is contributing to an understanding of epilepsy and will suggest new directions of inquiry toward unraveling the pathogenetic mechanisms of epilepsy.

Paroxysmal dyskinesias are episodic movement disorders that may be familial or sporadic. They share many features with epilepsy and there is some controversy whether they represent an unusual form of focal seizures. In addition to their episodic occurrence, paroxysmal dyskinesias and epilepsy share features with other disorders including the periodic paralyses/nondystrophic myotonias, episodic ataxias, startle disease, long-QT syndrome, and migraine headache.

These disorders have been studied clinically for many years. Clinical characterization has been very important in establishing a nosology that allows clinicians and scientists to communicate precisely about patients. Meticulous and exact nosology allows identification of more uniform patient populations when studying these disorders and may give clues to pathogenesis. However, this approach remains a descriptive one and does not help to distinguish between different causes yielding a similar clinical phenotype. Histological study of neurological disorders is another descriptive approach that is often important nosologically and diagnostically but does not lead to understanding their pathophysiology.

Advances over the last decade in brain imaging techniques have enabled similar descriptive approaches to neurological diseases *in vivo*. Some imaging techniques have been very important from the nosological and diagnostic perspective. As a research tool, however, brain imaging is very expensive technology and to date, has shed no light on pathophysiological mechanisms of disease.

Remarkable advances in the biochemical and physiological study of various diseases has relied on important descriptive work in the field of neurology, and particularly over the last several decades, have unraveled the fundamental causes of some neurological diseases. In some cases, this information has resulted in improved diagnostic and therapeutic possibilities for patients with diseases of the nervous system.

Tools and discoveries in the relatively new field of molecular biology have led to significant advances and, particularly in the last five years, have led to an understanding of the molecular basis of many rare, monogenic disorders. These advances in our understanding provide important clues to effective approaches toward further elucidating mechanisms of disease and developing better treatments.

Paroxysmal or episodic disorders of the nervous system form a large group of diseases where a molecular and genetic approach has defined the pathogenic basis of many disorders. This has already resulted in the reclassification of some of these diseases, led to understanding what causes them, and suggested novel therapeutic strategies for patients. Study of a group of diseases caused by abnormal ion channels, the 'channelopathies', is a newly recognized field that began with the original description of genetic disorders of voltage-gated ion channels in humans (Ptáček *et al.*, 1991; Rojas *et al.*, 1991). Consequently, a growing number of episodic disorders of the nervous system are being recognized as resulting from malfunction of ion channels in brain, nerve, and muscle.

The relationship of some of these episodic disorders will be reviewed. Special attention will be directed to the similarities and differences between the paroxysmal dyskinesias and epilepsy. Recent advances regarding the molecular basis of some of these disorders will also be discussed. Finally, future directions of such work will be examined, along with the impact that it will have on other episodic disorders.

The paroxysmal dyskinesias

Dyskinesias are hyperkinetic involuntary movements. These include movements that are brisk, small in amplitude, and 'dance-like' (chorea); slower and writhing (athetosis); large in amplitude and flailing (ballismus); and fixed posturing (dystonia). A large majority of patients have symptoms that are continuous or continual during wakefulness; these include chorea, dystonia, and tardive dyskinesias (Fahn, 1994). These abnormal movements may vary in intensity as a function of stress and relaxation or with other factors such as voluntary movements (e.g. action dystonia, intention myoclonus, intention tremor). In some patients, however, the hyperkinetic movements may occur as discrete episodic attacks, or paroxysms (Fahn, 1994). Therefore, these disorders are referred to as the paroxysmal dyskinesias.

The paroxysmal dyskinesias are a heterogeneous group of disorders

Paroxysmal dyskinesias can be classified clinically as either familial or acquired conditions (Goodenough *et al.*, 1978). Familial paroxysmal dyskinesias include choreoathetotic, dystonic, and mixed forms. Within the familial form, both kinesigenic (movement-induced) and non-kinesigenic types have been noted (Demirkiran & Jankovic, 1995; Fahn, 1994; Goodenough *et al.*, 1978; Kertesz, 1967; Mount & Reback, 1940). These disorders can be further classified on the basis of attack duration. Short attacks last from seconds to minutes while long attacks are defined as longer than 5 min (may last up to hours) (Demirkiran & Jankovic, 1995; Fahn, 1994). Both autosomal dominant and recessive forms are observed. Despite the clinical heterogeneity, the phenotype in any particular family is generally consistent. The classification of these disorders is confusing; whether this clinical heterogeneity reflects underlying genetic heterogeneity is not known. The clinical classification has evolved as additional phenotypes have been recognized. The classification of Demirkiran & Jankovic (1995) recognizes four main subgroups, each of which may be further subdivided based on attack duration (short or long) and aetiology (idiopathic or secondary):

> Paroxysmal kinesigenic dyskinesia – induced by sudden changes in movement
> Paroxysmal non-kinesigenic dyskinesia – spontaneous attacks
> Paroxysmal exertional dyskinesia – induced by periods of exertion (5–15 min)
> Paroxysmal hypnogenic dyskinesia – occurs during sleep

Another paroxysmal dystonia has been described but does not fit into the above classification. The main phenotypic feature is tonic upward deviation of the eyes associated with ataxia; 12 such patients have thus far been described (Ahn et al., 1989; Campistol et al., 1993; Deonna et al., 1990; Echenne & Rivier, 1992; Ouvrier & Billson, 1988). The long-term prognosis is favourable with no apparent neurological sequelae. Initially, this condition was thought to occur sporadically, perhaps because the phenotype resolves in childhood and is forgotten by the time the phenotype is manifest in members of the next generation. More recently, autosomal dominant segregation of the trait has been recognized (Campistol et al., 1993).

The clinical and pharmacological data in humans and animals suggest that these different dyskinesias have different pathophysiologies. Overlapping clinical features and the simultaneous occurrence of different types of paroxysmal dyskinesias in the same individual or family suggest a dysfunction involving different parts of the same neuronal circuits (Demirkiran & Jankovic, 1995). Moreover, the phenotype of all patients within a single family tends to be reasonably similar suggesting that specific mutations (probably involving distinct genes) are responsible for each phenotype. Better classification, and ultimately treatment, awaits genetic approaches that will help to characterize underlying pathogenic mechanisms responsible for these diseases.

Other episodic disorders

Periodic paralyses/non-dystrophic myotonias

The periodic paralyses include several conditions in which episodes of limb weakness occur spontaneously or are provoked by various stimuli including changes in plasma potassium, muscle cooling, and muscle activity. Some of these patients also exhibit myotonia, a form of abnormal electrical activity consisting of repetitive action potentials on electromyography associated with delayed relaxation of muscle after voluntary contraction or mechanical stimulation (Ptáček et al., 1993). A disabling feature of several of these periodic paralytic disorders is a progressive, fixed, inter-attack weakness seen in certain patients. The factors responsible for this fixed weakness are not known.

These disorders include hyperkalaemic periodic paralysis (hyperKPP) and hypokalaemic periodic paralysis (hypoKPP). The episodic weakness seen in these disorders is precipitated by high potassium in the former and low serum potassium in the latter. The reason for this potassium sensitivity is not known. Another striking difference between the hyperkalaemic and hypokalaemic forms of periodic paralysis is the occurrence of myotonia in most cases with hyperKPP, and the uniform absence of myotonia in hypoKPP.

A third disorder falling into this category is paramyotonia congenita, a condition with myotonia and episodic weakness that is precipitated by muscle cooling. There myotonia is paradoxical: repeated eye closure results in increasing myotonia rather that the 'warm up' phenomenon seen in myotonia congenita. In addition to the above mentioned phenotypes there are overlap syndromes of potassium- and temperature-sensitivity.

Myotonia congenita (MC) is a group of disorders characterized by myotonia. Some forms are precipitated by potassium loading while others are not. These patients uniformly show a phenomenon of 'warm up'. The stiffness that results from the myotonia improves as muscles are used. Among the non-potassium-sensitive forms of myotonia congenita there are both dominant (Thomsen's MC) and recessive (Becker's MC) types. Weakness is never seen in the potassium-sensitive and Thomsen's forms of myotonia congenita, but in the recessive Becker's form, brief episodes of transient weakness can be seen after periods of rest. Because of the clinical similarities and differences among all of these disorders, the clinical classification of these disorders has never been satisfactory.

Episodic ataxia

Episodic ataxia is a condition where patients develop intermittent incoordination associated with stress, fatigue and certain foods. The attacks may occur spontaneously. In some families, patients with episodic ataxia also have myokymia, a rippling of skeletal muscle arising from excessive excitability of peripheral nerves. Interestingly, paroxysmal kinesigenic dyskinesia is seen in some of these patients (Browne et al., 1994). In other families, an acetazolamide-responsive episodic ataxia is associated with cerebellar degeneration as patients age (Ophoff et al., 1994).

Startle disease

Hereditary hyperekplexia, or startle disease, is a condition where sudden auditory or tactile stimuli result in an exaggerated startle response and marked muscle rigidity of CNS origin. Electroencephalographic recordings are normal between attacks but reveal desynchronization and mild voltage attenuation upon startling (Shiang et al., 1993).

Cardiac muscle diseases

Long-QT syndrome (LQT) is a cardiac dysrhythmia syndrome where patients have prolonged QT interval on electrocardiograms. These patients are susceptible to life-threatening cardiac dysrhythmias such as torsade de pointe. Electrophysiologically, the findings in cardiac muscle share some similarity to the skeletal-muscle myotonia noted in many periodic paralysis patients. And like the periodic paralyses, cardiac tachydysrhythmias in LQT patients are very potassium sensitive. Interestingly, patients with Andersen's syndrome have both periodic paralysis and LQT with cardiac dysrhythmias (Tawil et al., 1994).

Epilepsy

Epilepsy is diagnosed when a patient has two or more unprovoked seizures. This is a common episodic disorder of the nervous system and is a genetically and phenotypically very complex group of disorders (Commission, 1989). Both genetic and environmental factors play important roles in epilepsy.

Migraine headaches

Headaches are yet another (very common) paroxysmal disorder of the nervous system in which certain precipitating factors lead to unilateral headache that may or may not be preceded by visual auras. The range of clinical phenotypes suggests that significant clinical and genetic heterogeneity exists (Headache Classification Committee, 1988). Hemiplegic migraine is a rare form of migraine in which a unilateral headache is followed by contralateral weakness (Joutel et al., 1994).

Similarities among paroxysmal disorders

All of these disorders have the shared feature of episodic occurrence. Other similarities include the factors that precipitate attacks in patients. For example, caffeine, chocolate, large carbohydrate meals, rest after exercise, and alterations in potassium (increases in some cases and decreases in others), precipitate paroxysmal events in subsets of the above-mentioned disorders. Many patients with these disorders (periodic paralysis, familial paroxysmal dyskinesia, epilepsy) have worsened symptoms with stress and fatigue. Menses can be associated with worsening of the familial paroxysmal dyskinesias, epilepsy, and migraine.

The sensory prodromata preceding attacks can be similar in different paroxysmal disorders. In paroxysmal kinesigenic dyskinesia patients, a prodrome is often seen and includes muscle tension, tingling, numbness, dizziness, or a combination of these symptoms; patients with paroxysmal non-kinesigenic dyskinesia frequently have a prodrome of diaphoresis, diplopia, headache, flushing, muscle tension, tingling, and/or dizziness (Demirkiran & Jankovic, 1995). What relationship such prodromes may have to auras in epilepsy or migraine is not known.

Interestingly, overlap of clinical features also exist among these disorders. Some patients with episodic ataxia also have paroxysmal kinesigenic dyskinesias (Browne et al., 1994). Paroxysmal hypnogenic dyskinesia has been regarded as a possible manifestation of epilepsy (Lugaresi & Cirigonotta, 1981). The absence of alteration of consciousness or post-ictal state in paroxysmal dyskinesias would not be typical of generalized epilepsies but is still consistent with partial epilepsy. The growing body of evidence supporting the relationship between paroxysmal hypnogenic dyskinesia and frontal epilepsy has only recently emerged (Meierkord et al., 1992; Oguni et al., 1992; Sellal & Hirsch, 1993; Tinuper et al., 1990). Some patients with paroxysmal hypnogenic dyskinesia, at least the patients with short attacks, probably are identical to patients who have been recognized more recently as having autosomal dominant nocturnal frontal lobe epilepsy (Demirkiran & Jankovic, 1995).

There is controversy regarding the relationship of the kinesigenic and non-kinesigenic paroxysmal dyskinesias to epilepsy (Burger et al., 1972; Demirkiran & Jankovic, 1995; Fahn, 1994; Fouad et al., 1996; Fukuyama & Okada, 1967; Goodenough et al., 1978; Gowers, 1964; Hirata et al., 1991; Lombroso, 1995; Spiller, 1927; Tibbles & Barnes, 1980). The earliest description of paroxysmal kinesigenic dyskinesia was reported as movement-induced seizures (Gowers, 1964). Some cases have been called subcortical epilepsy (Spiller, 1927) and reflex epilepsy (Burger et al., 1972; Fukuyama & Okada, 1967; Tibbles & Barnes, 1980).

Occasional patients with familial paroxysmal dyskinesia have abnormal electroencephalograms (Demirkiran & Jankovic, 1995; Fouad et al., 1996; Hirata et al., 1991; Lombroso, 1995). Several patients in a paroxysmal non-kinesigenic dyskinesia family that we have studied underwent electro-encephalography (EEG) between attacks and all were normal except one (Fouad et al., 1996). The EEG in this patient showed 4 Hz bilateral and synchronous spike-wave complexes with prevalence in the central brain region. It is not known whether this represents a causal or coincidental relationship. An epileptogenic mechanism is further suggested by observations that photic stimulation at low frequency performed close to the onset of the attack induces paroxysmal lateralized discharges from the hemisphere contralateral to the movements (Jacome & Risko, 1984). However, the dystonic and choreoathetoid nature of the attacks coupled with the absence of consistent EEG abnormalities during attacks argues against the hypothesis that these paroxysmal dyskinesias represent a form of epilepsy (Demirkiran & Jankovic, 1995). It is interesting to note that recently a syndrome associating benign familial infantile convulsions (BFIC) and variably expressed paroxysmal choreoathetosis in the same families has been described ('ICCA syndrome', Szepetowski et al., 1997).

Patients with paroxysmal kinesigenic dyskinesia generally respond well to anticonvulsants like phenytoin, carbamazepine, and valproic acid while paroxysmal non-kinesigenic dyskinesia patients do not. Benzodiazepines, like clorazepate, are very effective in treating many patients with paroxysmal non-kinesigenic dyskinesia. Phenytoin and other anticonvulsants, and some drugs commonly used to treat cardiac dysrhythmias (e.g. mexilitine, procainamide and tocainide), are often beneficial in treating myotonia in patients with a number of different muscle diseases (Ptáček et al., 1993). Carbonic anhydrase inhibitors benefit many patients with periodic paralysis and episodic ataxia, and some patients with epilepsy, but no information is available regarding the use of these drugs in patients with paroxysmal dyskinesias (Fouad et al., 1996; Griggs et al., 1978; Ptáček et al., 1993). Carbonic anhydrase catalyses the formation of bicarbonate and hydrogen ions. What the basis for therapeutic response is in patients treated with carbonic anhydrase inhibitors is not clear, but may be related to alterations to the redox potential of muscle or neuronal membranes.

The paroxysmal nature of the attacks, the response to anticonvulsants, the sensory prodromata preceding attacks, and the possible association with epilepsy are the chief reasons for linking the paroxysmal dyskinesias with epileptic disorders.

Rationale for a genetic approach to characterizing pathophysiology of paroxysmal nervous system disorders

The clinical phenotypes of the familial paroxysmal dyskinesias suggest that they result from abnormal membrane excitability of central nervous system neurons. There is a striking precedent for ion channel involvement in other periodic disorders of excitable tissues. *In vitro* and *in vivo* physiological data have demonstrated hyperexcitability of muscle or neuronal membranes in some of these disorders. Taken together, these data suggest that proteins regulating membrane excitability are excellent candidates as the site of defects. The periodic paralyses/nondystrophic myotonias were the first disorders in humans that were shown to be caused by mutations in voltage-gated ion channel genes (see below). Subsequently, many disorders have been shown to result from similar defects in other ion channel genes. The specific abnormality in paroxysmal dyskinesias or epilepsy, whether it is an increase in excitatory stimuli or a loss of inhibitory function of neurons, remains to be characterized. Proteins involved in membrane excitability include voltage-gated ion channels, ligand-gated channels, metabatropic receptors, ion exchangers and transporters.

Ion channels as the molecular basis of paroxysmal disorders

Sodium channel disorders

Hyperkalaemic periodic paralysis, paramyotonia congenita, and an *atypical form of myotonia congenita*, represent myotonic disorders due to episodic membrane hyperexcitability of skeletal muscle (Ptáček *et al.*, 1993). All are caused by mutations in the sodium channel gene SCN4A (McClatchey *et al.*, 1992; Ptáček *et al.*, 1992; Ptáček *et al.*, 1991; Rojas *et al.*, 1991). Physiological study of these mutations *in vitro* reveals abnormalities like those present in patient muscle and is leading toward understanding the pathophysiological basis of these diseases at the level of channel function and membrane excitability (Cannon & Strittmatter, 1993; Chahine *et al.*, 1994; Cummins *et al.*, 1993; Mitrovic *et al.*, 1994; Yang *et al.*, 1994). The cardiac homologue (SCN5A) of the skeletal muscle gene SCN4A, was later shown to cause an analogous syndrome in the heart muscle (Wang *et al.*, 1995).

Calcium channel disorders

Hypokalaemic periodic paralysis is another episodic weakness syndrome that results from mutations in a skeletal-muscle, voltage-gated, calcium channel gene, CACNL1A3 (Elbaz *et al.*, 1995; Fouad *et al.*, 1996; Jurkat Rott *et al.*, 1994; Ptáček *et al.*, 1994). The pathophysiological basis of this disorder is not yet understood. Subsequently, CACNL1A4, a brain homologue, has been shown to result in episodic ataxia (EA2) and hemiplegic migraine (Ophoff *et al.*, 1996).

Chloride channel disorders

Linkage analysis was used to demonstrate that both the Thomsen's and Becker's forms of myotonia congenita map to chromosome 7q near a voltage-gated chloride channel gene. Subsequently, identification of mutations in this gene has proven its pathophysiological role in these forms of myotonia congenita (Abdalla *et al.*, 1992; George *et al.*, 1993; Gronemeier *et al.*, 1994; Heine *et al.*, 1994; Koch *et al.*, 1992; Zhang *et al.*, 1996).

Potassium channel disorders

Mutations causing episodic ataxia with myokymia occur in a gene encoding a voltage-gated potassium channel (Browne *et al.*, 1994). Subsequently, mutations in three distinct voltage-gated potassium channel genes were shown to result in the LQT (Curran *et al.*, 1995; Wang *et al.*, 1996). Lastly, two novel voltage-dependent potassium channel genes, KCNQ2 and KCNQ3, have recently been described as mutated in benign familial neonatal convulsions (BFNC) families linked either to chromosome 20q13.3 or 8q24 (Biervert *et al.*, 1998; Charlier *et al.*, 1998; Singh *et al.*, 1998).

Ligand-gated channel disorders

The gene causing one form of inherited partial epilepsy, *autosomal dominant nocturnal frontal lobe epilepsy*, was mapped to chromosome 20q13 in a large Australian family. Subsequently, a mutation in the neuronal nicotinic acetylcholine receptor α4 subunit has been identified and is implicated as the molecular basis for the epilepsy in that family (Steinlein *et al.*, 1995). The biophysical effects of this mutation are beginning to be understood (see Chapters 19 and 20, this volume).

Hereditary hyperekplexia results from mutations in the inhibitory glycine receptor α1-subunit gene (Shiang *et al.*, 1993). This receptor is a hetero-oligomeric, ligand-gated chloride channel. Disease-causing mutations are hypothesized to result in a deficiency of functional glycine receptors (Shiang *et al.*, 1993).

Genetics of paroxysmal dyskinesias

An autosomal dominant *paroxysmal choreoathetosis syndrome associated with progressive spasticity* maps to the vicinity of a potassium channel gene cluster on chromosome 1p (Auburger *et al.*, 1996). These genes have not been identified and the pathogenesis of the disorder is not yet understood.

The familial form of paroxysmal non-kinesigenic dyskinesia has been mapped to chromosome 2q (Fink *et al.*, 1996; Fouad *et al.*, 1996). The gene causing this disease remains unknown. However, based on genetic localization, expression in appropriate regions of the brain, and a plausible physiological rationale, two genes located at the FPD1 locus are candidates as the site of defect in paroxysmal non-kinesigenic dyskinesia. We are examining both genes for mutations in patient DNA samples to test this hypothesis. One of these genes (AE3) maps to chromosome 2q31–36 and encodes an anion exchanger that is sodium-independent and functions as an alkali extruder (Kopito *et al.*, 1989; Linn *et al.*, 1992; Su *et al.*, 1994; Yannoukakos *et al.*, 1994). It is expressed most abundantly in the deep pontine gray matter, the tegmentum of the midbrain, and the medulla, but is widely expressed at lower levels in other regions of the brain (Kopito *et al.*, 1989). We hypothesize that, in conjunction with normal $GABA_A$ receptor function, AE3 mutations might lead to paroxysmal non-kinesigenic dyskinesia.

$GABA_A$ receptors are the principle mediators of synaptic inhibition in the brain; when activated, they allow preferential movement of chloride ions into the cell, thereby polarizing the membrane. However, dendritic $GABA_A$ receptors can depolarize neurons when intensely activated (Michelson & Wong, 1991). Carbonic anhydrase in the cell catalyses the formation of HCO_3^- from H_2O and CO_2 that diffuses across the membrane. Under the condition of intense stimulation, the HCO_3^- gradient is restored more quickly than the Cl^- gradient through the action of carbonic anhydrase. The result in an intensely stimulated cell is a greater outward HCO_3^- current than inward Cl^- current.

Staley and colleagues proposed that this GABA-mediated, activity-dependent depolarization could account for collapse of the chloride gradient, depolarization of the cell, and modulation of synaptic NMDA receptor activation (Staley *et al.*, 1995). We hypothesize that decreased electroneutral exchange of HCO_3^- through AE3 (exchanged 1:1 with Cl^-) could lead to increased electrogenic movement of HCO_3^- through $GABA_A$ receptors, thereby leading to hyperexcitability of neurons. We have obtained an AE3 genomic clone (Su *et al.*, 1994) and have characterized the boundaries of all exons which are contained within the clone (three through 24). We are analysing these exons in patient DNAs to test the hypothesis that AE3 mutations cause paroxysmal non-kinesigenic dyskinesia.

A second candidate, a serotonin receptor gene ($5HT_{2B}$), maps to the same region of chromosome 2 (Le Coniat *et al.*, 1996). The $5HT_{2B}$ receptors mediate many of the central and peripheral physiological functions of serotonin. The actions of serotonin receptors are very complex and we can only speculate about how mutations in this gene might lead to a paroxysmal movement disorder. However, the critical role of serotonin receptors in modulating membrane excitability in the central nervous system makes this gene a good candidate. We are currently testing this hypothesis by using primers from the published intron-exon boundaries (Schmuck *et al.*, 1994) to PCR-amplify patient DNA for mutational analysis.

In summary, genetic approaches to localizing and identifying genes are very powerful and have been used successfully. Numerous precedents now exist where genetic approaches were used to show that paroxysmal disorders result from mutations in voltage- or ligand-gated channels (Table 1). These discoveries have led to a new field – channelopathies – where an increasing number of disorders are being shown to result from mutations in ion channels. The prospect for application of these discoveries to more common (and genetically more complex) paroxysmal disorders such as epilepsy and migraine is excellent. Understanding of the genes, proteins, and biology of rare, single-gene disorders has been fundamental to these goals, and it is virtually certain that some idiopathic epilepsies, and various forms of migraine will be added to the growing list of channelopathies.

Table 1. Ion channels and paroxysmal human diseases

Disease	Genetic locus	Gene
Hyperkalaemic periodic paralysis	ch 17q23-q25	SCN4A
Paramyotonia congenita	ch 17q23-q25	SCN4A
Hypokalaemic periodic paralysis	ch 1q32	CACNL1A3
Episodic ataxia with myokymia (EA1)	ch 12p13	KCNA1
Episodic ataxia (EA2)	ch 19p13	CACNL1A4
Hemiplegic migraine	ch 19p13	CACNL1A4
Long-QT syndrome 1	ch 11p15.5	KVLQT1
Long-QT syndrome 2	ch 7q35-q36	HERG
Long-QT syndrome 3	ch 3p21-p24	SCN5A
Long-QT syndrome 4	ch 4	?
Long-QT syndrome 5	ch 21q22	minK
Startle disease	ch 5q32	GlyR 1
Autosomal dominant nocturnal frontal lobe epilepsy	ch 20q13	nAch 4
Benign familial neonatal convulsions (BFNC)	ch 20q13.3 ch 8q24	KCNQ2 KCNQ3
Paroxysmal choreoathetosis with spasticity	ch 1p	?
Non-kinesigenic paroxysmal dyskinesia	ch 2q33-q35	?
Familial infantile convulsions and paroxysmal choreoathetosis (ICCA)	ch 16	?

Acknowledgements: The author is grateful to Dr. Jong Rho for helpful discussions and critical reading of the manuscript. Investigations in the laboratory are supported by NIH grant NS32711; by the H.A. Benning Endowment; by a grant from the Muscular Dystrophy Association; and by the Charles E. Culpeper Foundation. Dr. Ptáček is a Charles E. Culpeper Foundation Scholar.

References

Abdalla, J.A., Casley, W.L., Cousin, H.K., Hudson, A.J., Murphy, E.G., Cornelis, F.C., Hashimoto, L. & Ebers, G.C. (1992): Linkage of Thomsen disease to the T-cell-receptor beta (TCRB) locus on chromosome 7q35. *Am. J. Hum. Genet.* **51**, 579–584.

Ahn, J.C., Hoyt, W.F. & Hoyt, C.S. (1989): Tonic upgaze in infancy. A report of three cases. *Arch. Ophthalmol.* **107**, 57–58.

Auburger, G., Ratzlaff, T., Lunkes, A., Nelles, H., Leube, B., Binkofski, F., Kugel, H. *et al.* (1996): A gene for autosomal dominant paroxysmal choreoathetosis/spasticity (CSE) maps to the vicinity of a potassium channel gene cluster on chromosome 1p, probable within 2 cM between D1S443 and D1S197. *Genomics* **31**, 90–94.

Biervert, C., Schroeder, B.C., Kubisch, C., Berkovic, S.F., Propping, P., Jentsch, T.J. & Steinlein, O.K. (1998): A potassium channel mutation in neonatal human epilepsy. *Science* **279**, 403–406.

Browne, D.L., Gancher, S.T., Nutt, J.G., Brunt, E.R., Smith, E.A., Kramer, P. & Litt, M. (1994): Episodic ataxia/myokymia syndrome is associated with point mutations in the human potassium channel gene, KCNA1 [see comments]. *Nat. Genet.* **8**, 136–140.

Burger, L., Lopez, R. & Elliott, F. (1972): Tonic seizures induced by movement. *Neurology* **22**, 656–659.

Campistol, J., Prats, J.M. & Garaizar, C. (1993): Benign paroxysmal tonic upgaze of childhood with ataxia. A neuro-ophthalmological syndrome of familial origin? *Dev. Med. Child Neurol.* **35**, 436–439.

Cannon, S.C. & Strittmatter, S.M. (1993): Functional expression of sodium channel mutations identified in families with periodic paralysis. *Neuron* **10**, 317–326.

Chahine, M., George, A.L., Jr., Zhou, M., Ji, S., Sun, W., Barchi, R.L. & Horn, R. (1994): Sodium channel mutations in paramyotonia congenita uncouple inactivation from activation. *Neuron* **12**, 281–294.

Charlier, C., Singh, N.A., Ryan, S.G., Lewis, T.B., Reus, B.E., Leach, R.J. & Leppert, M. (1998): A pore mutation in a novel KQT-like potassium channel gene in an idioipathic epilepsy family. *Nat. Genet.* **18**, 53–55.

Commission on the Classification and Terminology of the International League Against Epilepsy (1989): Proposal for revised classification of epilepsies and epileptic syndromes. *Epilepsia* **30**, 389–399.

Cummins, T.R., Zhou, J., Sigworth, F.J., Ukomadu, C., Stephan, M., Ptáček, L.J. & Agnew, W.S. (1993): Functional consequences of a Na+ channel mutation causing hyperkalemic periodic paralysis. *Neuron* **10**, 667–678.

Curran, M.E., Splawski, I., Timothy, K.W., Vincent, G.M., Green, E.D. & Keating, M.T. (1995): A molecular basis for cardiac arrhythmia: HERG mutations cause long QT syndrome. *Cell* **80**, 795–803.

Demirkiran, M. & Jankovic, J. (1995): Paroxysmal dyskinesias: clinical features and classification. *Ann. Neurol.* **38**, 571–579.

Deonna, T., Roulet, E. & Meyer, H.U. (1990): Benign paroxysmal tonic upgaze of childhood – a new syndrome. *Neuropediatrics* **21**, 213–214.

Echenne, B. & Rivier, F. (1992): Benign paroxysmal tonic upward gaze [see comments]. *Pediatr. Neurol.* **8**, 154–155.

Elbaz, A., Vale Santos, J., Jurkat Rott, K., Lapie, P., Ophoff, R.A., Bady, B., Links, T.P., Piussan, C., Vila, A., Monnier, N. *et al.* (1995): Hypokalemic periodic paralysis and the dihydropyridine receptor (CACNL1A3): genotype/phenotype correlations for two predominant mutations and evidence for the absence of a founder effect in 16 caucasian families. *Am. J. Hum. Genet.* **56**, 374–380.

Fahn, S. (1994): *The paroxysmal dyskinesias*, pp. 310–345. Oxford: Butterworth-Heinemann.

Fink, J.K., Rainier, S., Wilkowski, J., Jones, S.M., Kume, A., Hedera, P., Albin, R., Mathay, J., Girbach, L., Varvil, T., Otterud, B. & Leppert, M. (1996): Paroxysmal dystonic choreoathetosis: tight linkage to chromosome 2q. *Am. J. Hum. Genet.* **59**, 140–145.

Fouad, G., Dalakas, M., Servedei, S., Mendell, J.R., Van den Bergh, P., Angelini, C., Alderson, K., Griggs, R.C., Tawil, R., Gregg, R., Hogan, K., Powers, P.A., Weinberg, N., Malonee, W. & Ptáček, L.J. (1997): Genotype-phenotype correlations of DHP receptor alpha-1 gene mutations causing hypokalemic periodic paralysis. *Neuromusc. Disord.* **7**, 33–38.

Fouad, G.T., Servidei, S., Durcan, S., Bertini, E. & Ptáček, L.J. (1996): A gene for familial paroxysmal dyskinesia (FPD1) maps to chromosome 2q. *Am. J. Hum. Genet.* **59**, 135–139.

Fukuyama, S. & Okada, R. (1967): Hereditary kinesigenic reflex epilepsy: report of five families of peculiar seizures induced by sudden movements. *Adv. Neurol. Sci.* **11**, 168–197.

George, A.L., Jr., Crackower, M.A., Abdalla, J.A., Hudson, A.J. & Ebers, G.C. (1993): Molecular basis of Thomsen's disease (autosomal dominant myotonia congenita). *Nat. Genet.* **3**, 305–10.

Goodenough, D., Fariello, R., Annis, B. & Chun, R. (1978): Familial and acquired paroxysmal dyskinesias. *Arch. Neurol.* **35**, 827–831.

Gowers, W. (1964): *Epilepsy and other chronic convulsive diseases. Their causes, symptoms, and treatment*, pp. 75–76. New York: Dover (reprint of 1885 ed).

Griggs, R.C., Moxley, R.T., Lafrance, R.A. & McQuillen, J. (1978): Hereditary paroxysmal ataxia: Response to acetazolamide. *Neurology* **28**, 1259–1264.

Gronemeier, M., Condie, A., Prosser, J., Steinmeyer, K., Jentsch, T.J. & Jockusch, H. (1994): Nonsense and missense mutations in the muscular chloride channel gene Clc-1 of myotonic mice. *J. Biol. Chem.* **269**, 5963–5967.

Headache Classification Committee of the International Headache Society (1988): Classification and diagnostic criteria for headache disorders, cranial neuralgias and facial pain. *Cephalalgia* **8** Suppl. 7, 1–96.

Heine, R., George, A.L., Jr., Pika, U., Deymeer, F., Rudel, R. & Lehmann Horn, F. (1994): Proof of a non-functional muscle chloride channel in recessive myotonia congenita (Becker) by detection of a 4 base pair deletion. *Hum. Mol. Genet.* **3**, 1123–1128.

Hirata, K., Katayama, S., Saito, T., Ichihashi, K., Mukai, T., Katayama, M. & Otaka, T. (1991): Paroxysmal kinesigenic choreoathetosis with abnormal electroencephalogram during attacks. *Epilepsia* **32**, 492–494.

Jacome, D.E. & Risko, M. (1984): Photic induced-driven PLEDs in paroxysmal dystonic choreoathetosis. *Clin. Electroencephalogr.* **15**, 151–154.

Joutel, A., Ducros, A., Vahedi, K., Labauge, P., Delrieu, O., Pinsard, N., Mancini, J., Ponsot, G., Gouttiere, F., Gastaut, J.L., Maziaceck, J., Weissenbach, J., Bousser, M.G. & Tournier-Lasserve, E. (1994): Genetic heterogeneity of familial hemiplegic migraine. *Am. J. Hum. Genet.* **55**, 1166–1172.

Jurkat Rott, K., Lehmann Horn, F., Elbaz, A., Heine, R., Gregg, R.G., Hogan, K., Powers, P.A., Lapie, P., Vale Santos, J.E., Weissenbach, J. et al. (1994): A calcium channel mutation causing hypokalemic periodic paralysis. *Hum. Mol. Genet.* **3**, 1415–1419.

Kertesz, A. (1967): Paroxysmal kinesigenic choreoathetosis. *Neurology* **17**, 680–690.

Koch, M.C., Steinmeyer, K., Lorenz, C., Ricker, K., Wolf, F., Otto, M., Zoll, B., Lehmann Horn, F., Grzeschik, K.H. & Jentsch, T.J. (1992): The skeletal muscle chloride channel in dominant and recessive human myotonia. *Science* **257**, 797–800.

Kopito, R.R., Lee, B.S., Simmons, D.M., Lindsey, A.E., Morgans, C.W. & Schneider, K. (1989): Regulation of intracellular pH by a neuronal homolog of the erythrocyte anion exchanger. *Cell* **59**, 927–937.

Le Coniat, M., Choi, D.-S., Maroteaux, L., Launay, J.-M. & Berger, R. (1996): The 5-HT2B receptor gene maps to 2q36.3–2q37.1. *Genomics* **32**, 172–173.

Linn, S.C., Kudrycki, K.E. & Shull, G.E. (1992): The predicted translation product of a cardiac AE3 mRNA contains an N terminus distinct from that of the brain AE3 Cl-/HCO3- exchanger. Cloning of a cardiac AE3 cDNA, organization of the AE3 gene, and identification of an alternative transcription initiation site. *J. Biol. Chem.* **267**, 7927–7935.

Lombroso, C.T. (1995): Paroxysmal choreoathetosis: an epileptic or non-epileptic disorder? *Ital. J. Neurol. Sci.* **16**, 271–277.

Lugaresi, E. & Cirigonotta, F. (1981): Hypnogenic paroxysmal dystonia: epileptic seizures or a new syndrome? *Sleep* **4**, 129–138.

McClatchey, A.I., Van den Bergh, P., Pericak Vance, M.A., Raskind, W., Verellen, C., McKenna Yasek, D., Rao, K., Haines, J.L., Bird, T., Brown, R.H., Jr. et al. (1992): Temperature-sensitive mutations in the III-IV cytoplasmic loop region of the skeletal muscle sodium channel gene in paramyotonia congenita. *Cell* **68**, 769–774.

Meierkord, H., Fish, D.R., Smith, S.J., Scott, C.A., Shorvon, S.D. & Marsden, C.D. (1992): Is nocturnal paroxysmal dystonia a form of frontal lobe epilepsy? [see comments]. *Mov. Disord.* **7**, 38–42.

Michelson, H.B. & Wong, R.K. (1991): Excitatory synaptic responses mediated by $GABA_A$ receptors in the hippocampus. *Science* **253**, 1420–1423.

Mitrovic, N., George, A.L., Jr., Heine, R., Wagner, S., Pika, U., Hartlaub, U., Zhou, M., Lerche, H., Fahlke, C. & Lehmann Horn, F. (1994): K(+)-aggravated myotonia: destabilization of the inactivated state of the human muscle Na+ channel by the V1589M mutation. *J. Physiol. Lond.* **478** Pt 3, 395–402.

Mount, L. & Reback, S. (1940): Familial paroxysmal choreoathetosis. *Arch. Neurol. Psychiatry* **44**, 841–847.

Oguni, M., Oguni, H., Kozasa, M. & Fukuyama, Y. (1992): A case with nocturnal paroxysmal unilateral dystonia and interictal right frontal epileptic EEG focus: a lateralized variant of nocturnal paroxysmal dystonia? *Brain Dev.* **14**, 412–416.

Ophoff, R.A.M.T.G., Vergouwe, M.N., van Eijk, R., Oefner, P.J., Hoffman, S.M.G., Lamerdin, J.E., Mohrenweiser, H.W., Bulman, D.E., Ferrari, M., Haan, J., Lindhout, D., van Ommen, G.-J., Hofker, M.H., Ferrari, M.D. & Frants, R.R. (1996): Familial hemiplegic migraine and episodic ataxia type–2 are caused by mutations in the Ca2+ gene CACNL1A4. *Cell* **87**, 543–552.

Ophoff, R.A., van Eijk, R., Sandkuijl, L.A., Terwindt, G.M., Grubben, C.P.M., Haan, J., Lindhout, D., Ferrari, M.D. & Frants, R.R. (1994): Genetic heterogeneity of familial hemiplegic migraine. *Genomics* **22**, 21–26.

Ouvrier, R.A. & Billson, F. (1988): Benign paroxysmal tonic upgaze of childhood. *J. Child Neurol.* **3**, 177–180.

Ptáček, L.J., George, A.L., Jr., Barchi, R.L., Griggs, R.C., Riggs, J.E., Robertson, M. & Leppert, M.F. (1992): Mutations in an S4 segment of the adult skeletal muscle sodium channel cause paramyotonia congenita. *Neuron* **8**, 891–897.

Ptáček, L.J., George, A.L., Jr., Griggs, R.C., Tawil, R., Kallen, R.G., Barchi, R.L., Robertson, M. & Leppert, M.F. (1991): Identification of a mutation in the gene causing hyperkalemic periodic paralysis. *Cell* **67**, 1021–1027.

Ptáček, L.J., Johnson, K.J. & Griggs, R.C. (1993): Genetics and physiology of the myotonic muscle disorders. *N. Engl. J. Med.* **328**, 482–489.

Ptáček, L.J., Tawil, R., Griggs, R.C., Engel, A.G., Layser, R.B., Kwiecinski, H., McManis, P.G., Santiago, L., Moore, M., Fouad, G. *et al.* (1994): Dihydropyridine receptor mutations cause hypokalemic periodic paralysis. *Cell* **77**, 863–868.

Ptáček, L.J., Trimmer, J.S., Agnew, W.S., Roberts, J.W., Petajan, J.H. & Leppert, M. (1991): Paramyotonia congenita and hyperkalemic periodic paralysis map to the same sodium-channel gene locus. *Am. J. Hum. Genet.* **49**, 851–854.

Rojas, C.V., Wang, J.Z., Schwartz, L.S., Hoffman, E.P., Powell, B.R. & Brown, R.H., Jr. (1991): A Met-to-Val mutation in the skeletal muscle Na+ channel alpha-subunit in hyperkalaemic periodic paralysis. *Nature* **354**, 387–389.

Schmuck, K., Ullmer, C., Engels, P. & Lubbert, H. (1994): Cloning and functional characterization of the human 5-HT2B serotonin receptor. *FEBS Lett.* **342**, 85–90.

Sellal, F. & Hirsch, E. (1993): Nocturnal paroxysmal dystonia [letter; comment]. *Mov. Disord.* **8**, 252–253.

Shiang, R., Ryan, S.G., Zhu, Y.Z., Hahn, A.F. P.O.C. & Wasmuth, J.J. (1993): Mutations in the alpha 1 subunit of the inhibitory glycine receptor cause the dominant neurologic disorder, hyperekplexia. *Nat. Genet.* **5**, 351–358.

Singh, N.A., Charlier, C., Stauffer, D., DuPont, B.R., Leach, R.J., Melis, R., Ronen, G.B., Bjerre, I., Quattlebaum, T., Murphy, J.V., McHarg, M.L., Gagnon, D., Rosales, T.O., Peiffer, A., Anderson, V.E. & Leppert, M. (1998): A novel potassium channel gene, KCNQ2, is mutated in an inherited epilepsy of newborns. *Nat. Genet.* **18**, 25–29.

Spiller, W. (1927): Subcortical epilepsy. *Brain* **50**, 171–187.

Staley, K.J., Soldo, B.L. & Proctor, W.R. (1995): Ionic mechanisms of neuronal excitation by inhibitory GABA$_A$ receptors [see comments]. *Science* **269**, 977–981.

Steinlein, O.K., Mulley, J.C., Propping, P., Wallace, R.H., Phillips, H.A., Sutherland, G.R., Scheffer, I.E. & Berkovic, S.F. (1995): A missense mutation in the neuronal nicotinic acetylcholine receptor alpha 4 subunit is associated with autosomal dominant nocturnal frontal lobe epilepsy. *Nat. Genet.* **11**, 201–203.

Su, Y.R., Klanke, C.A., Houseal, T.W., Linn, S.C., Burk, S.E., Varvil, T.S., Otterud, B.E., Shull, G.E., Leppert, M.F. & Menon, A.G. (1994): Molecular cloning and physical and genetic mapping of the human anion exchanger isoform 3 (SLC2C) gene to chromosome 2q36. *Genomics* **22**, 605–609.

Szepetowski, P., Rochette, J., Berquin, P., Piussan, C., Lathrop, G.M. & Monaco, A.P. (1997): Familial infantile convulsions and paroxysmal choreoathetosis: a new neurological syndrome linked to the pericentromeric region of human chromosome 16. *Am. J. Hum. Genet.* **61**, 889–898.

Tawil, R., Ptáček, L.J., Pavlakis, S.G., DeVivo, D.C., Penn, A.S., Ozdemir, C. & Griggs, R.C. (1994): Andersen's syndrome: potassium-sensitive periodic paralysis, ventricular ectopy, and dysmorphic features [see comments]. *Ann. Neurol.* **35**, 326–330.

Tibbles, J. & Barnes, S. (1980): Paroxysmal dystonic choreoathetosis of Mount and Reback. *Pediatrics* **65**, 149–151.

Tinuper, P., Cerullo, A., Cirignotta, F., Cortelli, P., Lugaresi, E. & Montagna, P. (1990): Nocturnal paroxysmal dystonia with short-lasting attacks: three cases with evidence for an epileptic frontal lobe origin of seizures. *Epilepsia* **31**, 549–556.

Wang, Q., Curran, M.E., Splawski, I., Burn, T.C., Millholland, J.M., VanRaay, T.J., Shen, J., Timothy, K.W., Vincent, G.M., de Jager, T., Schwartz, P.J., Toubin, J.A., Moss, A.J., Atkinson, D.L., Landes, G.M., Connors, T.D. & Keating, M.T. (1996): Positional cloning of a novel potassium channel gene: KVLQT1 mutations cause cardiac arrhythmias. *Nat. Genet.* **12**, 17–23.

Wang, Q., Shen, J., Splawski, I., Atkinson, D., Li, Z., Robinson, J.L., Moss, A.J., Towbin, J.A. & Keating, M.T. (1995): SCN5A mutations associated with an inherited cardiac arrhythmia, long QT syndrome. *Cell* **80**, 805–811.

Yang, N., Ji, S., Zhou, M., Ptáček, L.J., Barchi, R.L., Horn, R. & George, A.L., Jr. (1994): Sodium channel mutations in paramyotonia congenita exhibit similar biophysical phenotypes *in vitro*. *Proc. Natl. Acad. Sci. USA* **91**, 12785–12789.

Yannoukakos, D., Stuart Tilley, A., Fernandez, H.A., Fey, P., Duyk, G. & Alper, S.L. (1994): Molecular cloning, expression, and chromosomal localization of two isoforms of the AE3 anion exchanger from human heart. *Circ. Res.* **75**, 603–614.

Zhang, J., George, A.L., Griggs, R.C., Fouad, G.T., Roberts, J., Kwiecinski, H., Connolly, A.M. & Ptáček, L.J. (1996): Mutations in the human skeletal muscle chloride channel gene (CLCN1) associated with dominant and recessive myotonia congenita. *Neurology* **47**, 993–998.

Chapter 22

Homeobox genes in the developing brain

Edoardo Boncinelli[1,2], Antonio Faiella[1], Silvia Brunelli[1], Renzo Guerrini[3]

[1]*DIBIT, Istituto Scientifico H.S.Raffaele, Via Olgettina 60, 20132 Milano, Italy;* [2]*Centro per lo Studio della Farmacologia Cellulare e Molecolare, CNR, Via Vanvitelli 32, 20129 Milano, Italy;* [3]*Istituto di Neuropsichiatria Infantile, I.R.C.C.S. Fondazione Stella Maris, Università di Pisa, 56018 Calambrone, Pisa, Italy*

During embryonic development, a great variety of cell types are produced in the neural tube from a relatively homogeneous population of precursor cells. In recent years, the cellular and molecular mechanisms by which specific types of neurons are generated and organized have been explored and a number of principles and developmental pathways have been discovered in the CNS. All events of differentiation and patterning at the level of single cells or groups of cells are preceded by developmental decisions that involve entire regions of the forming nervous system. Recently, some of these events have received particular attention – among them, the regionalization of the CNS along its anterior-posterior axis, the establishment and maintenance of a dorsal-ventral polarity of the neural tube, the process of segregation of the presumptive cerebral cortex from basal ganglia and the lamination of the cerebral cortex. Any alteration in one of these processes is likely to cause major developmental defects and generate pathology of the nervous system.

The regionalization of the CNS of vertebrates along the anterior-posterior body axis appears to be of paramount relevance for the specification of the identity of all regions along the body. In the neural tube of the developing vertebrate there are at least two levels of regionalization (Boncinelli, 1994). The first level is represented by the classical subdivision of the adult CNS into major structural regions like telencephalon, diencephalon, mesencephalon, metencephalon, myelencephalon and spinal cord. The subdivision of the adult brain can in turn be traced back to the initial subdivision of the developing brain into three early vesicles represented by forebrain, midbrain and hindbrain. Within some of the major regions of the developing neural tube there is a second level of regionalization, which gives rise to identifiable neuroepithelial domains, sometimes called neuromeres. Subsequent differentiation of the various neuroepithelial domains within each major region of the CNS results in neural structures of distinct histologies and anatomical complexity. In the past few years substantial progress has been made in deciphering the embryological and molecular mechanisms by which this pattern is generated, with a special emphasis on the establishment of the boundary between midbrain and hindbrain (Bally-Cuif & Wassef, 1995) and on the subdivision of the hindbrain (Guthrie, 1995). However, much less is known so far about how regional properties are established in other districts of the developing brain and in particular in the forebrain.

Regulatory genes in the developing CNS

A key role in the regionalization of the CNS and, more generally, in the specification of the various anatomical and functional neural domains, is played by regulatory genes – genes acting through the control of the expression of other genes laying hierarchically downstream from them and sometimes termed target genes. Regulatory genes generally code for transcription factors, i.e. nuclear proteins able to recognize specific DNA sequences, bind to them and modulate, through this specific binding, the level of expression of the corresponding target genes. A relatively large proportion of regulatory genes are indeed homeobox genes. Homeobox genes are regulatory genes characterized by the presence of a specific, evolutionary conserved, DNA sequence termed homeobox, able to code for a protein domain of some 60 amino acid residues, termed homeodomain. It is through the action of their homeodomain that the protein products of the homeobox genes, the homeoproteins, bind to the regulatory regions of specific genes and control their expression.

Among the vertebrate homeobox genes those belonging to the HOX family (Krumlauf, 1994 for reviews; McGinnis & Krumlauf, 1992), stand out as the true homologues of the *Drosophila* homeotic genes which provide biological information to specify the identity of the various body segments of this insect. Through the action of homeotic genes every segment along the body of the fly acquires its full endowment of anatomical structures, including appropriate appendages, and is put in condition to deploy its specific functionality. Mutations in these genes cause the transformation of a given body segment into a more or less perfect copy of a different body segment.

HOX genes are expressed in relatively extended expression domains along the major body axis of vertebrate embryos. These expression domains include discrete regions of the neural tube, in the spinal cord and hindbrain. Of particular interest is the situation in the developing hindbrain where some of these genes are expressed according to a specific pattern (Guthrie, 1995). Development of the hindbrain (rhombencephalon) is marked by the appearance of a series of periodic constrictions and bulges that subdivide the region into distinct areas, termed rhombomeres, r1 to r8 from anterior to posterior. Rhombencephalon appears to be the only primarily segmented region of the developing neural tube of vertebrates and several lines of evidence indicate that HOX genes play a pivotal role in its patterning. HOX gene expression in this embryonic region bears not only on the patterning of the neural tube but also on the formation and patterning of the entire branchial region. In fact, neural crest cells stemming from rhombencephalon also give rise to mesoderm and precisely to the cranio-facial mesoderm. The concerted expression of HOX genes, sometimes called the 'HOX code', in specific regions of the anterior neural tube also conveys biological information to the departing neural crest cells in order for them to pattern the branchial area properly.

Conversely, these genes do not seem to play any significant role in the head and brain regions anterior to the hindbrain. Actually, development of the anterior-most body domain corresponding to the anterior head has remained relatively obscure, even in flies (Finkelstein & Boncinelli, 1994). Nevertheless, in the last few years at least three genes have been identified that play a role in the development and regionalization of the *Drosophila* head: *empty spiracles* (*ems*), *orthodenticle* (*otd*) and *buttonhead* (*btd*).

The first two are homeobox genes and four vertebrate homologues of them have been isolated and characterized. These four genes are *Emx1* and *Emx2* (Simeone et al., 1992a, b), related to *ems*, and *Otx1* and *Otx2* (Finkelstein & Boncinelli, 1994; Simeone et al., 1992a, 1993), related to *otd*. The four vertebrate genes are expressed in extended regions of the developing rostral brain of mouse embryos, including the presumptive cerebral cortex and olfactory bulbs. We will summarize expression data and discuss the possible roles of the four genes in establishing cell identities and precise boundaries of the various brain regions, starting from their first specification in gastrulating embryos.

Regulatory homeobox genes in the developing brain

Expression of the four genes in E10 mouse embryos

At day 10 of development (E10) the neural tube of the mouse already shows recognizable regions corresponding to the future anatomical subdivisions. The entire neural tube consists of neuroepithelial cells in active proliferation and most of the specific differentiative events have not yet occurred. In E10 mouse embryos all four *Emx* and *Otx* genes are expressed. Their expression domains are continuous regions of the developing brain contained within each other in the sequence *Emx1*fs28 *Emx2*fs28 *Otx1*fs28 *Otx2* (Fig. 1). The *Emx1* expression domain includes the dorsal telencephalon with a posterior boundary slightly anterior to that between presumptive diencephalon and telencephalon. *Emx2* is expressed in dorsal and ventral neurectoderm of the presumptive forebrain with an anterior boundary slightly anterior to that of *Emx1* and a posterior boundary within the roof of presumptive diencephalon. This boundary most probably coincides with the boundary between the first and second thalamic segment, which will subsequently give rise to ventral thalamus and dorsal thalamus, respectively. The *Otx1* expression domain contains the *Emx2* domain. It covers a continuous region including part of the telencephalon, the diencephalon and the mesencephalon with an anterior boundary approximately coincident with that of *Emx2*. Finally, the *Otx2* expression domain contains the *Otx1* domain, both dorsally and ventrally, and practically covers the entire fore- and mid-brain, to the exclusion of the early optic area.

Expression of *Emx* and *Otx* genes identifies several regions in the forebrain. Some of these regions seem to correspond to presumptive anatomical subdivisions, whereas the significance of others remains to be assessed. Dorsally, for example, it is clear that the two *Emx* genes identify a presumptive cortical region, part of which will be neocortex and archicortex. *Emx2* expression also appears to define the boundary between future dorsal and ventral thalamus. On the other hand, it is notable that expression of these genes does not offer an unambiguous cue for the boundary between presumptive ventral thalamus and posterior dorsal telencephalon.

In summary, analysis of E10 brain shows a pattern of nested expression domains of the four genes in brain regions defining an embryonic rostral, or pre-isthmic, brain as opposed to hindbrain and spinal cord. The first appearance of the products of the four genes is also sequential during development:

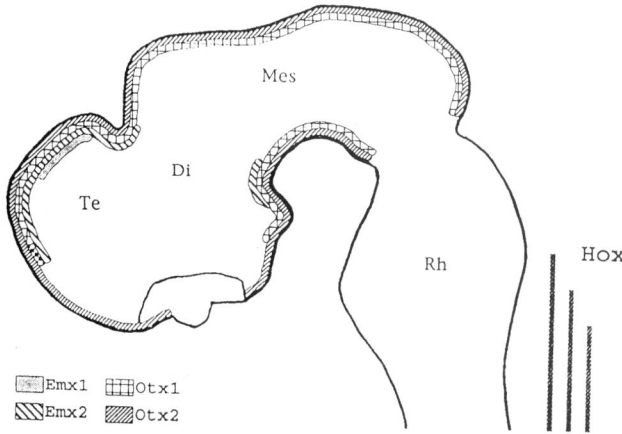

Fig. 1. Nested expression domains of Otx and Emx homeobox genes in the developing brain of E10 mouse embryos. Expression of members of the Hox gene family is also schematically indicated. Di, diencephalon; Mes, mesencephalon; Rh, rhomboencephalon; Te, telencephalon.

Otx2 is already expressed at least as early as at E5.5 (Simeone *et al.*, 1993), followed by *Otx1* and *Emx2* at E8–8.5 and finally by *Emx1* at E9.5 (Simeone *et al.*, 1992a). Thus, it seems reasonable to postulate a role of the four homeobox genes in establishing the identity of the various embryonic brain regions. In this line, the regionalization of the early rostral brain seems to be a centripetal process progressing through discrete steps and ultimately leading to the specification of dorsal telencephalon.

The vertebrate CNS, if not the entire vertebrate body axis, can be subdivided into at least five domains, on the basis of the regional expression of different families of regulatory genes (Fig. 2). There is increasing evidence that the five domains are specified and regionalized according to different developmental pathways that may turn out to be conceptually very distant. Domain 1, including fore- and mid-brain, represents the domain of action of *Otx* and *Emx* gene families. Domains 3, 4 and 5 subdivide the rhombencephalon posterior to rhombomere r1 and the spinal cord. This is the domain of *Hox* genes. It can be thought of as divided into three subdomains corresponding to the three subfamilies of the *Hox* gene family. Domain 2, essentially rhombomere r1 and the so-called met-mesencephalic boundary region, remains outside the domains of action of both the *Otx/Emx* gene families and the *Hox gene* family. It appears to represent something different from all the rest of the CNS and to follow unique developmental criteria, possibly owing to its relative evolutionary novelty.

Early expression of *Otx2*

Otx2 appears to play an early role in vertebrate gastrulation and first specification of anterior head and rostral brain. Its expression is already detectable in embryonic structures of the implanted mouse blastocyst since the prestreak stage at about day 5.5 of development (Simeone *et al.*, 1993). At that gestational age *Otx2* gene products are present in the embryonic ectoderm, or epiblast, but not in extra-embryonic ectoderm. The epiblast of the pre-gastrula mouse embryo represents the sole source of the tissues of the fetus. The same expression pattern is observed in early- to mid-streak E6.5-E7 embryos. Between day 7 and 7.5 of development the posterior boundary of the *Otx2* expression domain progressively recedes to anterior regions where it will remain confined throughout development. These regions correspond to neuroectoderm of presumptive prosencephalon and mesencephalon.

Essentially the same expression profile was observed in frog, chick and zebrafish embryos. Detailed expression analysis in these model systems reveals that *Otx2* is first expressed in cells of the invaginating axial mesendoderm, and precisely in its anteriormost region, sometimes termed prechordal plate, underlying the presumptive rostral brain. Around the period when the neural plate is induced and the first steps of its regionalization are laid down, *Otx2* gene products extend to the overlying neuroectoderm and presumably participate in the specification of rostral brain. This hypothesis found strong support from analysis of manipulated mouse (Acampora *et al.*, 1995; Ang *et al.*, 1996; Matsuo *et al.*, 1995), frog and chick embryos (Boncinelli & Mallamaci, 1996).

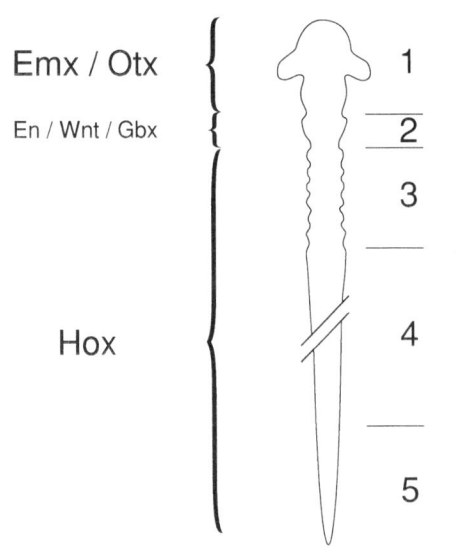

Fig. 2. *Schematic subdivision of the vertebrate CNS on the basis of the expression of specific families of regulatory genes. En and Gbx are two homeobox genes, whereas Wnt codes for growth factor.*

Transgenic mice carrying homozygous null mutations of *Otx2* fail to gastrulate and stop developing at early midgestation. The most conspicuous phenotype of these embryos is the deletion of rostral brain regions, including forebrain and midbrain, anterior to rhombomere r3. It is highly likely that the deletion of anterior neural structures is a consequence of the defective formation and migration of anterior axial mesendoderm cells. On the other hand, frog embryos deriving from zygotes where *Otx2* has been overexpressed show severely reduced trunk and tail structures and an expansion of anterior head structures including pharynx and forebrain (Boncinelli & Mallamaci, 1996).

Expression of *Otx* genes in the brain of midgestation mouse embryos

In midgestation mouse embryos the two *Otx* genes are expressed in dorsal and basal telencephalon, in diencephalon and mesencephalon (Simeone *et al.*, 1993). Their expression domains in mesencephalon show a sharp posterior boundary, both dorsally and ventrally, approximately at the level of rhombic isthmus. From E9.25 onward, the expression of both genes clearly marks the posterior boundary of mesencephalon to the exclusion of presumptive anterior cerebellar domains.

Otx1 and *Otx2* are also expressed in restricted regions of diencephalon: epithalamus, dorsal thalamus and mammillary region of posterior hypothalamus. In these regions, the hybridization signal is almost exclusively confined to cells of the ventricular zone. Their expression domain does not include the ventral thalamus. A two-layered narrow stripe of expression is detectable at the level of the boundary between dorsal and ventral thalamus, that is the zona limitans intrathalamica, the precursor of lamina medullaris externa and mammillo-thalamic tract. Other localizations are: fasciculus retroflexus, the precursor of habenulo-interpeduncular tract, stria medullaris, including the region surrounding the posterior commissure, primordium of mammillotegmental tract, epiphysis, fornix and sulcus lateralis hypothalami posterioris. Posterior to diencephalon, *Otx1* and *Otx2* are expressed in mesencephalic regions of tectum and tegmentum, possibly at the level of presumptive periventricular bundles.

Both *Otx* genes are also expressed in developing special sense organs, that is in the olfactory epithelium, as well as in the developing inner ear from early expression in the otic vesicle to epithelia in auricular ducts of sacculus and cochlea and in the developing eye, including the external sheaths of the optic nerve (Boncinelli *et al.*, 1993; Simeone *et al.*, 1993).

Areas and boundaries in the forebrain

Expression of *Otx* genes in diencephalon and mesencephalon of E12.5–14.5 embryos colocalizes with boundary regions and presumptive axon tracts, including anterior and posterior commissure (Boncinelli, 1994). This expression is confined to precursor cells surrounding these structures as if these cells could be used as borders of pathways for the pioneer axon tracts. This is particularly evident in posterior commissure and along the zona limitans intrathalamica. *Otx* gene expression in posterior commissure is limited to cells of ventricular epithelium, whereas primary fibres running on its surface are not labelled (Boncinelli *et al.*, 1993). Expression of *Otx* genes along the zona limitans intrathalamica might constitute a framework for the axon patterning of lamina medullaris and other structures physically separating the dorsal thalamus from the ventral thalamus. The existence of this barrier might account for the sharp dorsal boundary of the expression domain in ventral thalamus of some regulatory genes, such as those of the *Dlx* family (see Boncinelli,1994, for a review), and for the sharp ventral boundary of the expression domain in the dorsal thalamus of other genes. Both *Otx* genes are also expressed around the developing optic nerve. This localization is similar to that along the zona limitans intrathalamica in providing clues to axon pathfinding and patterning. In this light, expression of *Otx* genes might provide a global framework for the primary scaffold of specific axon pathways in the early neuroepithelium of the forebrain.

In this light, it is of interest to consider the possibility that *Otx* genes play a different role in the development of the head in at least two different stages. They first specify territories or areas in rostral brain of E8-E10 mouse embryos and provide later on a set of positional cues required for growing axons to follow specific pathways within the embryonic central nervous system. It is not clear whether the two functions are independent.

It has to be emphasized that *Otx* and *Emx* genes are by no means the only genes expressed in the developing brain. Many other regulatory or structural genes are also expressed here, even if not exclusively here (Rubenstein & Puelles, 1994; Rubenstein et al., 1994; Shimamura et al., 1995 and references therein). Partly on the basis of the expression domains of all of these genes, a model has been proposed for the subdivision of the developing rostral brain in neuromeres, namely the so-called prosomeric model (Rubenstein et al., 1994). It entails a subdivision of the embryonic forebrain into six neuromeres, termed prosomeres, p1 to p6, from posterior to anterior. Three of these, p1 to p3, subdivide the diencephalon and three subdivide what these authors call secondary prosencephalon, comprising telencephalon and hypothalamic regions.

Expression of *Otx* and *Emx* genes in the developing cerebral cortex

All four genes are expressed between E9.5 and E10.5 in the presumptive cerebral cortex. Starting from E10.75, *Otx2* expression progressively disappears from this region. This process is relatively quick and initiates in the central areas of both hemispheres. *Otx2* expression persists in the forming choroid plexus, an extremely specific *Otx2* localization (Boncinelli et al., 1993), and in septum and some regions of ganglionic eminence.

Emx1, *Emx2* and *Otx1* are expressed in presumptive cerebral cortex in an extended developmental period corresponding to major events in cortical neurogenesis (Simeone et al., 1992b). *Emx1* expression domain comprises cortical regions including primordia of neopallium, hippocampal and parahippocampal archipallium. *Emx1* expression seems characteristic of cortical regions, mainly but not exclusively hexalaminar in nature. In the same period, the *Emx2* expression domain comprises presumptive cortical regions including neopallium, hippocampal and parahippocampal archipallium and selected paleopallial localizations, but no basal internal grisea (Simeone et al., 1992b). *Otx1* expression domain in forebrain (Frantz et al., 1994; Gulisano et al., 1996; Simeone et al., 1993) includes dorsal telencephalon but also extends to basal regions.

It is interesting to consider the temporal pattern of expression of *Otx1* and the *Emx* genes in the various zones of the forming cerebral cortex (Frantz et al., 1994; Gulisano et al., 1996). Here, at least three major zones can be defined: the germinal neuroepithelium or ventricular zone, where cortical neurons proliferate, a transitional field, and finally the forming cortical plate from which the cortical gray matter will subsequently develop (Bayer & Altman, 1991). At the beginning and up to E12.5 the germinal neuroepithelium is practically the sole component of the prosencephalic wall. Then a transitional field appears. This includes the subventricular zone, a zone whose nature remains poorly known, and the intermediate zone whereto differentiating cortical cells translocate before migrating to outer regions. As development proceeds, the thickness of the cortical plate progressively increases. Both the transitional field and the cortical plate develop at the expense of the neuroepithelium according to specific spatial and temporal gradients within the forming cortex. Two major neurogenetic and morphogenetic gradients can be observed: one progressing anterior to posterior and a second progressing ventrolateral to dorsomedial. The various cortical layers are formed in an inside-out pattern (Bayer & Altman, 1991). Cell tracing experiments have shown that neurons destined to occupy the depth of the cortex are generated first and that the subsequently generated waves of neurons bypass the earlier ones by active migration and settle above them.

In mouse embryos of all stages *Emx2* expression coincides with cells of the germinal neuroepithelium (Gulisano et al., 1996) (Fig. 3). In E12.5 embryos, *Emx2* hybridization signal is uniformly distributed across the cortex without major differences, but starting from E13.5 it appears to be confined to the germinal neuroepithelium of the ventricular zone, excluding both the transitional field and the cortical plate. From day 14.5 on, *Emx2* cortical expression progressively declines in anterior and ventrolateral regions and by the end of gestation is solely confined to specific cell layers in the hippocampus. It is conceivable that *Emx2* plays a role in the control of proliferation of cortical neuroblasts, and thus, the regulation of their subsequent migration process, since it is known that these cells reach their final destination in the mature cortex according to their birthdate.

Otx1 is expressed in the ventricular zone and specifically in deeper layers of the telencephalic cortex since their birth. In the adult cortex *Otx1* is expressed in a subpopulation of neurons in layer 5 and overall in layer 6 (Frantz *et al.*, 1994; Gulisano *et al.*, 1996). Conversely, *Emx1* is expressed in most cortical neurons, whether proliferating, migrating, differentiating, or fully differentiated and organized in a mature cerebral cortex (Gulisano *et al.*, 1996). On the other hand, no *Emx1* expression is detectable in ventral forebrain regions and in particular in the developing basal ganglia. These observations suggest that *Emx1* may be involved in the definition of a specific cellular identity in the cerebral cortex.

A couple of final considerations are in order about the expression of the *Emx* genes in the developing cortex (Gulisano *et al.*, 1996). The adult cerebral cortex is subdivided into functional areas which reach maximal structural and functional complexity in humans. Very little is known about their specification. Two partially contrasting theories have been put forward to explain these events. According to one model (Rakic, 1988) this subdivision is largely specified on a genetic basis. A 'protomap' of the various functional areas is already present early in development, possibly in subplate cells (Shatz *et al.*,

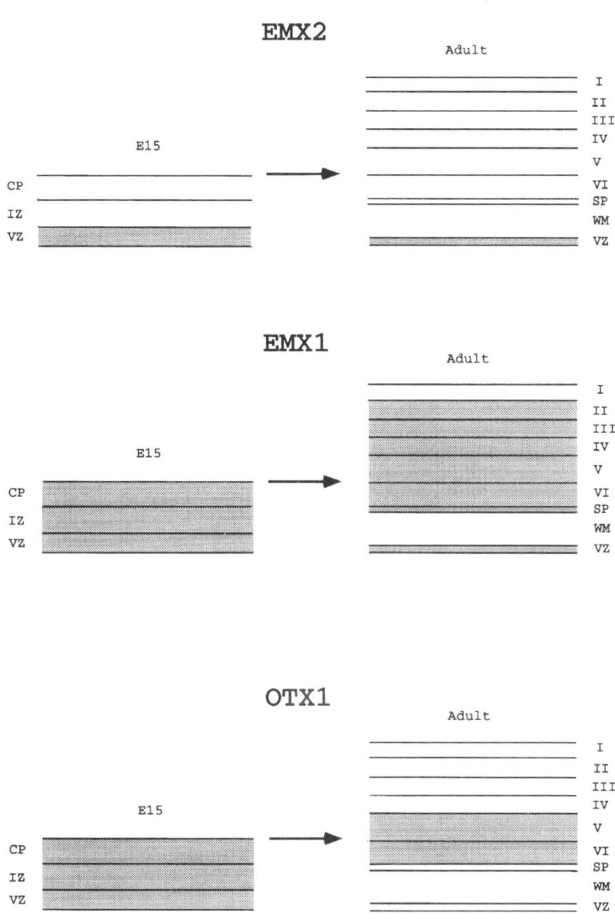

Fig. 3. Comparison of the expression domains of *Otx1*, *Emx1* and *Emx2* in the cerebral cortex of the mouse. Grey colour designates the zones where the corresponding gene is expressed. CP, cortical plate; IZ, intermediate zone; SP, subplate; VZ, ventricular zone; WM, white matter.

1988), and subsequently extends to the mature cortex through a point to point migration of cortical neurons along radial glial cells. According to a second model (O'Leary *et al.*, 1994), presumptive functional areas of the cortex are not defined in detail prior to the arrival of projections from subcortical, mainly thalamic, regions and these connections play a major role in their specification.

In this respect, it is interesting to note that *Emx2* is expressed in the ventricular zone of midgestation mouse embryos according to an anterior-posterior gradient of intensity, higher in posterior cortical regions than in anterior ones. This expression gradient of *Emx2* is suggestive of a contribution of *Emx2* to cortical polarization in the framework of an arealization process taking place in the ventricular zone (O'Leary *et al.*, 1994). As a regulatory gene encoding a transcription factor, *Emx2* is an ideal candidate for generating and/or maintaining a position-dependent signal within the cortex. *Emx1* is in turn highly expressed in at least a subset of subplate neurons. The subplate (Allendoerfer & Shatz,

1994) is a layer of early generated neurons lying just beneath the cortical plate. Subplate neurons seem to participate in early functional circuitry: they receive synaptic inputs from waiting thalamic afferents and make axonal projections on to the cortical plate. Some experiments suggest that the subplate shows basic features of cortical organization later projected onto the layers of the adult cerebral cortex. *Emx1* gene products might play a role in some of these crucial events.

Clues from the analysis of mutants

Preliminary data are available about the phenotypes exhibited by mice bearing null mutations in these four genes. We already noticed that transgenic mice lacking *Otx2* gene products are early embryonic lethal. Therefore, they do not provide useful information about the role of this gene in late brain development. Conversely, transgenic mice lacking the gene products of *Otx1*, *Emx1* and *Emx2* are born and their brain can be analysed. All of them show major disturbances in the architecture of various brain regions, including the cerebral cortex. Particularly noticeable is the altered patterning of hippocampus and the total absence of dentate gyrus in *Emx2* null mice (Pellegrini et al., 1996). A detailed anatomical and functional analysis of these mutants is underway. Plenty of useful information about the role of these genes may hopefully derive from this study even if it can be anticipated that these studies will require quite a long time, mainly due to the subtleties of the cortical functional architecture.

In the meantime, mutations in the human *Emx2* gene, more correctly designated EMX2, have been reported (Brunelli et al., 1996; Granata et al., 1997; Faiella et al., 1997) in sporadic cases of schizencephaly, a human congenital defect of the cerebral cortex. Schizencephaly is also defined as a genetic porencephaly distinct from encephaloclastic porencephaly (Harding, 1992). Schizencephaly is characterized by a full-thickness cleft of the cerebral hemisphere(s) with consequent communication between the ventricle and pericerebral subarachnoid spaces (Yakovlev & Wadsworth, 1946a, b). The malformation may be unilateral or bilateral, the latter being usually symmetric in location, but not in size (Guerrini et al., 1996). Based on the space separating the walls of the fissure, an open-lip form and a closed-lip form can be distinguished. The external opening is covered with cortex showing stellate convolutions with unlayered polymicrogyria (Ferrer, 1984), covering the lips of the fissure and proceeding down to the ventricular wall. The cortex is covered with a membrane resulting from the fusion between the pia and the ventricular ependyma (pia-ependymal seam). The cleft can be detected in any encephalic site, but it is far more frequent in the perisylvian area (Barkovich & Kjos, 1992). In 80 per cent of cases the septum pellucidum is absent (Chamberlain et al., 1990). Septo-optic dysplasia (agenesis of the septum pellucidum and optic nerve hypoplasia) is observed in about one third of cases (Barkovich & Norman, 1988; Hosley et al., 1992). Familial occurrence has been reported in two half-siblings of both sexes, indicating that autosomal inheritance, either dominant or recessive, is possible (Hosley et al., 1992).

Patients with bilateral clefts usually have microcephaly and severe developmental delay with spastic quadriparesis (Barkovich & Kjos, 1992; Granata et al., 1996). Open lip clefts result in more severe impairment, with seizures being present in most patients, usually beginning before 3 years of age. Unilateral clefts are accompanied by a much less severe clinical phenotype. Small, unilateral closed lip clefts may be discovered on MRI performed after the onset of seizures in otherwise normal individuals (Barkovich & Kjos, 1992). Epilepsy is estimated to occur in equal proportion in patients with unilateral or bilateral cleft (about 80 per cent) (Granata et al., 1996). However, early seizure onset and seizure intractability are much more frequent when the malformation is bilateral (81 per cent vs. 63 per cent and 50 per cent vs. 27 per cent, respectively). Epilepsy is always partial, and there are no distinctive electroclinical patterns. The presence of *Emx2* mutations in cases of schizencephaly lends support to the hypothesis that *Emx2* gene products are required for the correct formation of the human cerebral cortex.

Classification and molecular analysis of the various *Emx2* mutations implicated in schizencephaly is likely to provide useful information for both clinical practice and understanding of the pathogenesis of these types of diseases. Preliminary data (Brunelli *et al.*, 1996; Granata *et al.*, 1997; Faiella *et al.*, 1997) point in the direction of a correlation between the nature of the molecular defect, the severity of the phenotype and the presence of particular clinical features. In fact, serious molecular defects, like frameshift mutations or mutations affecting the splicing pattern are invariably associated with severe, open lip, bilateral schizencephaly, whereas subtle or leaky mutations are associated with mild, closed lip, seemingly unilateral schizencephaly (Table 1). In view of the difficulties of the differential diagnosis of schizencephaly versus similar cortical dysplasias, it would be extremely important to have a molecular tool available for an early and reliable diagnosis. Finally, it is conceivable to produce transgenic mice carrying specific *Emx2* mutations in order to investigate their cortical phenotype.

Table 1. Summary of cases analysed

Patient	Schizencephaly	Association	EMX2 mutation
BA	Severe, bilateral	call, sept	Frameshift
DZ	Severe, bilateral	call, sept	Missense
GM	Severe, bilateral	call, sept	Intron2 deletion
ME	Severe, bilateral	call, sept	Splicing defect
MI	Severe, bilateral	call, front	Splicing defect
MM	Severe, bilateral	call	Splicing defect
PN	Severe, bilateral	call, hydr	Splicing defect
Fa	Severe, bilateral	polymicrogyria?	–
BV	Mild, unilateral	Partial epilepsy	Synonymous*
DCS	Mild, unilateral	Partial epilepsy	Synonymous*
MB	Mild, unilateral	Partial epilepsy	Intron2
PB	Mild, unilateral	Partial epilepsy	Intron2
PC	Mild, unilateral	Partial epilepsy	Synonymous*
VF	Mild, unilateral	Partial epilepsy and mMR	Synonymous*
Rb	Mild, unilateral	Partial epilepsy	–
Mc	Mild, unilateral	Partial epilepsy	–
Od	Mild, unilateral	Partial epilepsy	–
CG	Mild, unilateral	Partial epilepsy	–

call, callosal dysgenesis; front, frontal lobe agenesis; hydr, hydrocephalus; mMR, mild mental retardation; sept, septo-optic dysplasia. – means no detectable mutations.
*Synonymous mutations found in patients BV, DCS, PC and VF are identical (synonymous mutation, that is mutation that do not change the nature of the encoded aminoacid residue).

Possible implications in cortical dysgenesis and epilepsies

Emx and *Otx* genes represent powerful tools for the study of the developing brain, and in particular of the developing cerebral cortex. Their expression patterns during mammalian embryogenesis allow us to follow closely major events in cortical neurogenesis and differentiation. It is also conceivable that mutational events, either germ line or somatic, in these genes or some of their targets underlie a number of brain defects and in particular cortical dysplasias (Guerrini *et al.*, 1996). Therefore, it seems useful to investigate the possible implication of mutations of these genes in pathological entities such as, for example, in various forms of gray matter heterotopia, agyria-pachygyria, polymicrogyria, hemimegalencephaly and focal cortical dysplasia. These defects are characterized by abnormal cortical architecture with either normal or dysplastic neurons in aberrant positions in turn implying abnormal connectivity.

Epileptic seizures are present in schizencephaly, as well as in most defects of cortical development (Guerrini *et al.*, 1996). It is still unknown whether seizure activity in the schizencephalic brain originates directly from intrinsic epileptogenic properties of cortical neurons bordering the cleft, from possible abnormalities in signaling systems (Eksioglu *et al.*, 1996) or abnormal connectivity and circuitry (Ferrer *et al.*, 1992). Seizure activity has been demonstrated to arise directly from abnormal neuronal aggregates in both gray matter heterotopia (Morrel, 1992; Munari, 1996) and focal cortical dysplasia. In the latter case, it has been related to intrinsic neuronal properties (Mattia *et al.*, 1995). However, unlike other non-dysplastic epileptogenic lesions in which epileptic activity originates from normal neurons bordering the abnormal tissue, in gray matter heterotopia and focal cortical dysplasia the seizure-generating neurons are those within the abnormal area. Therefore, the genetic abnormalities which may cause such malformations (Dobyns *et al.*, 1996; Eksioglu *et al.*, 1996; Robain, 1996) have a direct involvement in epileptogenesis as well. Whether these considerations also apply to schizencephaly is still unknown. Further insight into the epileptogenic properties of neurons forming the schizencephalic cleft may arise from electrocorticography or depth electrode studies in patients who are candidates for epilepsy surgery. Functional MRI or direct electrophysiological studies of tissue slices obtained from surgical specimens may provide additional information. Identification of epilepsy genes has profound implications for therapy as well as pathophysiology, but it has proven a difficult task mainly due to extreme genetic and phenotypic heterogeneity. For this reason it will be of interest to examine the structure and expression of specific developmental genes such as the *Otx* and *Emx* genes in these pathological entities causing human epilepsy. Results of this analysis are likely to be of primary relevance to not only these diseases, but also to our understanding of the genetic component of multifactorial congenital defects of the brain.

References

Acampora, D., Mazan, S., Lallemand, Y., Avantaggiato, V., Maury, M., Simeone, A. & Brulet P. (1995): Forebrain and midbrain regions are deleted in *Otx2-/-* mutants due to a defective anterior neuroectoderm specification during gastrulation. *Development* **121**, 3279–3290.

Allendoerfer, K.L. & Shatz, C.J. (1994): The subplate, a transient neocortical structure: its role in the development of connection between thalamus and cortex. *Annu. Rev. Neurosci.* **17**, 185–218.

Ang, S.-L., Jin, O., Rhinn, M., Daigle, N., Stevenson, L. & Rossant, J. (1996): A targeted mouse *Otx2* mutation leads to severe defects in gastrulation and formation of axial mesoderm and to deletion of rostral brain. *Development* **122**, 243–252.

Bally-Cuif, L. & Boncinelli, E. (1997): Transcription factors and head formation in vertebrates. *Bioessays* **19**, 127–135.

Bally-Cuif, L. & Wassef, M. (1995): Determination events in the nervous system of the vertebrate embryo. *Current Opinion in Genetics and Development* **5**, 450–458.

Barkovich, A.J. & Kjos, B.O. (1992): Schizencephaly: correlation of clinical findings with MR characteristics. *AJNR.* **13**, 85–94

Barkovich, A.J. & Norman, D. (1988): MR of schizencephaly. *AJNR.* **9**, 297–302.

Bayer, S.A. & Altman, J. (1991): *Neocortical development.* New York: Raven Press.

Boncinelli, E. (1994): Early CNS development: *Distal-less* related genes and forebrain development. *Current Opinion in Neurobiology* **4**, 29–36.

Boncinelli, E., Gulisano, M. & Broccoli, V. (1993): Emx and Otx genes in the developing mouse brain. *J. Neurobiol.* **24**, 1356–1366.

Boncinelli, E. & Mallamaci, A. (1995): Homeobox genes in vertebrate gastrulation. *Current Opinion in Genetics and Development* **5**, 619–627.

Brunelli, S., Faiella, A., Capra, V., Nigro, V., Simeone, A., Cama, A. & Boncinelli, E. (1996): Germline mutations in the homeobox gene EMX2 in patients with severe schizencephaly. *Nat. Genet.* **12**, 94–96.

Chamberlain, M.C., Press, G.A., Bejar, R.F. (1990): Neonatal schizencephaly: comparison of brain imaging. *Pediatr. Neurol.* **6**, 382–387.

Dobyns, W.B., Andermann, E., Andermann, F., Czapansky-Beilman, D., Dubeau, F., Dulac, O., Guerrini, R., Hirsch, B., Ledbetter, D.H., Lee, N.S., Motte, J., Pinard, J.-M., Radtke, R.A., Ross, M.E., Tampieri, D., Walsh, C.A. & Truwit, C.L. (1996): X-linked malformations of neuronal migration. *Neurology* **47**, 331–339.

Eksioglu, Y.Z., Scheffer, I.E., Cardenas, P., Knoll, J., DiMario, F., Ramsey, G., Berg, M., Kamuro, K., Berkovic, S.F., Duyk, G.M., Parisi, J., Huttenlocher, P.R. & Walsh, C.A. (1996): Periventricular heterotopia: an X-linked dominant epilepsy locus causing aberrant cerebral cortical development. *Neuron* **16**, 77–78.

Faiella, A., Brunell1, S., Granata, T., D'Incerti, L., Cardini, R., Lenti, C., Battaglia, G. & Boncinelli, E. (1997): A number of schizencephaly patients including two brothers are heterozygous for germline mutations in the homeobox gene EMX2. *Eur. J. Hum. Genet.* **5**, 186–190.

Ferrer, I. (1984): A Golgi analysis of unlayered polymicrogyria. *Acta Neuropathol.* **65**, 69–76.

Ferrer, I., Pineda, M., Tallada, M., Olivier, B., Russi, A., Oller, L., Noboa, R., Zujar, M.J. & Alcantara, S. (1992): Abnormal local circuit neurons in epilepsia partialis continua associated with focal cortical dysplasia. *Acta Neuropathol.* **83**, 647–652.

Finkelstein, R. & Boncinelli, E. (1994): From fly head to mammalian forebrain: the story of *Otd* and *Otx. Trends Genet.* **10**, 310–315.

Frantz, G.D., Weimann, J.M., Levine, M.E. & McConnell, S.K. (1994): *Otx1* and *Otx2* define layers and regions in developing cerebral cortex and cerebellum. *J. Neurosci.* **14**, 5725–5740.

Granata, T., Battaglia, G., D'Incerti, L., Franceschetti, S., Spreafico, R., Savoiardo, M. & Avanzini, G. (1996): Schizencephaly: clinical findings. In: *Dysplasias of cerebral cortex and epilepsy*, Guerrini, R., Andermann, F., Canapicchi, R., Roger, J., Zifkin, B. & Pfanner, P. (eds), pp. 407–415. Philadelphia-New York: Lippincott-Raven.

Granata, T., Farina, L., Faiella, A., Cardini, R., D'Incerti, L., Boncinelli, E. & Battaglia, G. (1997): Familial schizencephaly associated with EMX2 mutation. *Neurology* **48**, 1403–1406.

Guerrini, R., Andermann, F., Canapicchi, R., Roger, J., Zifkin, B. & Pfanner, P. (eds) (1996): *Dysplasias of cerebral cortex and epilepsy*. Philadelphia: Lippincott-Raven.

Gulisano, M., Broccoli, V., Pardini, C. & Boncinelli, E. (1996): *Emx1* and *Emx2* show different patterns of expression during proliferation and differentiation of the developing cerebral cortex. *Eur. J. Neurosci.* **8**, 1037–1050.

Guthrie, S. (1995): The status of the neural segment. *Trends Neurosci.* **18**, 74–79.

Harding, B.N. (1992): Malformations of the nervous system. In: *Greenfieldís neuropathology*, Adams, J.H. & Duchen, L.W. (eds), pp. 521–638. London, Melbourne, Auckland: Edward Arnold.

Hosley, M.A., Abroms, I.F. & Ragland, R.L. (1992): Schizencephaly: case report of familial incidence. *Pediatr. Neurol.* **8**, 148–150.

Krumlauf, R. (1994): *Hox* genes in vertebrate development. *Cell* **78**, 191–201.

Matsuo, I., Kuratani, S., Kimura, C., Takeda, N. & Aizawa, S. (1995): Mouse *Otx2* functions in the formation and patterning of rostral head. *Genes Dev.* **9**, 2646–2658.

Mattia, D., Olivier, A. & Avoli, M. (1995): Seizure-like discharges recorded in the human dysplastic neocortex maintained *in vitro. Neurology* **45**, 1391–1395.

McGinnis, W. & Krumlauf, R. (1992): Homeobox genes and axial patterning. *Cell* **68**, 283–302.

Morrell, F., Whisler, W. & Hoeppner, T. (1992): Electrophysiology of heterotopic gray matter in the 'double cortex' syndrome. *Epilepsia* **33** (Suppl. 3), 76.

Munari, C., Francione, S., Kahane, P., Tassi, L., Hoffmann, D., Garrel, S. & Pasquier, B. (1996): Usefulness of stereo EEG investigations in partial epilepsy associated with cortical dysplastic lesions and gray matter heterotopia. In: *Dysplasias of cerebral cortex and epilepsy*, Guerrini, R., Andermann, F., Canapicchi, R., Roger, J., Zifkin, B. & Pfanner, P. (eds), pp. 383–394. Philadelphia-New York: Lippincott-Raven.

O'Leary, D.D.M., Schlaggar, B.L. & Tuttle, R. (1994): Specification of neocortical areas and thalamocortical connections. *Ann. Rev. Neurosci.* **17**, 419–439.

Pellegrini, M., Mansouri, A., Simeone, A., Boncinelli, E. & Gruss, P. (1996): Dentate gyrus formation requires *Emx2. Development* **122**, 3893–3898.

Rakic P. (1988): Specification of cerebral cortical areas. *Science* **183**, 170–176.

Robain, O. (1996): Introduction to the pathology of cerebral cortical dysplasia. In: *Dysplasias of cerebral cortex and epilepsy*, Guerrini, R., Andermann, F., Canapicchi, R., Roger, J., Zifkin, B.G. & Pfanner, P. (eds), pp. 1–9. Philadelphia-New York: Lippincott-Raven.

Rubenstein, J.L.R., Martinez, S., Shimamura, K. & Puelles, L. (1994): The embryonic vertebrate forebrain: The prosomeric model. *Science* **266**, 578–580.

Shatz, C.J., Chun, J.J.M. & Luskin, M.B. (1988): The role of the subplate in the development of the mammalian telencephalon. In: *Cerebral Cortex*, Peters, A. & Jones, E.G. (eds), vol. 7, pp. 35–38. New York: Plenum.

Shimamura, K., Hartigan, D.J., Martinez, S., Puelles, L. & Rubenstein, J.L.R. (1995): Longitudinal organization of the anterior neural plate and neural tube. *Development* **121**, 3923–3933.

Simeone, A., Acampora, D., Gulisano, M., Stornaiuolo, A. & Boncinelli, E. (1992): Nested expression domains of four homeobox genes in developing rostral brain. *Nature* **358,** 687–690.

Simeone, A., Acampora, D., Mallamaci, A., Stornaiuolo, A., D'Apice, M.R., Nigro, V. & Boncinelli, E. (1993): A vertebrate gene related to *orthodenticle* contains a homeodomain of the *bicoid* class and demarcates anterior neuroectoderm in the gastrulating mouse embryo. *EMBO J.* **12,** 2735–2747.

Simeone, A., Gulisano, M., Acampora, D., Stornaiuolo, A., Rambaldi, M. & Boncinelli, E. (1992): Two vertebrate homeobox genes related to the *Drosophila empty spiracles* gene are expressed in the embryonic cerebral cortex. *EMBO J.* **11,** 2541–2550.

Yakovlev, P. & Wadsworth, R.C. (1946a): Schizencephalies: a study of the congenital clefts in the cerebral mantle, I. Clefts with fused lips. *J. Neuropathol. Exp. Neurol.* **5,** 116–130.

Yakovlev, P.L. & Wadsworth, R.C. (1946b): Schizencephalies: a study of congenital clefts in the cerebral mantle, II. Clefts with hydrocephalus and lips separated. *J. Neuropathol. Exp. Neurol.* **5,** 169–206.

Part VII
Animal models

Chapter 23

Genetics of the EL mouse: a multifactorial epilepsy model

Thomas N. Seyfried, Michael J. Poderycki and Mariana Todorova

Department of Biology, Boston College, Chestnut Hill, MA 02035, USA

Multifactorial disorders are quantitative traits where the action of more than one gene together with environmental factors contribute to the disease phenotype. In contrast to polygenic traits where many genes with minor effects make an additive and equal contribution to the phenotype, multifactorial traits are significantly influenced by gene-gene (epistasis) and genotype-environmental interactions (Falconer, 1960). As a result, multifactorial disorders do not usually follow simple Mendelian modes of inheritance. This problem has hindered progress in identifying genes responsible for both human and murine multifactorial disorders. In contrast to simple Mendelian traits where the phenotype is largely determined by the genotype, environmental factors play a significant role in the determination of the phenotype for multifactorial disorders. Although the genotype may render a predisposition or susceptibility to disease, it is the environment that modifies the degree of gene penetrance and expressivity.

Both external and internal environmental factors can influence the expression of multifactorial disorders (Strickberger, 1985). In the case of epilepsy, external environmental factors can include temperature, light, sound, nutrition, head trauma, infectious agents and maternal effects. Internal environmental factors, on the other hand, can include age, gender, circadian rhythms, hormones and seizure history. Besides these and other environmental factors, epigenetic factors, e.g. genomic imprinting, may also influence the expression of multifactorial disorders (Banko *et al.*, 1997). Since the most common forms of human idiopathic epilepsy are expressed as multifactorial disorders (Andermann, 1982), multifactorial mouse epilepsy models will be useful for characterizing the mechanisms by which genes and environmental factors interact to influence seizure susceptibility.

The EL mouse as an experimental epilepsy model

Seizure phenotype and developmental expression

The EL (epilepsy) mouse has been one of the most extensively studied mouse models of idiopathic epilepsy. The mouse was originally called Ep and was discovered by Imaizumi in 1954 in an outbred DDY (formally ddy) mouse colony (Naruse & Kurokawa, 1992). Both the seizure susceptible EL mice and non susceptible DDY mice are now maintained as inbred strains (Saito *et al.*, 1992; Frankel *et al.*, 1995a). The seizures in EL mice appear to originate in or near the parietal lobe and then spread quickly to the hippocampus and to other brain regions (Suzuki *et al.*, 1991; Kasamo *et al.*, 1992; Ishida

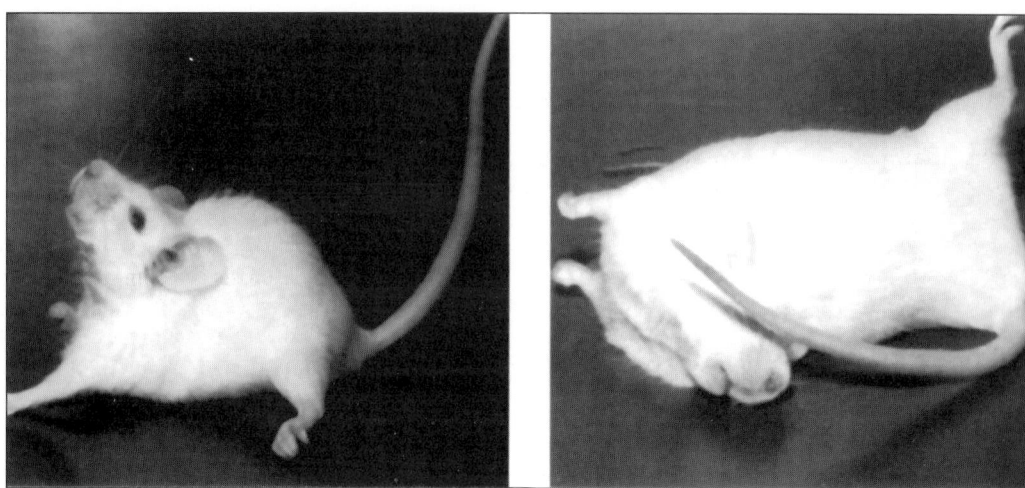

Fig. 1. EL mice experience seizures that are similar to complex partial seizures with secondary generalization in humans. The seizures in EL mice can occur during routine handling associated with cage changing or can be induced with vestibular stimulation such as mechanical tossing. The seizures induced from repeated mechanical tossing are phenotypically identical to those observed during routine handling.

et al., 1993). The appearance of an erect forward-arching Straub tail (Fig. 1) is indicative of spinal cord activation (Hasegawa et al., 1990). The seizures are also accompanied by EEG abnormalities (synchronized spike wave complexes at 3–4 c/s), vocalization (squeaking), incontinence, loss of postural equilibrium, excessive salivation, and head, limb and chewing automatisms (Kurokawa et al., 1966; Suzuki, 1976; Suzuki & Nakamoto, 1977; Naruse & Kurokawa, 1992; Seyfried et al., 1992). Phenytoin and phenobarbital, the anticonvulsant drugs of choice for treatment of human partial epilepsies, inhibit the seizures in EL mice (Suzuki & Nakamoto, 1977; Matsumoto et al., 1983; Nagatomo et al., 1996). Based on these observations, the EL mouse is considered a genetic model for human complex partial seizures with secondary generalization (Seyfried et al., 1992).

The seizures in EL mice begin at about 80 to 100 days of age and usually occur during routine handling associated with cage changing. The incidence of seizures increases with age. Rhythmic vestibular stimulation, e.g. tossing, rotation or rocking, is often used to induce seizures in young EL mice (around 45 to 55 days) (Kurokawa et al., 1966; Fueta et al., 1983; Brigande et al., 1992; Naruse & Kurokawa, 1992; Frankel et al., 1995a). Although vestibular stimulation was believed to trigger the EL seizures (Kurokawa et al., 1966; Naruse & Kurokawa, 1992), EL mice older than 150 days will sometimes seize without handling or vestibular stimulation, e.g. from removing the cage top. It is important to mention that EL mice do not seize spontaneously (Todorova et al., 1997). The trigger for seizure induction may be stress or fear which can arise from numerous environmental factors including vestibular stimulation. Furthermore, the stress-related seizure threshold decreases as the EL mice age (Todorova et al., 1997).

Besides an enhanced susceptibility to handling-induced seizures, susceptibility to metrazol-induced seizures is also greater in EL mice than in non-epileptic control DDY mice (Sugaya et al., 1986; Fueta & Mita, 1992). It is not yet known, however, whether a common genetic mechanism is responsible for the handling- and metrazol-induced seizures in EL mice. Although EL mice are also more susceptible to olfactory bulb kindling than DDY mice, they are less susceptible than non-epileptic C57BL/6 (B6) mice (Green & Seyfried, 1991). These findings suggest that different genetic mechanisms contribute to these seizure susceptibilities (Green et al., 1993).

Neuropathology

The seizures in EL mice are not associated with gross neurostructural changes in the CNS (Suzuki et al., 1983; Mizukawa & Mori, 1992; Naruse & Kurokawa, 1992). Nevertheless, an intense reactive gliosis occurs in the hippocampus of EL mice (Brigande et al., 1992). Both the number of glial fibrillary acidic protein (GFAP) positive cells and the relative GFAP concentration are significantly greater in EL mice than in age-matched seizure resistant C57BL/6J (B6) mice or young EL mice that have yet to seize (Tables 1 and 2). Since GFAP expression is a good marker for reactive glia in neurological disease, these findings indicate that the seizure activity in EL mice is associated with hippocampal gliosis. Although hippocampal gliosis or Ammon's horn sclerosis is a common finding in humans with complex partial seizures, there is considerable controversy as to whether the gliosis arises as a cause or an effect of the seizures (Babb & Brown, 1987; Ribak, 1991). Our results suggest that the gliosis in EL mice is associated with the effects rather than the cause of seizure activity (Brigande et al., 1992). The EL mouse can serve as a useful natural model for examining the association between epilepsy and reactive gliosis.

Table 1. Number of GFAP-positive cells per square millimeter of hippocampus in adult EL mice and in young non seizing control EL and adult B6 mice[a]

Age and strain	n[d]	Number of GFAP-positive cells per mm^2 hippocampus ($\pm$ SEM)
Experiment 1[b]		
Young EL	4	42.5 ± 2.0
Adult B6	4	7.2 ± 6.0
Adult EL	4	291.0 ± 68.0*
Experiment 2[c]		
Young EL	3	0.0
Adult B6	9	6.5 ± 1.0
Adult EL	9	98.0 ± 18.0*

[a]Data derived as described previously (Brigande et al. 1992);
[b]Adult EL and B6 mice did not receive vestibular stimulation and were sacrificed at 240–370 days of age (these EL mice, however, had many spontaneous seizures);
[c]Adult EL and B6 mice received vestibular stimulation and were killed at 130–160 days of age (these EL mice received an average of 43 seizures each);
[d]n = the number of independent samples.
*Significantly different from young EL and adult B6 mice at $P < 0.01$ (analysed using Mann-Whitney U-test).

Table 2. Hippocampal and cerebellar GFAP content in adult EL and control B6 mice[a]

Brain region	Strain	n	Relative GFAP content, υg/ mg total tissue protein
Hippocampus	B6	3	3.5 ± 0.9
	EL	3	9.6 ± 1.4*
Cerebellum	B6	3	2.5 ± 0.4
	EL	3	1.8 ± 0.4

[a]The relative GFAP content was estimated by scanning densitometry of peroxidase stained western blots as we described (Brigande et al., 1992). n, the number of separate samples analysed
*Significantly different from B6 value at $P < 0.01$ (analysed using two-tailed Student's t-test).

In contrast to human hippocampal sclerosis, where seizures and gliosis are associated with significant neuronal loss (Babb & Brown, 1987), the gliosis in EL mice is not associated with obvious neuronal loss (Suzuki et al., 1983; Brigande et al., 1992). Using the silver impregnation method, Mizukawa & Mori found a slight, but non significant, reduction in the number of hippocampal pyramidal cells (Mizukawa & Mori, 1992). Furthermore, no reduction was found for the concentration of hippocampal gangliosides in EL mice (Brigande et al., 1992). Gangliosides are complex sialoglycosphingolipids that are enriched in neural cell membranes and can serve as cell-surface markers for changes in neuronal cytoarchitecture that accompany brain development or disease. Neither the total ganglioside concentration, a sensitive index for neuronal content, nor the concentration of GD1a, a major disialoganglioside enriched in dendritic and synaptic membranes, was reduced in EL hippocampus (Brigande et al., 1992).

These findings are markedly different from those in human complex seizures where total hippocampal ganglioside and GD1a content were significantly reduced in association with gliosis and neuronal loss (Yu et al., 1987). The reason for the difference between man and mouse in seizure-associated neuronal loss is not clear, but may reflect a species difference in either neuronal or glial response to seizures. It is possible that mouse hippocampal neurons are more resistant to seizure-associated damage than human neurons or that mouse glia are more protective of neurons than human glia. The EL mouse may facilitate identification of factors that protect or buffer neurons from seizure-induced excitotoxity.

Neurochemical studies

Despite over three decades of intensive neurochemical research on EL mice conducted in both Japan and the United States, the biochemical defects underlying the EL seizures are unclear (Kurokawa et al., 1966; Mori, 1988; Mita et al., 1991; Seyfried et al., 1992). Difficulties in distinguishing innate neurochemical changes associated with seizure susceptibility from changes occurring as a consequence of repeated seizure activity have obscured underlying biochemical defects. Additional complicating factors also arise from the various methods used to induce the EL seizures. Some of these methods, e.g. vestibular stimulation or mechanical tossing, may produce neurochemical changes that are unrelated to either seizure susceptibility or to the effects of seizures (Kohsaka et al., 1978; Hiramatsu, 1981; Tsuda et al., 1993). Furthermore, there is no ideal genetic control for the EL mouse. Although the DDY strain is more closely related to the EL strain than to other mouse strains, the EL and DDY mice differ in about 25–30 per cent of their genes (Frankel et al., 1995a). Consequently, it is necessary that several mouse groups be used to control for the effects of genetic background, age, number of prior seizures, and for the seizure testing procedure itself. Unfortunately, many of the neurochemical and physiological studies conducted on EL mice have not employed all of the control groups necessary to determine whether a particular neurochemical change is related to the cause of seizures or to the effects of seizures or the seizure test.

Table 3. *The calcium-dependent potassium-evoked release of aspartate, glutamate, and GABA from hippocampal slices in epileptic EL mice and non epileptic B6 and DDY mice*[a]

Strain	Age (days)	Released neurotransmitter[b]		
		Aspartate	Glutamate	GABA
B6	320	3.3 ± 0.7 (5)	15.4 ± 3.6 (5)	12.7 ± 1.4 (5)
EL	320	6.6 ± 0.7 (5)*	18.2 ± 2.6 (5)	17.3 ± 2.9 (4)
B6	38	8.5 ± 1.4 (4)	23.0 ± 2.0 (4)	23.5 ± 0.7 (4)
DDY	38	8.4 ± 0.7 (4)	32.3 ± 5.8 (4)	19.5 ± 3.2 (4)
EL	38	15.8 ± 0.8 (3)*	25.9 ± 2.6 (3)	21.8 ± 3.2 (3)

[a]Data from 300 days are from (Flavin et al. 1991) and from 38 says from (Flavin & Seyfried, 1994).
[b]Values are expressed as the mean pmol amino acid released/ml/min incubation/slice $\pm$ S.E.M. The number of independent samples analysed is indicated in parentheses.
*Indicates that the EL aspartate release is significantly higher than that of B6 mice ($P < 0.02$; unpaired, two-tailed t-test).

One neurochemical defect that may be causally related to the EL seizures involves the calcium-dependent release of aspartate. Aspartate is an important excitatory neurotransmitter in the mammalian CNS that may be involved in some epilepsies (Flavin et al., 1991). Although the amount of releasable amino acid represents only a small portion of the total tissue amino acid content, this is the physiological pool most relevant to neuronal signal transmission and epilepsy. We found that the endogenous release of aspartate, but not of glutamate or GABA, was significantly higher in hippocampal slices of EL mice than in seizure resistant C57BL/6J or DDY control mice at both young and adult ages (Table 3). Enhanced aspartate release may be related to the cause rather than to the effects of seizure activity, since the enhanced release was apparent in young EL mice that neither had seizures nor were tested for seizures (Flavin et al., 1991; Flavin & Seyfried, 1994). Endogenous aspartate release from cortical slices was also greater in seizing than in non-seizing EL mice (Hiramatsu et al., 1992). The aspartate findings are interesting in view of the hippocampal gliosis in EL mice and the postulated excitotoxicity hypothesis of epilepsy (Ribak, 1991).

In addition to the possible involvement of aspartate in EL seizures, GABAergic abnormalities may also play some role in EL seizure susceptibility. GABA concentration and glutamic acid decarboxylase activity were significantly higher in hippocampus of adult EL mice than in control DDY mice (Murashima et al., 1992). In contrast to hippocampus, these parameters were significantly reduced in a specifically localized region of the EL parietal cortex. The authors suggest that the spatial and temporal GABAergic abnormalities in EL brain are likely involved in epileptogenesis (Murashima et al., 1992).

In addition to alterations in aspartergic and GABAergic mechanisms, several other abnormalities have been reported in EL mice that may relate to global metabolic disturbance or to the effects of seizures. The ATP-dependent uptake of glutamate into synaptic vesicles is higher in EL than in non-epileptic control strains (Lewis et al., 1997). This was attributed to the development or maintenance of seizures rather than to the cause of seizures. Other abnormalities in EL mice involve metals (Sutoo et al., 1987; Fukahori et al., 1988; Mori, 1988), biogenic amines (Sutoo et al., 1992), RNA synthesis (Mui et al., 1991), and the developmental properties of primary cultured EL neurons (Sugaya et al., 1992). It will be interesting to determine how the neurochemical and physiological abnormalities in EL mice are related to the expression of specific seizure genes.

Genetic studies

Early studies suggested that the inheritance of seizures in EL mice was dominant and complex (Fueta et al., 1986; Naruse & Kurokawa, 1992). To better define the genetic basis of the EL seizures, we outcrossed EL mice to two seizure resistant strains, ABP/Le (ABP) and DBA/2J (D2) and followed the inheritance of seizures and genetic markers in backcrosses to the seizure resistant ABP and D2 parental strains (Rise et al., 1991). Although D2 mice are susceptible to audiogenic seizures, they do not experience handling seizures as seen in EL mice. All of the animals used in these genetic studies were tested for seizure susceptibility using a tossing procedure in a mechanical shaker as shown in Fig. 1 (Seyfried et al., 1992). The mice were tested twice per week beginning at thirty days of age and the mean seizure frequency per a total of 20 tests was calculated for each mouse. The results from these genetic studies indicated that seizure susceptibility in EL mice was inherited as an incompletely dominant multifactorial trait (Rise et al., 1991).

Using several statistical tests to analyse the association between seizure susceptibility and the various genetic markers in the backcrosses, we mapped three genes that influenced seizure susceptibility in EL mice. One gene, designated *El1*, was found on the distal region of mouse chromosome 9 near the dilute/short ear locus and another, designated *El2*, was found on chromosome 2 near the microsatellite marker *D2Mit30* (Rise et al., 1991; Frankel et al., 1995a). In contrast to *El1* and *El2*, which were present in the EL genome, we also found a recessive 'modifier' gene in the D2 genome that enhanced seizure susceptibility. This modifier mapped on chromosome 4 near the brown (*b*) coat colour locus. This chromosomal region also contains *Asp2*, a previously identified enhancer of audiogenic seizure susceptibility (Neumann & Seyfried, 1990). We suggested that this *b*-linked seizure modifier may enhance both tossing-induced seizures in EL mice and audiogenic seizures in D2 mice (Rise et al., 1991).

Besides these seizure genes, several additional seizure frequency quantitative trait loci (QTL) were recently identified on chromosomes 10 (*El3*), 9 (*El4*), 14 (*El5*) and 11 (*El6*) (Frankel et al., 1995a; Frankel et al., 1995b). The effects of these genes, however, were dependent upon the genetic background (the mouse strain to which EL is crossed) and upon the type of cross (backcrosses or F2 intercrosses). For example, *El1* and *El2* accounted for much of the variation in seizure-frequency in a backcross to ABP, while *El3* and *El4* had the largest effects in the F2 intercross. In crosses between EL and DDY, a seizure-resistant mouse strain related to EL, *El5* was the major QTL detected in the F2 intercross, but was undetectable in the backcross to DDY (Frankel et al., 1995a). Similar to the *b*-linked recessive enhancer from the D2 background described above, *El6* is a recessive enhancer on the DDY background. The authors concluded that no single *El* locus was essential for high seizure frequency and that the seizures in EL mice resulted from complex epistatic interactions between many nonallelic *El* seizure genes (Frankel et al., 1995a; Frankel et al., 1995b).

Besides epistasis, environmental factors also contribute to this complexity. This comes from findings that much of the phenotypic variance associated with tossing-induced seizures in genetic crosses involving EL mice is of environmental origin (Rise et al., 1991; Frankel et al., 1995a; Frankel et al., 1995b). Furthermore, a significant gender effect was observed in crosses between EL and the DDY strains, where females were more seizure prone than males (Frankel et al., 1995a). Besides gender, other environmental factors that could complicate the inheritance of seizures include age, seizure history, and the seizure testing procedure itself. Age is a significant factor since the frequency, duration, and intensity of the EL seizures increases gradually with age. Consequently, the effect of some seizure modifier genes may be greater at one age than at another. The seizure frequency in some mice may also depend in part on the influence of prior seizures. This follows from Gowers' dictum that 'seizures beget seizures' (Gowers, 1901; Wasterlain & Shirasaka, 1994). Such a phenomenon could cause the phenotypic misclassification of some mice.

Another environmental factor that could influence the inheritance of the EL seizures includes the seizure testing procedure. This test involves tossing the mice (1–4 cm) in a mechanical shaker at a high frequency (250–280 tosses per min) for a total of 30 s or until the animal seizes (Seyfried et al., 1992). The animals are usually tested once every three days for a total of 20 tests (Rise et al., 1991; Seyfried et al., 1992; Frankel et al., 1995a). It was generally assumed that the tossing procedure could identify animals that would normally experience handling-induced seizures. Little consideration was given, however, to the possibility that various tossing procedures might complicate the genetics of the seizure phenotype (Seyfried et al., 1992).

In a recent study involving 200 day-old ABP backcross mice, we found that the strength of the associations between genetic markers and seizures was strongly dependent on the number of tests that the animals received (Poderycki et al., 1998). For example, the association between seizures and *El1* decreased with increasing number of tests, whereas the opposite was the case for *El2*. These findings indicate that the seizure phenotype is not independent of the seizure test, suggesting that gene-environmental interactions contribute to the complexity of the seizure phenotype.

We suggest that the gene-environmental interactions may arise in part from the physical and emotional trauma of the testing procedure and/or from the seizures themselves. Recent findings suggest that repeated tossing may induce brain trauma (Todorova et al., 1997), and can alter brain neurochemistry independent of the seizures in EL and in non-epileptic control strains (Kohsaka et al., 1978; Hiramatsu, 1981; Tsuda et al., 1993). Gene-environmental interactions might alter the neurochemical properties of the CNS and thereby enhance seizure frequency in some genotypes or reduce seizure frequency in others. Furthermore, these interactions could also produce phenocopies (false positives or false negatives), the most extreme form of environmental influence.

Evidence for phenocopies comes from our previous findings and those of others that the testing procedure can induce a low, but significant number of seizures in the non-epileptic parental strains, i.e. ABP, D2 and DDY (Rise et al., 1991; Frankel et al., 1995a). Although these strains rarely express seizures induced by routine handling as seen in EL mice, their tossing-induced seizure phenotype is indistinguishable from that observed in EL mice. Evidence for false negatives comes from recent findings that tossing procedures might inhibit the formation of spontaneous seizures (Muraguchi & Serikawa, 1995). We also found that handling-induced seizures in EL X ABPF$_1$ hybrids could inhibit the formation of tossing-induced seizures. It is therefore likely that some mice in segregating populations (backcrosses and intercrosses) are phenocopies.

Considering the influence of environmental factors on the seizure phenotype and that different genetic mechanisms may be responsible for the different types of seizures in EL mice (Green & Seyfried, 1991; Muraguchi & Serikawa, 1995), it is not clear whether the previously mapped *El* 'epilepsy' genes are relevant to idiopathic epilepsy or to symptomatic epilepsy caused by tossing-induced brain trauma. Repeated mouse tossing over several weeks may obscure the boundaries between idiopathic and symptomatic aetiologies and produce a phenomenon that is multifactorial, continuous, and extremely complex (Poderycki *et al.*, 1998). The development of new seizure testing methods, that avoid brain trauma and do not induce seizures in non-epileptic control strains, may facilitate epilepsy gene mapping in EL mice (Todorova *et al.*, 1997).

Mapping epilepsy genes in man and mouse

Although positional cloning has been successful for the localization and isolation of many single locus neurological mutations in man and mouse, this genetic strategy has had less success with complex multifactorial disorders. This comes largely from the uncertainty in phenotypic assessment due to the influence of environmental factors and to the segregation of nonallelic modifier genes which can lead to the misclassification of some individuals as either susceptible or nonsusceptible. These gene-gene and gene-environmental interactions can distort map distances between genetic markers and the QTLs for multifactorial disorders. If there is a 'fast track' to mapping genes for complex convulsive disorders in man it will likely involve candidate gene analysis and luck. Some epilepsy QTLs could map in regions with cloned genes which could then be screened for defects in probands and their relatives. Interspecific candidate gene analysis may also be helpful. Since about 37 per cent of the mouse autosomal genome is syntenic with the human autosomal genome, mapping mouse genes can predict the chromosomal location of similar genes in man (Nadeau, 1989; Copeland *et al.*, 1993). Hence, the mapping of epilepsy genes in EL mice could increase the likelihood for identification of a candidate gene for a human multifactorial epilepsy.

Acknowledgements: This work was supported by NIH grant (NS23355) and from the Boston College Research Expense fund.

References

Andermann, E. (1982): Multifactorial inheritance of generalized and focal epilepsy. In: *Genetic basis of the epilepsies*, Anderson, V.E., Hauser, W.A., Penry, J.K. & Sing, C.F. (eds), pp. 355–376. New York: Raven Press.

Babb, T.L. & Brown, W.J. (1987): Pathological findings in epilepsy. In: *Surgical treatment of the epilepsies*, Engel, J. (ed.), pp. 101–114. New York: Raven Press.

Banko, M.L., Allen, K., Dolina, S., Neumann, P.E. & Seyfried, T.N. (1997): Genomic imprinting and audiogenic seizures in mice. *Behav. Genet.* **27**, 465–475.

Brigande, J.V., Wieraszko, A., Albert, M.D., Balkema, G.W. & Seyfried, T.N. (1992): Biochemical correlates of epilepsy in the E1 mouse: analysis of glial fibrillary acidic protein and gangliosides. *J. Neurochem.* **58**, 752–760.

Copeland, N.G., Jenkins, N.A., Gilbert, D.J., Eppig, J.T., Maltais, L.J., Miller, J.C., Dietrich, W.F., Weaver, A., Lincoln, S.E., Steen, R.G. *et al.* (1993): A genetic linkage map of the mouse: current applications and future prospects. *Science* **262**, 57–66.

Falconer, D.S. (1960): *Introduction to quantitative genetics*. New York: Ronald Press.

Flavin, H.J. & Seyfried, T.N. (1994): Enhanced aspartate release related to epilepsy in (EL) mice. *J Neurochem* **63**, 592–595.

Flavin, H.J., Wieraszko, A. & Seyfried, T.N. (1991): Enhanced aspartate release from hippocampal slices of epileptic (El) mice. *J. Neurochem.* **56**, 1007–1011.

Frankel, W.N., Johnson, E.W. & Lutz, C.M. (1995b): Congenic strains reveal effects of the epilepsy quantitative locus, *El2*, separate from other *El* loci. *Mamm. Genome* **6**, 839–843.

Frankel, W.N., Valenzuela, A., Lutz, C.M., Johnson, E.W., Dietrich, W.F. & Coffin, J.M. (1995a): New seizure frequency QTL and the complex genetics of epilepsy in EL mice. *Mamm. Genome* **6**, 830–838.

Fueta, Y., Matsuoka, S. & Mita, T. (1986): Crossbreeding analysis of the mouse epilepsy. *Sangyo Ika Daigaku Zasshi* **8**, 417–424.

Fueta, Y. & Mita, T. (1992): Susceptibility to pentylenetetrazole-induced convulsion of developing and adult EL mice. *Neurosciences* **18** (Suppl. 2), 163–169.

Fueta, Y., Mita, T. & Matsuoka, S. (1983): Experimental animal epilepsy. A new device for the induction of epileptic seizures in the murine, El mouse. *Sangyo Ika Daigaku Zasshi* **5**, 359–364.

Fukahori, M., Itoh, M., Oomagari, K. & Kawasaki, H. (1988): Zinc content in discrete hippocampal and amygdaloid areas of the epilepsy (El) mouse and normal mice. *Brain Res.* **455**, 381–384.

Gowers, W.R. (1901): *Epilepsy and other chronic convulsive diseases: their causes, symptoms and treatment*. Brinklow, MD: Old Hickory Bookshop.

Green, R.C., Rees, H.D. & Feller, D.J. (1993): Olfactory bulb kindling in mice susceptible and resistant to ethanol withdrawal. *Epilepsia* **34**, 416–419.

Green, R.C. & Seyfried, T.N. (1991): Kindling susceptibility and genetic seizure predisposition in inbred mice. *Epilepsia* **32**, 22–26.

Hasegawa, Y., Kurachi, M. & Otomo, S. (1990): Dopamine D2 receptors and spinal cord excitation in mice. *Eur. J. Pharmacol.* **184**, 207–212.

Hiramatsu, M. (1981): Brain monoamine levels and El mouse convulsions. *Folia Psychiat. Neurol. Japon* **35**, 261–266.

Hiramatsu, M., Kinno, I., Kanakura, K., Sato, K. & Mori, A. (1992): Increased aspartate release from brain slices of epileptic experimental animals and effect of valproate on it. *Jpn. J. Psychiatry Neurol.* **46**, 541–543.

Ishida, N., Kasamo, K., Nakamoto, Y. & Suzuki, J. (1993): Epileptic seizure of El mouse initiates at the parietal cortex: depth EEG observation in freely moving condition using buffer amplifier. *Brain Res.* **608**, 52–57.

Kasamo, K., Ishida, N., Murashima, Y.L., Ozawa, N., Nakamoto, Y. & Suzuki, J. (1992): The depth EEG and the multiunit activity in the hippocampal CA1 region during the epileptic seizure of an El mouse: involvement of the hippocampal neurons in seizure manifestations. *Neurosciences* **18** (Suppl. 2), 129–136.

Kohsaka, M., Hiramatsu, M. & Mori, A. (1978): Brain catecholamine concentrations and convulsions in El mice. *Adv. Biochem. Psychopharmacol.* **19**, 389–392.

Kurokawa, M., Naruse, H. & Kato, M. (1966): Metabolic studies on ep mouse, a special strain with convulsive predisposition. *Prog. Brain Res.* **21**, 112–129.

Lewis, S.M., Lee, F.S., Todorova, M., Seyfried, T.N. & Ueda, T. (1997): Synaptic vesicle glutamate uptake in epileptic (EL) mice. *Neurochem. Int..* **31**, 581–585.

Matsumoto, Y., Hiramatsu, M. & Mori, A. (1983): Effects of phenytoin on convulsions and brain 5-hydroxytryptamine levels of El mice. *IRCS Med. Sci.* **11**, 837.

Mita, T., Sashihara, S., Aramaki, I., Fueta, Y. & Hirano, H. (1991): Unusual biochemical development of genetically seizure-susceptible El mice. *Brain Res. Dev. Brain Res.* **64**, 27–35.

Mizukawa, K. & Mori, A. (1992): Cytoarchitecture of hippocampal formation of El mouse: silver impregnation investigation and quantitative analysis. *Neurosciences* **18** (Suppl. 2), 137–141.

Mori, A. (1988): El Mice: Neurochemical approach to the seizure mechanism. *Neurosciences* **14**, 275–285.

Mui, K., Yamagami, S., Kioka, T., Onishi, H. & Kawakita, Y. (1991): Sequence complexity of polyadenylated RNA from seizure-susceptible El mouse brain polysomes. *Epilepsy Res.* **10**, 134–141.

Muraguchi, T. & Serikawa, T. (1995): Strain differences for tossing-up induced seizures and pentylenetetrazol-induced convulsions in CXB RI strains. *Mouse Genome* **93**, 1035–1037.

Murashima, Y.L., Kasamo, K. & Suzuki, J. (1992): Developmental abnormalities of GABAergic system are involved in the formation of epileptogenesis in the EL. *Neurosciences* **18** (Suppl. 2), 63–73.

Nadeau, J.H. (1989): Maps of linkage and synteny homologies between mouse and man. *Trends Genet.* **5**, 82–86.

Nagatomo, I., Akasaki, Y., Nagase, F., Nomaguchi, M. & Takigawa, M. (1996): Relationships between convulsive seizures ans serum and brain concentrations of phenobarbital and zonisamide in mutant inbred strain EL. *Brain Res.* **731**, 190–198.

Naruse, H. & Kurokawa, M. (1992): The beginnings of studies on EL mice. *Neurosciences* (Suppl. 2) **18**, 1–3.

Neumann, P.E. & Seyfried, T.N. (1990): Mapping of two genes that influence susceptibility to audiogenic seizures in crosses of C57BL/6J and DBA/2J mice. *Behav. Genet.* **20**, 307–323.

Poderycki, M.J., Simoes, J.M., Todorova, M., Neumann, P.E. & Seyfried, T.N. (1998): Environmental influences on epilepsy gene mapping in EL mice. *J. Neurogenetics* **12**, 67–86.

Ribak, C.E. (1991): Epilepsy and the cortex. In: *Cerebral cortex*, Peters, A. (ed.), pp. 427–483. New York: Plenum.

Rise, M.L., Frankel, W.N., Coffin, J.M. & Seyfried, T.N. (1991): Genes for epilepsy mapped in the mouse. *Science* **253**, 669–673.

Saito, M., Endo, S., Hioki, K. & Nomura, T. (1992): Rearing and maintenance of EL mice as laboratory animals. *Neurosciences* **18** (Suppl. 2), 5–8.

Seyfried, T.N., Brigande, J.V., Flavin, H.J., Frankel, W.N., Rise, M.L. & Wieraszko, A. (1992): Genetic and biochemical correlates of epilepsy in the EL mouse. *Neurosciences* **18** (Suppl. 2), 9–20.

Strickberger, M.W. (1985): *Genetics*. New York: MacMillan Publishing.

Sugaya, E., Ishige, A., Sekiguchi, K., Iizuka, S., Ito, K., Sugimoto, A., Aburada, M. & Hosoya, E. (1986): Pentylenetetrazol-induced convulsion and effect of anticonvulsants in mutant inbred strain El mice. *Epilepsia* **27**, 354–358.

Sugaya, E., Sugaya, A., Yuyama, N., Tsuda, T., Kajiwara, K., Kubota, K., Katoh, K., Hosoya, S., Takagi, T. & Motoki, M. (1992): Developmental defects of primary cultured neurons from the cerebral cortex of the El mouse and their amelioration with a herbal mixture formulation, TJ–960. *Neurosciences* **18** (Suppl. 2), 111–128.

Sutoo, D., Akiyama, K. & Takita, H. (1987): The relationship between metal ion levels and biogenic amine levels in epileptic mice. *Brain Res.* **418**, 205–213.

Sutoo, D., Akiyama, K. & Takita, H. (1992): Abnormal behavior in epileptic El mice related to a calcium-dependent-catacholamine synthesis disorder of the central nervous system. *Neurosciences* **18** (Suppl. 2), 55–62.

Suzuki, J. (1976): Paroxysmal discharges in the electroencephalogram of the E1 mouse. *Experientia* **32**, 336–338.

Suzuki, J., Kasamo, K., Ishida, N. & Murashima, Y.L. (1991): Initiation, propagation and generalization of paroxysmal discharges in an epileptic mutant animal. *Jpn. J. Psychiatry Neurol.* **45**, 271–274.

Suzuki, J., Matsushita, M. & Nakamoto, Y. (1983): Histopathological alterations in the hippocampus of an El mouse. *Folia Psychiatr. Jpn.* **37**, 362–363.

Suzuki, J. & Nakamoto, Y. (1977): Seizure patterns and electroencephalograms of E1 mouse. *Electroencephalogr Clin. Neurophysiol.* **43**, 299–311.

Todorova, M.T., Burwell, T.J. & Seyfried, T.N. (1997): New procedure for seizure induction in epileptic EL mice. *Epilepsia* **38**, 37.

Tsuda, H., Ito, M., Oguro, K., Mutoh, K., Shiraishi, H., Shirasaka, Y. & Mikawa, H. (1993): Age- and seizure-related changes in noradrenaline and dopamine in several brain regions of epileptic El mice. *Neurochem. Res.* **18**, 111–1117.

Wasterlain, C.G. & Shirasaka, Y. (1994): Seizures, brain damage and brain development. *Brain Dev.* **16**, 279–295.

Yu, R.K., Holley, J.A., Macala, L.J. & Spencer, D.D. (1987): Ganglioside changes associated with temporal lobe epilepsy in the human hippocampus. *Yale J. Biol. Med.* **60**, 107–117.

Chapter 24

Evidence for supernumerary GABAergic neurons and disinhibition in the hippocampus of seizure-sensitive gerbils

Gary M. Peterson[1] and Charles E. Ribak[2]

[1]*Department of Anatomy & Cell Biology, East Carolina University School of Medicine, Greenville, North Carolina 27858, USA; and* [2]*Department of Anatomy & Neurobiology, University of California, Irvine, Irvine, California 92717, USA*

Mongolian gerbils (*Meriones unguiculatus*) provide a useful animal model for the study of epilepsy because they exhibit clonic-tonic seizures which resemble human secondarily generalized seizures (Thiessen *et al.*, 1968; Loskota *et al.*, 1974) with a focal onset. Seizures are induced by a number of sensory stimuli but exposure to a novel environment seems to be the best inducer (Loskota *et al.*, 1974; Ludvig *et al.*, 1991). The intensity of seizure varies within the gerbil population but is relatively constant for individual animals so that it is therefore possible to correlate a known history of seizure intensity with morphological observations. A typically intense seizure lasts several minutes and begins with whisker twitching, eye blinking, and flattening of the pinnae. This rapidly evolves into lordosis, followed by wild jumping and running and then by loss of righting, whole body tonus, and clonic movements of the forelimbs. After 1–2 min, the animal rights itself but maintains a frozen posture while exhibiting facial movements. This postictal phase lasts for at least another 2 min. Within the wild-type population seizures occur in about 50 per cent of gerbils, but the frequency can be increased by selective breeding. The animals used in our studies had been bred phenotypically to produce two strains, one which is seizure-sensitive and one which is seizure-resistant. Since the onset of seizure activity does not begin until about 50 days of age (Loskota *et al.*, 1974), it is possible to examine the brains of young 'seizure-predisposed' progeny of seizure-sensitive animals prior to the occurrence of seizure activity to determine if the differences between seizure-sensitive and seizure-resistant brains occur prior to seizure onset or are the result of seizure activity.

Abnormalities within the GABAergic system have been implicated in the seizure sensitivity of gerbils. For example, when GABA levels are increased in seizure-sensitive gerbils by the administration of GABA agonist drugs, seizure susceptibility is reduced and the dose required for this effect is significantly smaller than that required for other genetically predisposed animals or animals with chemically- or electrically-induced seizures (Löscher, 1984; Löscher *et al.*, 1983). Furthermore, all three categories of GABA mimetic drugs (GABA agonists, GABA-T inhibitors, and inhibitors of

GABA uptake) are highly effective in suppressing seizures in gerbils. This efficacy suggests that the seizure susceptibility results, at least in part, from impairment of GABA-mediated neurotransmission.

Several lines of evidence indicate that the hippocampus is involved in seizure activity. These include electroencephalographic recording, alterations in seizure following lesions to hippocampal pathways, and morphological changes within the hippocampus after seizure activity. Majkowski & Donadio (1984) showed hippocampal electrographic activity during the clonic–tonic phase of the seizure, but concluded that the seizure began in the frontal cortex. The role of the hippocampal formation in seizure activity was also examined following lesions of its input and output. Bilateral transection of the perforant path, which provides the hippocampal formation with its primary excitatory input, results in the abolition of the behavioural expression of seizure activity whereas unilateral transection of the perforant path or bilateral transection of the fornix resulted in no change or an increase in seizure intensity (Table 1; Ribak & Khan, 1987). A reduction in the number of pyramidal cells (Mouritzen Dam et al., 1981) and diminished density of spines on the proximal portion of their apical dendrites (Paul et al., 1981) was shown. In the latter study, the examined dendritic region is known to be contacted by mossy fibre terminals arising from the dentate granule cells. We (Peterson et al., 1985) subsequently showed that the terminals of these mossy fibres (mossy tufts) were dramatically depleted of synaptic vesicles, had increased numbers of cisternae of agranular reticulum, and had numerous mitochondria in close proximity to the synaptic zone immediately after seizure (Fig. 1). Because these features are indicative of a high rate of synaptic activity (Nitsch & Rinne, 1981) we suggested that the granule cells in seizure-sensitive gerbils are more active, perhaps due to disinhibition. Our light and electron microscopic examination of GABAergic neurons and their terminals in the dentate gyrus and Ammon's horn was designed to test this hypothesis.

Table 1. *Effects of transection of the major input and output pathways of the hippocampal formation on seizure expression. Note that bilateral transection of the perforant path, the major input pathway, completely abolished behavioural evidence of seizure (data from Ribak & Khan, 1987).*

Lesion	Mean seizure score	
	Before	After
Bilateral fornix + perforant path	3.2	0
Bilateral perforant path	2.5	0
Bilateral fornix	1.7	2.6
Unilateral perforant path	2.7	3.3
Sham	3.1	3.3

Methods

Animals

The adult gerbils used in our studies were provided by Scheibel & Paul and originated from the colony of Lomax & Loskota (see Loskota et al., 1974). The seizure-sensitive animals had been selectively bred for seizure sensitivity for over 15 generations and the seizure-resistant gerbils had been selectively bred for seizure resistance for at least 10 generations. Adult animals of both sexes and strains were tested once a week for seizure sensitivity and intensity of seizure. The testing procedure involved placing the animals, one at a time, into an empty stainless steel box for 5 min or until they had a seizure. Seizure intensity was rated on a five point scale from 0 to 4 that was modified from

Chapter 24 Supernumerary GABAergic neurons and disinhibition in the hippocampus of gerbils

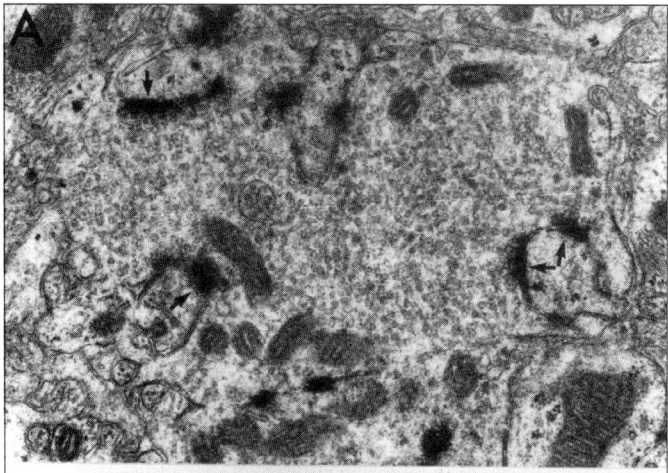

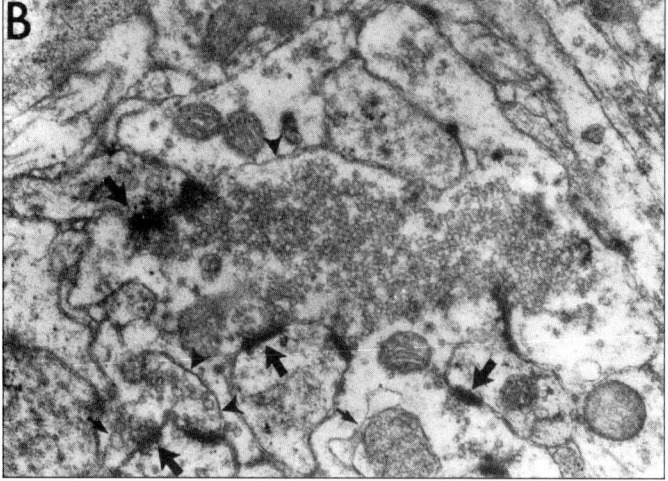

Fig. 1. A: Electron micrograph of a mossy tuft from a seizure-resistant brain. Round synaptic vesicles fill most of this terminal that forms typical asymmetric axospinous synapses (arrows). 21,000X. B: A mossy tuft from a seizure-sensitive brain. This terminal displays a depletion of synaptic vesicles, membrane infoldings derived from active sites (arrowheads) and cisternae of agranular reticulum (arrows). These features are typical for 'active' terminals. Asymmetric axospinous synapses (large arrows) are also formed by seizure-sensitive mossy tufts. 24,000X. (Reproduced from Peterson et al., 1985, with permission of the publisher.)

Loskota *et al.* (1974). A zero score was given when no seizure was observed. A score of one indicated a mild seizure in which vibrissae twitching and some flattening and flicking of the pinna were observed. A score of 2 was given if the twitching of vibrissae and pinnae occurred with motor arrest. A 3 indicated a gerbil with the same features as in 2 but with myoclonic jerks. Lastly, a 4 indicated a severe seizure in which the animal manifested clonic–tonic forepaw movements (forelimb jerking, followed by tonic extension), head bobbing, extreme lordosis and falling, followed by righting, wild running and jumping. None of the gerbils died following a seizure. After a seizure, the gerbils would often enter a post-ictal state for 2 min or more during which they exhibited behaviour characteristic of limbic seizures. The progeny of seizure-sensitive gerbils, the 'seizure-prone' gerbils, were not subjected to this testing because they were analysed with histological methods at 25 to 30 days of age, an age prior to the onset of seizure activity.

Histology

Animals were deeply anesthetized with pentobarbital and transcardially perfused for fixation of brain tissue. For light microscopic examination, fixation was by buffered 4 per cent paraformaldehyde. After cryoprotection in buffered 25 per cent sucrose, brains were cut in the coronal plane at a thickness of 40 µm and collected into five sets of a one-in-five series. One set of sections was stained with cresyl violet to provide Nissl staining and an adjacent set was stained immunocytochemically for glutamic acid decarboxylase (GAD; Oertel *et al.*, 1981a, b) as a marker for GABAergic neurons. Details of the staining procedures have been described previously (Peterson & Ribak, 1987). When possible, seizure-sensitive, seizure-resistant and seizure-prone brain sections were processed simultaneously. For electron microscopic examination, fixation was according to the method of Friedrich & Mugnaini (1981) as described by Farias *et al.* (1992).

Cell counting

The number of GAD-immunoreactive neurons in various regions was determined within individual sections. GAD-immunoreactive somata were counted in six seizure-sensitive, four seizure-resistant and three seizure-prone brains in the hippocampus, dentate gyrus, motor cortex, substantia nigra and nucleus reticularis thalami. Within the hippocampus, counts were made in six subdivisions: three in regio superior (CA1; strata oriens, pyramidale and radiatum-lacunosum-moleculare) and three in regio inferior (CA2,3; strata oriens, pyramidale and lucidum-radiatum-lacunosum-moleculare). The dentate gyrus was subdivided into five parts: the hilar region and the supra- and infrapyramidal blades of strata granulosum and moleculare, respectively. In the hippocampus and dentate gyrus every fifth section along the entire septotemporal axis was analysed. To standardize the data for variations in the sizes of strata granulosum and moleculare of the dentate gyrus, area measurements were made by tracing each of the lamina onto the digitizing tablet of a Bioquant Image Analysis System (R & M Biometrics) and relative cell counts were converted to cell densities. Since these data were not used to estimate the total number of neurons in any of the brain regions studied but rather the relative number per section, it was not necessary to use a split-cell correction factor. The size of GAD-immunoreactive somata within the dentate gyrus and hippocampus was calculated by computer-assisted image analysis (Bioquant, R & M Biometrics). Counts of GAD-immunoreactive neurons were also made in the motor cortex throughout all cortical layers from several traverses between the pial surface and the white matter. In addition, cell counts were made throughout the rostral 1000 µm of the substantia nigra, and cell density measurements for the reticular nucleus of the thalamus were made from equivalent regions of known area.

Synaptic interactions

In addition to the counts of GAD-immunoreactive neuronal somata, GAD-immunoreactive puncta (the presumed light microscopic analog of synaptic terminals (Ribak *et al.*, 1981; Oertel *et al.*, 1981b)) were counted in thick and semi-thin sections of the dentate gyrus stratum granulosum using a 100x oil immersion objective and an eye-piece grid reticule. A region approximately 100 µm lateral to the crest of stratum granulosum was sampled in both the supra- and infrapyramidal blades approximately 1200 µm caudal to the septal pole of the dentate gyrus which was within the septal third of its long axis. Similar regions were sampled for electron microscopic examination and counts were made of asymmetric and symmetric synapses on somata of GAD-immunoreactive basket cells and non-immunoreactive granule cells.

Statistics

To determine whether significant differences existed between the data groups obtained from seizure-sensitive, seizure-resistant and seizure-prone gerbils, a one way analysis of variance for these groups was initially used. When the sample populations were small, a non-parametric test, the Kruskal-Wallis method, was employed. If significant differences were found between the groups, then an unpaired t-test or a Mann-Whitney U-test was used to determine which groups were responsible for the differences. Differences were expressed relative to the seizure-resistant gerbils which are generally considered a control group.

Results

Analysis of GABAergic neurons

Dentate gyrus

The size and distribution of GAD-immunoreactive somata in the seizure-resistant dentate gyrus was similar to that in the rat; the spacing between adjacent cells was usually 80–140 µm and they were only rarely found in close proximity to one another. In contrast, GAD-immunoreactive somata in the

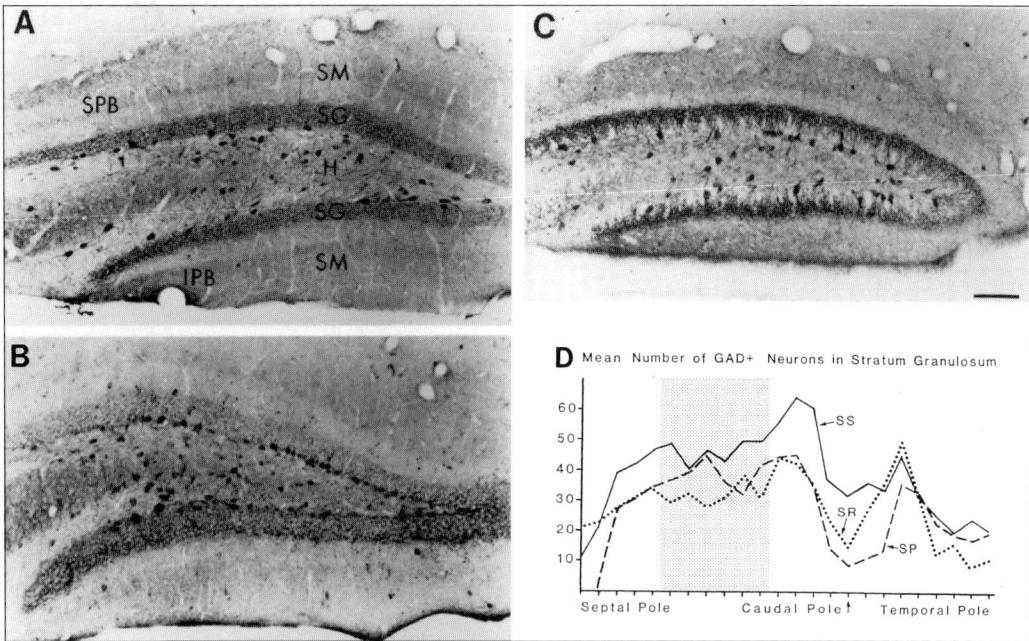

Fig. 2. Coronal sections which were incubated in antiserum to GAD to show the somal distribution of GABAergic neurons in the gerbil dentate gyrus. GABAergic pyramidal basket cells in the seizure-resistant dentate gyrus (A) are found at the border between the stratum granulosum (SG) and the hilus (H) in both the suprapyramidal (SPB) and infrapyramidal (IPB) blades. SM = stratum moleculare. Both seizure-sensitive (B) and seizure-prone (C) dentate gyri display more GABAergic neurons at this location than those from seizure-resistant brains. Counts from the hilus and stratum moleculare also showed increases in the seizure-sensitive brains (see text). Scale bar = 100 μm. D. Graphic representation of the mean number of GAD-immunoreactive neurons in the dentate gyrus of seizure-sensitive, seizure-resistant and seizure-prone gerbils. The septotemporal axis has been displayed in a linear fashion so that variations in cell number along this axis can be identified. The position of the septal, caudal and temporal poles of the dentate gyrus are indicated. Only the data for the suprapyramidal blade are shown. The shading indicates the septal region where the differences between seizure-sensitive and seizure-resistant gerbils were most substantial. (A, B, and C are reproduced from Peterson et al., 1985, with permission of the publisher. D is reproduced from Peterson & Ribak, 1987, with permission of the publisher.)

seizure-sensitive dentate gyrus often formed groups of three or four where some appeared to contact each other. In addition, the average size of the GAD-immunoreactive somata in the seizure-sensitive dentate gyrus was 30 per cent smaller than in the seizure-resistant dentate gyrus ($\bar{x}_{\text{seizure-sensitive}} = 112.6$ μm^2, $\bar{x}_{\text{seizure-resistant}} = 144.1$ μm^2, $P < 0.01$, Student's t-test). The most striking difference between the seizure-resistant and seizure-sensitive dentate gyri was the number of GAD-immunoreactive somata, especially those contained within or having processes passing through the stratum granulosum (Fig. 2). In some cases there were nearly twice as many cells in the suprapyramidal blade of the seizure-sensitive brains as compared to the corresponding region of seizure-resistant brains. Across all animals there was a statistically significant 35 per cent increase in the total number of GAD-immunoreactive neurons in the suprapyramidal blade of seizure-sensitive brains as compared to seizure-resistant brains ($P < 0.05$, Mann-Whitney U-Test). The difference was most substantial and consistent in the septal half of the dentate gyrus (Fig. 2D) in which significant differences were also observed (unpaired t-test, seizure-sensitive vs. seizure-resistant, $P < 0.05$ and seizure-sensitive vs. seizure-prone, $P < 0.05$). Within the infrapyramidal blade the number of GAD-immunoreactive neurons was approximately the same in both the seizure-sensitive and seizure-resistant brains. Regression analysis showed that the number of GAD-immunoreactive neurons in the suprapyramidal blade of the stratum granulosum was positively correlated with the intensity score of the individual animal's seizure record ($r = 0.725$). As in stratum granulosum, stratum moleculare had more GAD-immunoreactive neurons in seizure-sensitive brains than in seizure-resistant brains and again the difference was most pronounced in the suprapyramidal blade. Even the number of GAD-immunoreactive cells in the seizure-sensitive hilus was approximately 20 per cent greater than in the seizure-resistant. Thus, seizure-sensitive brains displayed more GAD-immunoreactive somata than did seizure-resistant brains in all three regions of the dentate gyrus. This difference was maintained even when cell counts were standardized by converting counts to cell density (number of GAD-immunoreactive somata/mm^2).

In general, the brains of the young offspring of seizure-sensitive gerbils, the seizure-prone group, displayed more GAD-immunoreactive neurons than the seizure-resistant brains but somewhat less than the seizure-sensitive brains. After correcting for differences in size by converting raw cell counts to cell densities some of the seizure-prone brains were found to have similar GABAergic neuronal densities to the seizure-sensitive brains. Furthermore, with this calculation, all seizure-prone brains had densities greater than the seizure-resistant brains. The variation in seizure-prone data may reflect the variation that is known to occur in the seizure records of the offspring of seizure-sensitive gerbils.

Ammon's horn

GAD-immunoreactive neurons were found in all subregions within the hippocampus except the alveus and they varied in size, ranging from 13 to 20 µm in diameter. Those cells that showed staining of the proximal dendrites could be characterized as either multipolar or fusiform. The major difference in the number of GAD-immunoreactive somata in the hippocampus occurred in the CA2,3 region where an overall increase of 42 per cent was observed in seizure-sensitive gerbils as compared to seizure-resistant gerbils. The most pronounced difference and the only one that was statistically significant between groups ($P < 0.05$, Kruskal-Wallis method) occurred between seizure-sensitive and seizure-resistant gerbils (65 per cent, $P < 0.05$, unpaired t-test) and was observed in the CA2,3 apical dendritic field which consisted of the strata lucidum, radiatum and lacunosum-moleculare. The CA1 region of seizure-sensitive brains showed a small (10–15 per cent) increase in the number of GAD-immunoreactive cells, but it was not statistically significant. In seizure-prone gerbil brains an overall increase of 10 per cent was observed in the number of GAD-immunoreactive neurons in all regions of the hippocampus when compared with seizure-resistant brains. This difference was not statistically significant. Again, the greatest difference (23 per cent) was noted in the apical dendritic field of the CA2,3 pyramidal cells. In general, the numbers for seizure-prone gerbils were intermediate between the counts for seizure-sensitive and seizure-resistant gerbils.

Other brain regions

GAD-immunoreactive neurons were examined in the substantia nigra, reticular nucleus of the thalamus, and motor cortex from seizure-sensitive and seizure-resistant gerbils. These regions represent areas which are either rich in GABAergic neurons or have been implicated in seizure activity or both. No differences in terminal or somal staining were noted between seizure-sensitive and seizure-resistant gerbils, nor did the number or size of GAD-immunoreactive neurons differ between the two strains in any of these regions.

Analysis of synaptic contacts between GABAergic cells in the dentate gyrus

The distribution of GAD-immunoreactive puncta (previously shown to correspond to axon terminals) within the seizure-resistant dentate gyrus was similar to that reported in the rat (Barber & Saito, 1976; Ribak *et al.*, 1981; Goldowitz *et al.*, 1982; Seress & Ribak, 1983). Thus, the outer third of stratum moleculare was moderately dense and the density of puncta in stratum granulosum was uniform

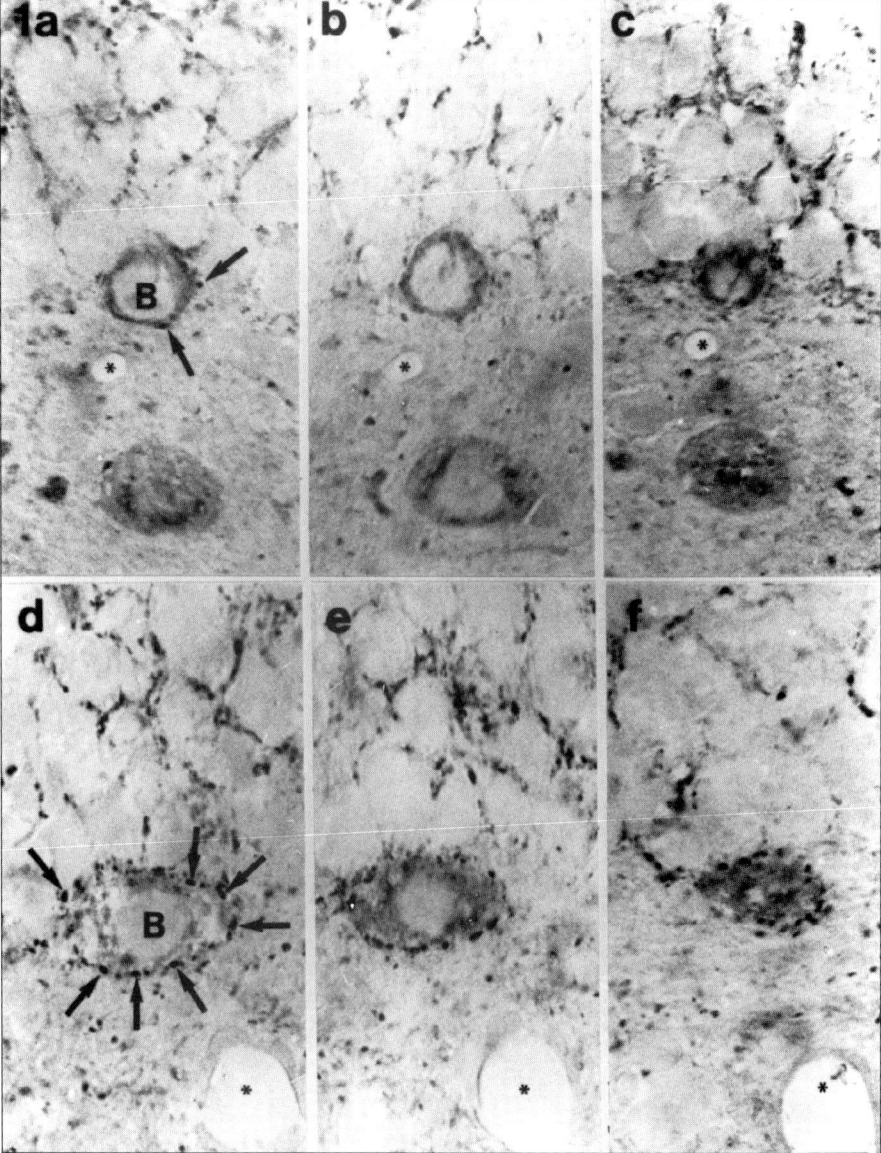

Fig. 3. Photomicrographs of serial semithin sections (1 μm thick) that show GAD-immunoreactive basket cells (B) in the dentate gyrus of seizure-resistant (a–c) and seizure-sensitive (d–f) gerbils. The somata of these GABAergic basket cells are found on the hilar border with the granule cell layer. The number of GAD-immunoreactive puncta (arrows) adjacent to the seizure-resistant basket cell body (a) is less than that for the seizure-sensitive gerbil basket cell (d). Note that few, if any, GAD-immunoreactive puncta are found on the basal surface of seizure-resistant basket cell somata (a–c). In contrast, the seizure-sensitive gerbil basket cell (d–f) displays many GAD-immunoreactive puncta apposed to its basal surface. The number of GAD-immunoreactive puncta around the somata of granule cells located above the basket cells (B) appears to be similar for both types of gerbil. A capillary (*) is indicated for orientation in each set of three panels. Scale bar = 10 μm. (Reproduced from Farias et al., 1992, with permission of the publisher.)

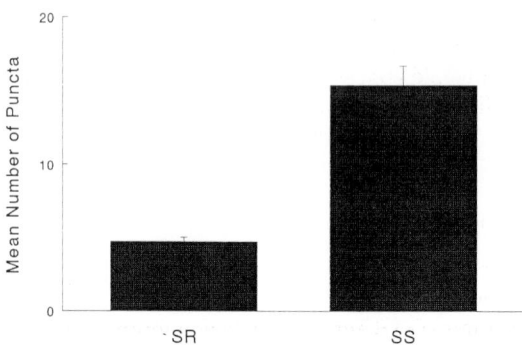

Fig. 4. Histogram showing the mean number of GAD-immunoreactive puncta around GAD-immunoreactive basket cells in the dentate gyrus of seizure-resistant and seizure-sensitive gerbils. In seizure-resistant brains 460 GAD-immunoreactive puncta were found around 97 GAD-immunoreactive basket cells. In seizure-sensitive brains 618 GAD-immunoreactive puncta were found around 39 GAD-immunoreactive basket cells. The difference is significant at $P < 0.0005$ (unpaired t-test with 135 df).
Data are from Farias et al. (1992).

between the infra- and suprapyramidal blades. In contrast, the density of GAD-immunoreactive puncta in the seizure-sensitive dentate gyrus was approximately three times greater in the infrapyramidal blade of stratum granulosum than in the suprapyramidal blade. The density of puncta in both blades of the seizure-sensitive dentate gyrus was significantly greater than in the seizure-resistant ($P < 0.01$; Student's t-test), and the GAD-immunoreactive terminals appeared to be both larger and more densely stained in the seizure-sensitive brains, especially in the infrapyramidal blade. No differences were observed in the density of GAD-immunoreactive puncta within stratum moleculare either between blades or between strains.

Light microscopic analysis of semi-thin sections showed that GAD-immunoreactive cells in the suprapyramidal blade from seizure-resistant gerbils had relatively few GAD-immunoreactive puncta adjacent to their somata (Figs. 3a–c, 4). In contrast, sections from seizure-sensitive gerbils showed numerous GAD-immunoreactive puncta surrounding GAD-immunoreactive somata (Figs. 3d–e, 4). These differences were partially confirmed by electron microscopic analysis of numbers of asymmetric (excitatory, non-GABAergic) and symmetric (inhibitory, GABAergic) synapses on to the somata of GAD-immunoreactive basket cells and non-immunoreactive granule cells. The basket cells ($n = 9$) from seizure-sensitive gerbils had more symmetric synapses per unit length of somal surface than those ($n = 4$) from seizure-resistant gerbils. In contrast, there were no differences in the numbers of asymmetric synapses between basket cells from seizure-sensitive and seizure-resistant gerbils. Granule cell somata from seizure-sensitive ($n = 42$) and seizure-resistant ($n = 26$) gerbils showed no differences in the number of either asymmetric or symmetric synapses.

Discussion

Taken together, our data suggest that the hippocampal formation of seizure-sensitive gerbils has an abnormal circuitry that is involved in the generation and/or propagation of epileptic activity. Not only is the number of GABAergic neurons increased, but the number of GABAergic synapses on to GABAergic somata is also increased in both seizure-sensitive and seizure-prone gerbils. Furthermore, the increased numbers of GABAergic neurons have been observed only in the dentate gyrus and hippocampus, and these appear to be interconnected in an aberrant fashion.

The differences between the seizure-sensitive and seizure-resistant hippocampus do not appear to be the result of compensatory changes following seizure activity because the hippocampus of young seizure-sensitive progeny (seizure-prone) which had not had seizures also showed increased numbers of GABAergic cells. Thus, it would appear that the differences between the two strains is genetically related. Another important finding was the correlation between the number of GABAergic neurons in the dentate gyrus and the individual gerbil's seizure intensity. This correlation suggests that the severity of seizure activity is related to this abnormality.

Hippocampal disinhibition hypothesis

We have proposed an hypothesis of disinhibition which explains the apparent contradiction between the occurrence of seizure activity including vesicle depletion in mossy terminals and the increased numbers of inhibitory structures (GABAergic somata and terminals) in the hippocampal formation. GABAergic basket cells in the hippocampal formation receive collateral input from the excitatory granule and pyramidal cells (Frotscher, 1985; Ribak & Seress, 1983). The GABAergic cells in turn form pericellular basket plexuses around the granule cell somata and form axosomatic connections (Ribak & Seress, 1983; Seress & Ribak, 1985). Thus, the GABAergic cells provide feed-back inhibition to the granule cells of the dentate gyrus and pyramidal cells of the hippocampus (Andersen, 1975). In the non-epileptic hippocampal formation feed-back inhibition is responsible for controlling the output of the granule and pyramidal cells. Our morphological observations have shown that the number of GABAergic neurons and the number of inhibitory synaptic connections onto GABAergic somata are increased in the dentate gyrus of the seizure-sensitive gerbils. The normal feed-back circuit and our proposed abnormal circuitry is illustrated in Fig. 5. Activation of such a circuit by the collateral input from the excitatory cells would cause one of the inhibitory neurons to inhibit the other, thereby effectively blocking the feed-back inhibition or inducing *dis*inhibition.

The observation that increased GABA levels suppress seizures in epileptic gerbils (Löscher, 1984; Löscher *et al.*, 1983) would appear to be contradictory to our hypothesis of disinhibition within the

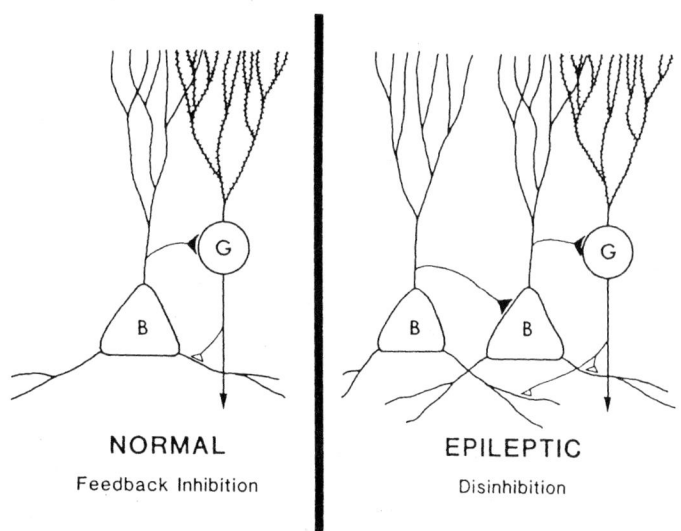

Fig. 5. Schematic diagram of the circuitry between granule and basket (GABAergic) cells in the dentate gyrus from seizure-resistant (left) and seizure-sensitive (right) gerbils. In seizure-resistant gerbils, axon collaterals of granule cells (G) form excitatory synapses with the basal dendrites of basket cells (B), which send inhibitory axons to the soma of the granule cell. This circuitry provides a normal feedback inhibition. In contrast, the seizure-sensitive gerbils have additional basket cells (B) that inhibit other basket cells that contact the granule cells (G), thereby resulting in disinhibition of the granule cells.

dentate gyrus. According to our hypothesis, increased GABA levels (at the synapses between GABAergic cells) would be predicted to increase disinhibition and thereby increase excitation (and presumably seizure activity). It is likely, however, that the systemic administration of GABA agonists and GABA mimetics used in the studies of Löscher and colleagues affects all regions of the brain and not just the contacts between GABAergic cells in the dentate gyrus. Thus, even though disinhibition might be increased within the dentate gyrus, the overall effect of these drugs on cortical and limbic brain structures would be increased inhibition resulting in reduced susceptibility to seizure.

Although GABA is usually associated with postsynaptic hyperpolarization and inhibition (Mody et al., 1994), GABA has been shown to evoke excitatory responses in a subpopulation of neurons in the dentate hilus (Michelson & Wong, 1991, 1994). It is conceivable that the aberrant synaptic contacts that we have shown between GABAergic neurons in the dentate gyrus of the seizure-sensitive gerbil may be coupled by such excitatory synaptic contacts. However, the GABAergic cells which we have shown to be interconnected are within the granule cell layer whereas those studied by Michelson & Wong are in the hilus; furthermore, they studied guinea pig rather than gerbil. Finally, in their studies, they found that the net result of GABA-mediated excitation of hilar interneurons was synchronized and large amplitude inhibitory postsynaptic potentials in granule and pyramidal cells. Since electrophysiological data for GABAergic basket cells in gerbils are lacking, we assumed the traditional inhibitory effect in advancing our disinhibition hypothesis, i.e. the physiological effect of the supernumerary synapses with basket cells is to inhibit the basket cells and thus disinhibit granule cells. Consistent with this proposal is the finding by Farias et al. (1992) that removal of the entorhinal excitatory drive to this abnormal circuit in seizure-sensitive gerbils is associated with quiescent or normal looking mossy fibre terminals. In fact, electrophysiological data on the gerbil hippocampus (Buckmaster & Schwartzkroin, 1994) indicate that the dentate gyrus displays hyperexcitability. More detailed analyses are required to confirm the disinhibition hypothesis.

Acknowledgements: This work was supported by NS15669 to C.E.R. The authors wish to acknowledge the efforts of several collaborators and former students including Kim Anderson, Paul Farias, Dr. Sana Khan, Savina Low and Dr. Nandor Ludvig.

References

Andersen, P. (1975): Organization of hippocampal neurons and their connections. In: *The hippocampus, Vol 1*, Isaacson, R.L. & Pribram, K.H. (eds), pp. 155–175. New York: Plenum Press.

Barber, R. & Saito, K. (1976): Light microscopic visualization of GAD and GABA-T in immunocytochemical preparations of rodent CNS. In: *GABA in nervous system function*, Roberts, E., Chase, T.N. & Tower, D.B. (eds), pp. 113–132. New York: Raven Press.

Buckmaster, P.S. & Schwartzkroin, P.A. (1994): Hyperexcitability in the dentate gyrus of the epileptic Mongolian gerbil. *Epilepsy Res.* **18**, 23–28.

Farias, P.A., Low, S., Peterson, G.M. & Ribak, C.E. (1992): Morphological evidence for altered synaptic organization and neural activity in the hippocampal formation of seizure sensitive gerbils. *Hippocampus* **2**, 229–246.

Friedrich, V.L., Jr. & Mugnaini, E. (1981): Electron microscopy: Preparation of neural tissues for electron microscopy. In: *Neuroanatomical tract-tracing methods*, Heimer, L. & Robards, M.J. (eds), pp. 345–376. New York: Plenum Press.

Frotscher, M. (1985): Mossy fibers form synapses with identified pyramidal basket cells in the CA3 region of the guinea pig hippocampus: a combined Golgi-electron microscopic study. *J. Neurocytol.* **14**, 245–259.

Goldowitz, D., Vincent, S.R., Wu, J.-Y. & Hökfelt, T. (1982): Immunohistochemical demonstration of plasticity in GABA neurons of the adult rat dentate gyrus. *Brain Res.* **238**, 413–420.

Löscher, W. (1984): Evidence for abnormal sensitivity of the GABA system in gerbils with genetically determined epilepsy. In: *Neurotransmitters, seizures and epilepsy II*, Fariello, R.G., Lloyd, K.G., Morselli, P.L., Quesney, L.F. & Engel, J. (eds), pp. 179–188. New York: Raven Press.

Löscher, W., Frey, H.-H., Reiche, R. & Schultz, D. (1983): High anticonvulsant potency of γ-aminobutyric acid (GABA) mimetic drugs in gerbils with genetically determined epilepsy. *J. Pharmacol. Exp. Therap.* **226**, 839–844.

Loskota, W.J., Lomax, P. & Rich, S.T. (1974): The gerbil as a model for the study of the epilepsies. *Epilepsia* **15**, 109–119.

Ludvig, N., Farias, P.A. & Ribak, C.E. (1991): An analysis of various environmental and specific sensory stimuli on the seizure activity of the Mongolian gerbil. *Epilepsy Res.* **8**, 30–35.

Majkowski, J. & Donadio, M. (1984): Electro-clinical studies of epileptic seizures in Mongolian gerbils. *Electroencephalogr. Clin. Neurophysiol.* **57**, 369–377.

Michelson, H.B. & Wong, R.K.S. (1991): Excitatory synaptic responses mediated by $GABA_A$ receptors in the hippocampus. *Science* **253**, 1420–1423.

Michelson, H.B. & Wong, R.K.S. (1994): Synchronization of inhibitory neurons in the guinea-pig hippocampus *in vitro*. *J. Physiol.* **477.1**, 35–45.

Mody, I., DeKoninck, Y., Otis, T.S. & Soltesz, I. (1994): Bridging the cleft at GABA synapses in the brain. *Trends Neurosci.* **17**, 517–525.

Mouritzen Dam, A., Bajorek, J.C. & Lomax, P. (1981): Hippocampal neuron density and seizures in the Mongolian gerbil. *Epilepsia* **22**, 667–674.

Nitsch, C. & Rinne, U. (1981): Large dense-core vesicle exocytosis and membrane recycling in the mossy fibre synapses of the rabbit hippocampus during epileptiform seizures. *J. Neurocytol.* **57**, 201–219.

Oertel, W.H., Schmechel, D.E., Weise, V.K., Ranson, D.H., Tappaz, M.L., Krutzsch, H.C. & Kopin, I.J. (1981a): Comparison of cysteine sulphinic acid decarboxylase isoenzymes and glutamic acid decarboxylase in rat liver and brain. *Neuroscience* **6**, 2701–2714.

Oertel, W.H., Schmechel, D.E., Mugnaini, E., Tappaz, M.L. & Kopin, I.J. (1981b): Immunocytochemical localization of glutamate decarboxylase in rat cerebellum with a new antiserum. *Neuroscience* **6**, 2715–2735.

Paul, L.A., Fried, I., Watanabe, K., Forsythe, A.B. & Scheibel, A.B. (1981): Structural correlates of seizure behaviour in the Mongolian gerbil. *Science* **213**, 924–926.

Peterson, G.M. & Ribak, C.E. (1987): Hippocampus of the seizure-sensitive gerbil is a specific site for anatomical changes in the GABAergic system. *J. Comp. Neurol.* **261**, 405–422.

Peterson, G.M., Ribak, C.E. & Oertel, W.H. (1985): A regional increase in the number of hippocampal GABAergic neurons and terminals in the seizure-sensitive gerbil. *Brain Res.* **340**, 384–389.

Ribak, C.E. & Khan, S.U. (1987): The effects of knife cuts of hippocampal pathways on epileptic activity in the seizure-sensitive gerbil. *Brain Res.* **418**, 146–151.

Ribak, C.E. & Seress, L. (1983): Five types of basket cell in the hippocampal dentate gyrus: a combined Golgi and electron microscopic study. *J. Neurocytol.* **12**, 577–597.

Ribak, C.E., Vaughn, J.E. & Barber, R.P. (1981): Immunocytochemical localization of GABAergic neurones at the electron microscopical level. *Histochem. J.* **13**, 555–582.

Seress, L. & Ribak, C.E. (1983): GABAergic cells in the dentate gyrus appear to be local circuit and projection neurons. *Exp. Brain Res.* **50**, 173–182.

Seress, L. & Ribak, C.E. (1985): A combined Golgi-electron microscopic study of non-pyramidal neurons in the CA1 area of the hippocampus. *J. Neurocytol.* **14**, 717–730.

Thiessen, D.D., Lindzey, G. & Friend, H.D. (1968): Spontaneous seizures in the Mongolian gerbil. *Psychon. Sci.* **11**, 227–228.

Chapter 25

Genetic predisposition to partial (focal) seizures and to generalized tonic/clonic seizures: interactions between seizure circuitry of the forebrain and brainstem

P.C. Jobe[1], P.K. Mishra[1], J.W. Dailey[1], K.H. Ko[2] and M.E.A. Reith[1]

Department of Biomedical and Therapeutic Sciences, University of Illinois College of Medicine, Box 1649, Peoria, Illinois 61656, USA; and [2]Department of Pharmacy, College of Pharmacy, Seoul National University, Centre for Biofunctional Molecules, Postech, Korea

Seizure predisposition denotes the capacity of epileptic mammals to exhibit seizures in response to exogenous stimuli or endogenous neuronal events that do not cause such episodes in normal subjects. Three types of seizure predisposition have been identified (Jobe *et al.*, 1994b).

Type 1   Susceptibility to seizures evoked by endogenous and exogenous stimuli that, regardless of magnitude or dose, fail to produce seizures in normal subjects.

Type 2   Exaggerated seizure severity in response to stimuli which also provoke seizures in normal subjects.

Type 3   Abnormally low seizure thresholds to stimuli which in higher doses also precipitate seizures in non-epileptic subjects.

The genetically epilepsy-prone rats (GEPRs) are characterized by all three types of seizure predisposition (Jobe *et al.*, 1994b). Studies in other species including humans and other primates also support the concept that seizure predisposition is a characteristic of epilepsy (Buchhalter, 1993; Davis & King, 1967; Green & Seyfried, 1991; Jobe *et al.*, 1991; Killam & Killam, Jr., 1984; Killam *et al.*, 1967; King, Jr. & LaMotte, 1989; Ludvig *et al.*, 1985; Marley *et al.*, 1986; Menini & Silva Barrat, 1990; Porter, 1993; Sugaya *et al.*, 1986). Type 1 seizure predisposition is well known in human epilepsy. Many people suffering from epilepsy exhibit 'spontaneous seizures' which are primarily generalized and occur in response to variations in endogenous neuronal events. In most but not all instances, these seizures occur in the absence of a known environmental stimulus (Tassinari *et al.*, 1990). Types 2 and 3 seizure predisposition have also been documented in human epilepsy, albeit few such studies have been undertaken (Cure *et al.*, 1948; Garretson *et al.*, 1966; Gastaut, 1950; Kaufman *et al.*, 1947; Wieser *et al.*, 1979).

Seizure predisposition represents a fundamental distinction between epilepsy and normality (Jobe *et al.*, 1991, 1994b). The occurrence of a seizure does not distinguish normal mammals from their counterparts with epilepsy because both exhibit seizures in response to convulsant stimuli.

Brainstem and forebrain seizure circuitry

The concept of a different circuitry for brainstem and forebrain convulsive seizures has been established via neuroanatomical, behavioural and neurochemical studies (Browning, 1994). In some genetically epileptic animals, seizure predisposition is a characteristic both of forebrain and brainstem seizure circuitry (Cure *et al.*, 1948; Jobe *et al.*, 1991; Porter, 1993). Mounting evidence supports the concept that partial seizures are driven by forebrain circuitry, whereas generalized tonic/clonic seizures are driven by brainstem circuitry (Coffey *et al.*, 1996; McNamara, 1986). This topic will be explored in greater depth in subsequent portions of this chapter.

Forebrain convulsive seizures are driven by activity within and between limbic nuclei and in some instances the circuitry extends rostrally to the cerebral cortex and caudally to the substantia nigra and the superior colliculus (Browning, 1994; Gale, 1992; Handforth & Ackermann, 1988; Patel, 1988). Brainstem seizures appear to be driven by a network of interacting substrates, including the reticular formation of the brainstem, inferior colliculus and superior colliculus (Batini *et al.*, 1996; Browning, 1994; Burnham & Browning, 1987; Faingold & Naritoku, 1992; Randall & Faingold, 1995; Riaz & Faingold, 1994; Wang *et al.*, 1993).

Table 1. Convulsions driven by forebrain seizures

Class	Behaviours
0	Immobility
1	Facial clonus
2	Class 1 plus neck clonus
3	Class 2 plus forelimb clonus
4	Class 3 plus rearing
5	Class 4 plus falling

Table 2. Convulsions driven by brainstem seizures

Class	Initial running/bouncing episode	Subsequent convulsion
1	Present	None
3	Long duration	Brainstem generalized clonus with loss of righting capacity. Neck clonus is superimposed on a dominant dorsiflexion of the neck. (Clonus of the limbs is superimposed on tonic flexion of the shoulder, hip, elbow and knee joints. The tonic posture gives way to high amplitude clonus of the pelvic limbs. The postictal state is characterized by catatonia)
5	Intermediate duration	Brainstem clonus of pelvic limbs coupled with tonic vetriflexion of the trunk and neck and tonic extension of the forelimbs.
7	Shorter duration	Same as class 5 except hip and knee joints are extended. Ankle joints are flexed.
9	Very short duration	Same as 7 except pelvic limbs are fully extended.
10	Massive myoclonic thrusts of the limbs occur in lieu of a running episode.	Same as 9

Behaviours resulting from forebrain and brainstem seizures have been described and sub-classified (Jobe *et al.*, 1973, 1992, 1994a; Racine, 1972; Racine *et al.*, 1973). The behaviours driven by forebrain seizures are summarized in Table 1. The behaviours caused by brainstem seizures are summarized in Table 2. Forebrain seizure behaviours are distinctly different and readily differentiable by observation from the behaviours of brainstem seizures. In some instances, the same word might be chosen to describe some of the behaviours in brainstem and forebrain seizures. For example, clonus occurs in both cases. Nevertheless, as can be seen in Tables 1 and 2 the clonic behaviours of forebrain seizures are different than those of brainstem seizures.

Both brainstem and forebrain circuitry may exhibit seizures simultaneously. When both sets of circuitry are operative, the forebrain seizure behaviours are obscured by behaviours driven by brainstem circuitry (Browning *et al.*, 1990; Jobe *et al.*, 1995). Accordingly, when both systems are active, rhythmic spike or spike/wave discharges in the cortical EEG cannot be used to exclude brainstem circuitry as the dominant driving source of the behavioural components of the seizures (Jobe *et al.*, 1995).

Forebrain seizure predisposition in GEPRs

Forebrain seizure predisposition in GEPRs was documented in a limbic kindling study (Savage *et al.*, 1986). Compared to non-epileptic rats, the rate of kindling to a class 5 forebrain seizure is accelerated in GEPRs. Moreover, this accelerated rate of kindling is greater in GEPR–9s than in GEPR–3s, a distinction that is compatible with other observations showing that seizure predisposition is more marked in GEPR–9s than in GEPR–3s (Jobe *et al.*, 1994a). Subsequently, Browning and colleagues (1990) demonstrated that in response to transcorneal electroshock the threshold for forebrain seizures is lowest in GEPR–9s, intermediate in GEPR–3s and highest in non-epileptic controls.

Brainstem seizure predisposition in GEPRs

Several studies have shown that GEPRs are characterized by brainstem seizure predisposition. For example, both GEPR–3s and GEPR–9s exhibit seizures driven by brainstem circuitry in response to an acoustical stimulus, whereas non-epileptic rats do not exhibit this trait (Jobe *et al.*, 1992). Other studies have shown that brainstem seizure thresholds for electrical stimuli are abnormally low in GEPRs, with the magnitude of the deficit being more pronounced in GEPR–9s than in GEPR–3s (Browning *et al.*, 1990).

Relationship of forebrain to brainstem seizure thresholds in GEPRs

Comparison of forebrain to brainstem seizure thresholds for corneal electroshock yields an interesting result. Accordingly, for non-epileptic control rats and for GEPR–3s, the ratio of the thresholds for forebrain and brainstem seizures is less than unity (Browning *et al.*, 1990). In contrast, the ratio is greater than unity for GEPR–9s. These findings support the concept that the threshold for triggering brainstem seizure discharge is lower than the threshold for triggering forebrain seizure discharge in GEPR–9s, whereas the reverse relationship exists in normal rats and in GEPR–3s. Other observations with different seizure inducing modalities support these concepts (Jobe *et al.*, 1994a).

Forebrain seizure predisposition occurs as a genetic trait and as a response to repeated brainstem seizures

Recently, Coffey and colleagues (1996) showed that amygdala kindling of forebrain seizures occurs both in presumptive seizure-naïve GEPR–9s and in brainstem seizure experienced GEPR–9s. These authors observed that seizure-naïve GEPR–9s kindle more rapidly than non-epileptic rats. Also, they found that brainstem seizure-experienced GEPR–9s kindled faster than their seizure-naïve counterparts. These observations support the hypothesis that both genetically determined seizure predisposition and previous brainstem seizure experience accelerate limbic kindling. However, they should not be interpreted to imply that genetically determined brainstem seizure predisposition *a priori* results in forebrain seizure predisposition in every form of convulsive epilepsy. Accordingly, the coexistence of these traits in GEPRs contrasts with the absence of dual predisposition in Strasbourg audiogenic seizure susceptible rats. In these French rats, accelerated limbic kindling occurs upon repetition of sound-induced brainstem seizures, but not in audiogenic seizure-naïve subjects (Maton *et al.*, 1992). Thus, at least some components of these two traits appear to be under separate genetic control. In more general terms, the GEPR data combined with the Strasbourg data support the concept that some epilepsies are characterized by the combination of genetically determined forebrain seizure and brainstem seizure predispositions. Moreover, in these cases, brainstem seizures will exacerbate forebrain seizure predisposition, thereby increasing the probability of a forebrain seizure. In contrast, other epilepsies are characterized by genetically determined seizure predisposition only in the seizure circuitry of either the forebrain or the brainstem.

Ignition of forebrain seizure circuitry by brainstem seizures

Several studies demonstrate that, under defined conditions, brainstem seizure activity has the capacity to ignite forebrain seizure circuitry. Hirsch *et al.* (1992) and Maton *et al.* (1992) showed this phenomenon in adult Strasbourg audiogenic seizure susceptible rats. Also, Naritoku *et al.* (1992) documented the caudal to rostral activation in adult GEPRs. Accordingly, upon initial exposure of GEPR–9s to an acoustical stimulus, brainstem seizures occur behaviourally without evidence of cortical EEG seizure activity. Upon repetition of audiogenic convulsions, the EEG seizure encompasses both the cortex and the brainstem (Jobe *et al.*, 1995; Naritoku *et al.*, 1992). In a subsequent study, Garcia-Cairasco *et al.* (1994) observed that, in adult GEPRs exposed to an audiogenic seizure repetition protocol (18–22 exposures), brainstem seizures became progressively less severe and class 1–5 limbic forebrain seizures eventually emerged as sequela to the brainstem seizures.

Prior to these observations, Reigel *et al.* (1989) reported behavioural evidence of brainstem seizure-induced activation of forebrain seizures in GEPR–3 pups. At postnatal day 15, an initial sound-induced brainstem seizure secondarily activated class 4 forebrain seizures in 5 per cent of the pups. On postnatal day 15, secondary class 4 forebrain seizures occurred in 100 per cent of the GEPR–3 pups. In each of these instances, the forebrain seizures occurred a few seconds following the end of the brainstem convulsion.

Ignition of brainstem seizure circuitry by forebrain seizures

A high percentage of GEPR–9s being kindled in the amygdala exhibit forebrain seizure-induced brainstem seizures; whereas, non-epileptic rats do not exhibit brainstem seizures in response to forebrain seizures (Coffey *et al.*, 1996). These brainstem seizures are severe, with 67 per cent falling between class 6 and 9 in the classification system of Jobe *et al.* (1973). The high incidence of forebrain seizures is essentially the same both in previously brainstem seizure-naïve GEPR–9s and in brainstem seizure experienced GEPR–9s. Moreover, brainstem seizures occur in response to initial forebrain seizures and the incidence of brainstem seizures remains unchanged with progression of kindling. Thus, in GEPR–9s, the brainstem seizure circuitry is innately susceptible to activation by forebrain seizures.

Mechanisms of seizure initiating interactions between the forebrain and brainstem circuitry

Several processes may enable seizure initiating interactions between the rostral and caudal circuitry of the brain in GEPR–9s. Some structures of the brain may be common to both types of seizure or some parts of the brain may serve as an interface between the rostral and caudal seizure circuitry (Coffey *et al.*, 1996). Also, abnormalities in specific neurotransmitter systems may play an important role in the generalization from the rostral to the caudal seizure circuitry. Deficits in noradrenergic, serotonergic and GABAergic transmission in GEPRs play key roles as determinants of seizure predisposition both in the rostral and caudal circuitry (Faingold & Naritoku, 1992; Jobe et al., 1991, 1994b). Such deficits are potentially responsible for the susceptibility of GEPR–9s to activation of brainstem seizures by forebrain seizures. Similarly, they may also play a role in the susceptibility of GEPRs to brainstem seizure-induced forebrain seizures. We suggest that these deficits are tantamount to an open gate through which seizure impulses from one set of circuitry pass to ignite seizure activity in the other circuitry. In non-epileptic mammals or in some epileptic animals with a sufficiently restricted seizure predisposition, seizure discharges from the forebrain may be suppressed before they reach the seizure-initiating regions of the brainstem. Thus, a seizure in the brainstem circuitry would not occur even in response to a severe forebrain seizure. This process of suppression, whether discretely localized or diffusely represented, would be tantamount to a closed gate.

As an alternative hypothesis, the gate may be open both in epileptic and non-epileptic brains. A sufficiently low seizure threshold in either circuitry might predispose to seizure ignition by seizure activity in the other circuitry. This concept is compatible with observations showing that GEPR–9s have markedly reduced thresholds to electrically induced forebrain and brainstem seizures (Browning et al., 1990).

Table 3. *The behavioural manifestations of human complex seizures are analogous to the behaviours driven by forebrain seizures in GEPRs and other rats*

Region	Humans[a]	Rats[b]
Whole body	Arrest reaction or motionless stare	Immobility
Face	Palpebral & other facial clonus, smacking, chewing, salivation, grimacing	Palpebral clonus & spasm, jaw clonus, mouth opening
Neck	Head turning sometimes with a clonic component	Neck clonus
Thoracic limbs	Picking at clothes, scratching, rubbing of hands, boxing, flailing, hand elevation as head turns	Scratching, alternating & synchronous forelimb clonus sometimes with increasing shoulder flexion & head turning
Trunk and legs	Lateral incurvation, flexion or turning of the trunk; sitting up; loss of postural tone & slumping slowly to floor	Rearing with turning of the trunk, plus loss of postural tone & slowly falling to floor

[a]Aicardi, 1986a; 1986b; Engel, Jr. 1989; [b]Racine, 1972; Coffey et al. 1996; Savage et al. 1986

GEPR–9s as a model for secondary generalization of human partial seizures

Recently, we proposed that brainstem seizures induced by forebrain seizures in GEPR–9s provide a model of human partial seizures that secondarily generalize to tonic/clonic seizures (Coffey et al., 1996). Three lines of evidence underlie this hypothesis. First, a large body of evidence supports limbic kindled seizures in rodents as a model for human complex partial seizures (McNamara, 1986). Table 3 summarizes the behavioural similarities between kindled seizures in rats and complex partial seizures in humans. Second, the concept is also supported by the fact that partial seizures in humans frequently evolve into secondarily generalized tonic/clonic seizures (Engel, Jr., 1989). Third, evidence shows that class 9 brainstem seizures in GEPR–9s are analogous to tonic/clonic seizures in humans (Jobe et al., 1995). Accordingly, in many GEPR–9s, class 9 seizure behaviours begin with a very brief running episode which rapidly translates into a tonic/clonic convulsion. In other GEPR–9s, the initial behaviour is characterized by myoclonic thrusts of the limbs and trunk in lieu of a running episode. This type of brainstem seizure (defined in Table 2 as class 10) closely mimics behavioural and EEG phases of human tonic/clonic seizures (Fig. 1).

The EEG data reported in Fig. 2 provides additional support for a point made earlier in this manuscript; namely, that generalized tonic clonic seizures are driven by brainstem seizure circuitry. Accordingly,

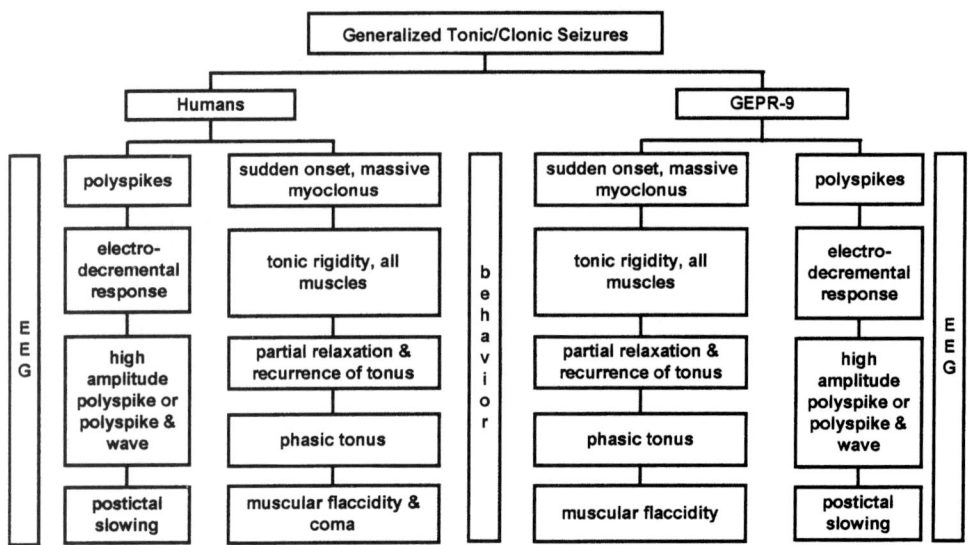

Fig. 1. Correspondence between EEG and behavioural components of generalized tonic/clonic seizures in humans with epilepsy and in GEPR–9s exhibiting class 10 brainstem seizures in response to acoustical stimuli. Human behaviours are from Engel (1989). Data on GEPR–9s are from Jobe et al. (1995) and Naritoku et al. (1992). The figure is from Jobe et al. (1995) with permission.

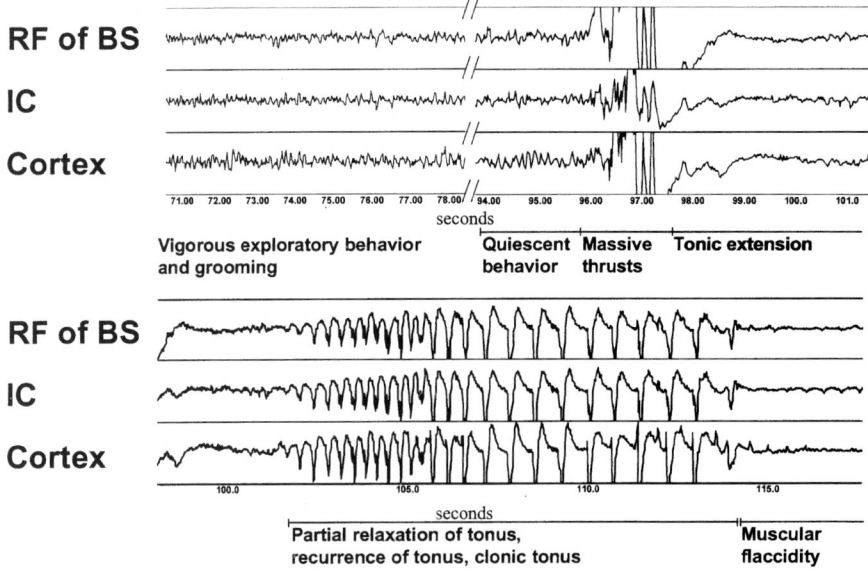

Fig. 2. Intracerebral electroencephalographic manifestations of a class 10 brainstem seizure in a freely moving unanesthetized GEPR–9. The seizure was induced by auditory input initiated at 90 s.
RF of BS indicates the reticular formation of the brainstem. IC denotes the inferior colliculus. Monopolar electrodes were inserted stereotactically into each of these structures approximately a week prior to the recording. The recording was made from a GEPR–9 which had experienced three audiogenic seizures in weeks prior to the recording.

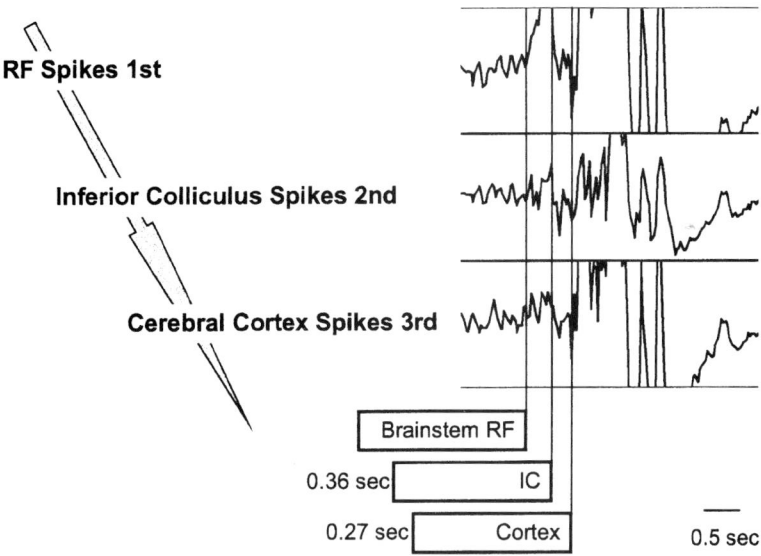

Fig. 3. High amplitude polyspikes occur in the reticular formation of the brainstem before they appear in the inferior colliculus and then in the cerebral cortex. The view shown in this figure is a magnification of the initial parts of the seizure shown the Fig. 2. RF refers to the reticular formation of the brainstem. IC refers to the inferior colliculus.

Fig. 2 depicts simultaneous recordings made in the reticular formation of the brainstem, the inferior colliculus and the cerebral cortex. A temporal comparison of the initiation of high amplitude spikes in these three brain areas is presented in Fig. 3. These tracings reveal that the seizure circuitry of the brainstem ignites prior to the rostral circuitry of the brain. More specifically, high amplitude spikes occur initially in the reticular formation of the brainstem. Subsequently, they appear in the inferior colliculus and then in the cerebral cortex.

Notes added to proof

Soon to be published observations from the current GEPR–9 colony show that the time differences between the initial EEG spikes in the different parts of the brain are no longer detectable with conventional EEG technology (Moraes, M., Mishra, P.K., Cairasco, N., Dailey, J.W. & Jobe, P.C., in preparation). Moreover, these studies show that, with newly developed localization technologies, the brainstem continues to be the site of origin of the initial spikes. These recent results were obtained from the GEPR–9 colony during a 12-month period in the years 1997 and 1998. The earlier results were obtained from the less highly developed GEPR–9 colony of 1993. We attribute the electrographic differences between the current and earlier GEPR–9s to a progressive exacerbation of the epileptic condition of the animals that has resulted from continued inbreeding for seizure predisposition.

Summary and conclusions

Two distinct sets of convulsive seizure circuitry have been identified. One circuitry resides in the forebrain, the other in the brainstem. Forebrain seizures in GEPRs and other rodents correspond in important ways to partial seizures in humans. Some classes of brainstem seizures in rodents correspond to generalized tonic/clonic seizures in humans. Accordingly, class 10 brainstem convulsions in GEPR–9s mimic many behavioural and EEG phases of human tonic/clonic seizures.

Seizure predisposition, which represents a fundamental distinction between epilepsy and normality, occurs as a genetic trait and as a consequence of prior seizures. Seizure predisposition in one convulsive seizure circuitry does not imply predisposition in the other. At least some components of these two traits appear to be under separate genetic control. Nevertheless, both forebrain and brainstem seizure predisposition coexist in some forms of epilepsy.

Seizure predisposition occurs as a consequence of genetic determinants. Seizure experience superimposed on genetically determined seizure predisposition may result in a further exacerbation of the epilepsy. Albeit in some paradigms seizure experience may, at least temporarily, cause some degree of seizure suppression.

In epileptic brains, seizure igniting interactions between forebrain and brainstem seizure circuitry occur. An especially intriguing form of such interaction occurs in the GEPR–9 which is characterized by marked seizure predisposition of both the rostral and caudal circuitry. In these animals a limbic seizure will ignite the brainstem seizure circuitry. Current data provide strong initial support for the concept that genetic predisposition is a prerequisite for secondary generalization of partial seizures to tonic/clonic seizures in adult subjects. In this new GEPR–9 kindling model, the secondary tonic/clonic seizures are as spontaneous as those of humans because both are precipitated by a seizure occurring in the forebrain.

References

Aicardi, J. (1986a): Epilepsies with affective-psychic manifestations and complex partial seizures. In: *Epilepsy in children*, Anonymous, pp. 79–99. New York: Raven Press.

Aicardi, J. (1986b): Epilepsies characterized by simple partial seizures. In: *Epilepsy in children*, French, J., Prichard, J.S., Rapin, I., Familusi, J., Fukuyama, Y., Mattyus, A., Cantlon, B., Logan, W. & Aicardi, J. (eds), pp. 112–139. New York: Raven Press.

Batini, C., Teillet, M.A., Naquet, R. & Le Douarin, N.M. (1996): Brain chimeras in birds – application to the study of a genetic form of reflex epilepsy. *Trends Neurosci.* **19**, 246–252.

Browning, R.A., Wang, C., Lanker, M.L. & Jobe, P.C. (1990): Electroshock- and pentylenetetrazol-induced seizures in genetically epilepsy-prone rats (GEPRs): differences in threshold and pattern. *Epilepsy Res.* **6**, 1–11.

Browning, R.A. (1994): Anatomy of generalized convulsive seizures. In: *Idiopathic generalized epilepsies*, Malafosse, A., Genton, P., Hirsch, E., Marescaux, C., Broglin, D. & Bernasconi, R. (eds), pp. 399–413. London: John Libbey.

Buchhalter, J.R. (1993): Animal models of inherited epilepsy. *Epilepsia* **34** Suppl. 3, S31–S41.

Burnham, W.M. & Browning, R.A. (1987): The reticular core and generalized convulsions: a unified hypothesis. In: *Epilepsy and the reticular formation: The role of the reticular core in convulsive seizures*, Fromm, G.H., Faingold, C.L., Browning, R.A. & Burnham, W.M. (eds), pp. 193–201. New York: Alan R. Liss.

Coffey, L.L., Reith, M.E.A., Chen, N.H. & Jobe, P.C. (1996): Amygdala kindling of forebrain seizures and the occurrence of brainstem seizures in genetically epilepsy-prone rats. *Epilepsia* **37**, 188–197.

Cure, D., Rasmussen, T. & Jasper, H. (1948): Activation of seizures and electroencephalographic disturbances in epileptic and in control subjects with 'metrazol'. *Arch. Neurol. Psychiatry* **59**, 691–717.

Davis, W.M. & King, W.T. (1967): Pharmacogenetic factor in the convulsive responses of mice to flurothyl. *Experientia* **23**, 214–215.

Engel, J., Jr. (1989): Epileptic seizures. In: *Seizures and epilepsy*, Vol. 6, pp. 137–178. Philadelphia: F.A. Davis Company.

Faingold, C.L. & Naritoku, D.K. (1992): The genetically epilepsy-prone rat: neuronal networks and actions of amino acid neurotransmitters. In: *Drugs for the control of epilepsy: Actions on neuronal networks involved in seizure disorders*, Faingold, C.L. & Fromm, G.H. (eds), pp. 277–308. Boca Raton, Florida: CRC Press.

Gale, K. (1992): Subcortical structures and pathways involved in convulsive seizure generation. *J. Clin. Neurophysiol.* **9**, 264–277.

Garcia-Cairasco, N., Terra, V.C., Mishra, P.K., Dailey, J.W. & Jobe, P.C. (1994): Neuroethology of brainstem-induced forebrain seizure kindling in genetically epilepsy-prone rats (GEPRs). *Soc. Neurosci. Abstr.* **20**, 406(Abstract).

Garretson, H., Gloor, P. & Rasmussen, T. (1966): Intracarotid amobarbutal and metrazol test for the study of epileptiform discharges in man: A note on its technique. *Electroenceph. Clin. Neurophysiol.* **21,** 607–610.

Gastaut, H. (1950): Combined photic and metrazol activation of the brain. *Electroenceph. Clin. Neurophysiol.* **2,** 249–261.

Green, R.C. & Seyfried, T.N. (1991): Kindling susceptibility and genetic seizure predisposition in inbred mice. *Epilepsia* **32,** 22–26.

Handforth, A. & Ackermann, R.F. (1988): Electrically induced limbic status and kindled seizures. In: *Anatomy of epileptogenesis,* Meldrum, B.S., Ferrendelli, J.A. & Wieser, H.G. (eds), pp. 71–87. London: John Libbey.

Hirsch, E., Maton, B., Vergnes, M., Depaulis, A. & Marescaux, C. (1992): Positive transfer of audiogenic kindling to electrical hippocampal kindling in rats. *Epilepsy Res.* **11,** 159–166.

Jobe, P.C., Picchioni, A.L. & Chin, L. (1973): Role of brain norepinephrine in audiogenic seizure in the rat. *J. Pharmacol. Exp. Ther.* **184,** 1–10.

Jobe, P.C., Mishra, P.K., Ludvig, N. & Dailey, J.W. (1991): Scope and contribution of genetic models to an understanding of the epilepsies. *CRC Crit. Rev. Neurobiol.* **6,** 183–220.

Jobe, P.C., Mishra, P.K. & Dailey, J.W. (1992): Genetically epilepsy-prone rat: Actions of antiepileptic drugs and monoaminergic neurotransmitters. In: *Drugs for the control of epilepsy: Actions on neuronal networks involved in seizure disorders,* Faingold, C. & Fromm, G.H. (eds), pp. 253–275. Boca Raton, Florida: CRC Press.

Jobe, P.C., Mishra, P.K., Adams-Curtis, L.E., Ko, K.H. & Dailey, J.W. (1994a): The GEPR model of the epilepsies. In: *Idiopathic generalized epilepsies: Clinical, experimental and genetic aspects,* Malafosse, A., Genton, P., Hirsch, E., Marescaux, C., Broglin, D. & Bernasconi, R. (eds), pp. 385–398. London: John Libbey.

Jobe, P.C., Mishra, P.K., Browning, R.A., Wang, C.D., Adams-Curtis, L.E., Ko, K.H. & Dailey, J.W. (1994b): Noradrenergic abnormalities in the genetically epilepsy-prone rat. *Brain Res. Bull.* **35,** 493–504.

Jobe, P.C., Mishra, P.K., Adams-Curtis, L.E., Deoskar, V.U., Ko, K.H., Browning, R.A. & Dailey, J.W. (1995): The genetically epilepsy-prone rat (GEPR). *Ital. J. Neurol. Sci.* **16,** 91–99.

Kaufman, I.C., Marshall, C. & Walker, A.E. (1947): Activated electroencephalography. *Arch. Neurol. Psychiatry* **58,** 533–549.

Killam, E.K. & Killam, K.F., Jr. (1984): Evidence for neurotransmitter abnormalities related to seizure activity in the epileptic baboon. *Fed. Proc.* **43,** 2510–2515.

Killam, K.F., Killam, E.K. & Naquet, R. (1967): An animal model of light sensitive epilepsy. *Electroencephalogr. Clin. Neurophysiol.* **22,** 497–513.

King, J.T., Jr. & LaMotte, C.C. (1989): El mouse as a model of focal epilepsy: a review. *Epilepsia* **30,** 257–265.

Ludvig, N., Gyorgy, L., Folly, G. & Vizi, E.S. (1985): Yohimbine can not exert its anticonvulsant action in genetically audiogenic seizure-prone mice. *Eur. J. Pharmacol.* **115,** 123–124.

Marley, R.J., Gaffney, D. & Wehner, J.M. (1986): Genetic influences on GABA-related seizures. *Pharmacol. Biochem. Behav.* **24,** 665–672.

Maton, B., Hirsch, E., Vergnes, M., Depaulis, A. & Marescaux, C. (1992): Dorsal tegmentum kindling in rats. *Neurosci. Lett.* **134,** 284–287.

McNamara, J.O. (1986): Kindling model of epilepsy. *Adv. Neurol.* **44**P, 303–318.

Menini, C. & Silva Barrat, C. (1990): Value of the monkey Papio papio for the study of epilepsy. *Pathol. Biol.* **38,** 205–213.

Naritoku, D.K., Mecozzi, L.B., Aiello, M.T. & Faingold, C.L. (1992): Repetition of audiogenic seizures in genetically epilepsy-prone rats induces cortical epileptiform activity and additional seizure behaviours. *Exp. Neurol.* **115,** 317–324.

Patel, S. (1988): Chemically indeuced limbic seizures in rodents. In: *Anatomy of epileptogenesis,* Meldrum, B.S., Ferrendelli, J.A. & Wieser, H.G. (eds), pp. 89–106. London: John Libbey.

Porter, R.J. (1993): The absence epilepsies. *Epilepsia* 34 Suppl. 3, S42-S48.

Racine, R.J. (1972): Modification of seizure activity by electrical stimulation: II. Motor seizure. *Electroencephalogr. Clin. Neurophysiol.* **32,** 281–294.

Racine, R.J., Burnham, W.M., Gartner, J.G. & Levitan, D. (1973): Rates of motor seizure development in rats subjected to electrical brain stimulation: strain and inter-stimulation interval effects. *Electroencephalogr. Clin. Neurophysiol.* **35,** 553–556.

Randall, M.E. & Faingold, C.L. (1995): Aberrant neuronal firing patterns in deep layers of superior colliculus subserve audiogenic seizure expression in genetically epilepsy-prone rats. *Soc. Neurosci. Abstr.* **21,** 1961(Abstract).

Reigel, C.E., Jobe, P.C., Dailey, J.W. & Savage, D.D. (1989): Ontogeny of sound-induced seizures in the genetically epilepsy-prone rat. *Epilepsy Res.* **4,** 63–71.

Riaz, A. & Faingold, C.L. (1994): Seizures during ethanol withdrawal are blocked by focal microinjection of excitant amino acid antagonists into the inferior colliculus and pontine reticular formation. *Alcoholism Clin. Exp. Res.* **18,** 1456–1462.

Savage, D.D., Reigel, C.E. & Jobe, P.C. (1986): Angular bundle kindling is accelerated in rats with a genetic predisposition to acoustic stimulus-induced seizures. *Brain Res.* **376,** 412–415.

Sugaya, E., Ishige, A., Sekiguchi, K., Iizuka, S., Ito, K., Sugimoto, A., Aburada, M. & Hosoya, E. (1986): Pentylenetetrazol-induced convulsion and effect of anticonvulsants in mutant inbred strain El mice. *Epilepsia* **27,** 354–358.

Tassinari, C.A., Rubboli, G. & Michelucci, R. (1990): Reflex epilepsy. In: *Comprehensive epileptology,* Dam, M. & Gram, L. (eds), pp. 233–246. New York: Raven Press.

Wang, C., Mishra, P.K., Yan, Q.S., Dailey, J.W., Browning, R.A. & Jobe, P.C. (1993): Electrographic activity in the inferior colliculus or medullary reticular formation during audiogenic seizures in severe seizure genetically epilepsy-prone rats (GEPR–9s). *Soc. Neurosci. Abstr.* **19,** 602(Abstract).

Wieser, H.G., Bancaud, J., Talairach, J., Bonis, A. & Szikla, G. (1979): Comparative value of spontaneous and chemically and electrically induced seizures in establishing the lateralization of temporal lobe seizures. *Epilepsia* **20,** 47–59.

Chapter 26

Transgenic animal models of epilepsy

Miklos Toth

Department of Pharmacology, Cornell University Medical College, New York, NY 10021, USA

Transgenic animal models can reconstruct cellular, biochemical and molecular alterations associated with human diseases. These animal models may not point to those genes most frequently mutated in human disease, but may identify key mechanisms acting in the same pathway. Recently, a number of null mutant (knock-out) mice have been described which display recurrent seizures. The aim of this summary is to analyse how these mouse mutants contributed to our understanding of the molecular and cellular mechanisms underlying epileptic seizures.

A number of single gene mutations lead to seizures in mice

The pathophysiological pathways that lead to epilepsy are complex, and disease-causing mutations can occur at many different steps. Based on the present knowledge of epileptogenesis, a large number of candidate genes can be selected. For example, epileptiform activity in individual neurons may be generated by mutations in ion channels and receptors, synchronization of local circuitries can be initiated with mutations affecting extra and intracellular environment, and assembly of neuronal networks could be altered by developmental defects. Indeed, in the last two years (1995–96), a number of genetically manipulated mouse strains have been described that are characterized by seizures or seizure-like phenotype.

Table 1. Seizure displaying knock-out mouse models

Inactivated gene	Reference
Serotonin$_{2C}$ receptor	Tecott *et al.*, 1995
Synapsin I and II	Rosahl *et al.*, 1995
Calcium calmodulin kinase IIα	Butler *et al.*, 1995
Jerky	Toth *et al.*, 1995
Glutamate RB receptor subunit	Brusa *et al.*, 1995
Inositol triphosphate receptor	Matsumoto *et al.*, 1996
Neuropeptide Y	Erickson *et al.*, 1996

Most of these mouse strains were generated by targeted gene inactivation. Homologous recombination between DNA sequences residing in the chromosome and newly introduced, cloned DNA sequences

GENETICS OF FOCAL EPILEPSIES

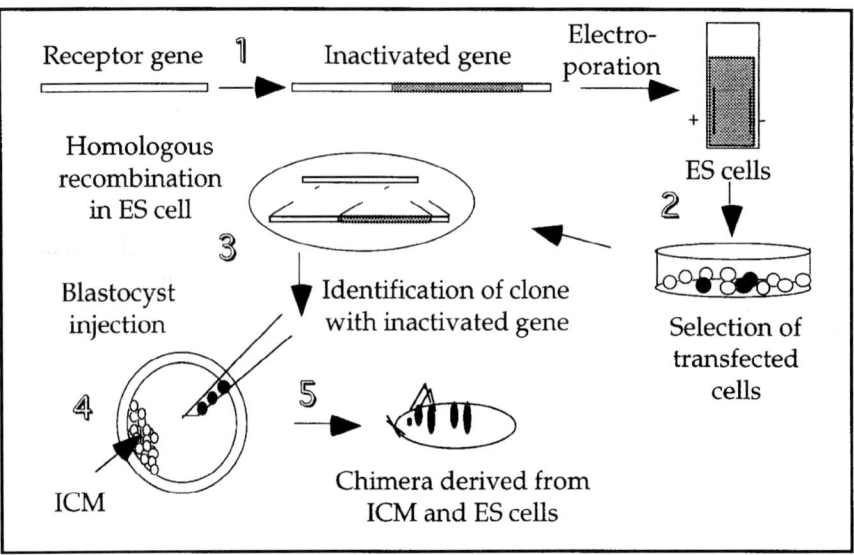

Fig. 1. Generation of transgenic animals with an inactivated gene.
1. The coding region of the gene of interest is disrupted by a DNA insertion represented by the shaded area on the gene. 2. The disrupted gene is introduced into pluripotent ES cells by electroporation, and the construct integrates into the genome. 3. Selection procedure enrich clones derived from transfected cells. The presence of flanking regions of the gene facilitates homologous recombination within ES cells. 4. Clones underwent homologous recombination are identified by PCR and/or Southern hybridization and injected into 3.5 day old mouse blastocysts. 5. Blastocysts are implanted into foster mothers resulting in chimeras. Germline chimeras are bred to obtain hetero- and homozygotes for the mutated allele.

allows the transfer of any modification, such as inactivation of the cloned gene, into the genome of pluripotent, embryo-derived stem (ES) cells (Fig. 1). Transfer of these modifications into a living mouse is possible by generating chimeras from the manipulated ES cells (Evans & Kaufman, 1981; Thomas & Capecchi, 1987; Zijlstra et al., 1989; Joyner et al., 1989; Capecchi, 1989). Disruption of a gene also occurs when a transgene integrates into a cellular gene, impairing its function (insertional mutagenesis, see Toth et al., 1995).

Table 1 lists seven seizure-displaying mouse strains generated by gene disruption. The first transgenic animal with a seizure phenotype was published in 1995, followed by a number of other mutations in the same year. Publications on transgenic animals up to the end of 1996 are summarized here with a specific emphasis on the nature of the molecular defects and possible pathogenic pathways involved in seizure induction.

Serotonin2C (5-HT$_{2C}$) receptor deficient mice

The 5-HT$_{2C}$ receptor is a prominent member of the serotonin receptor family. The 5-HT$_{2C}$ receptor is coupled to a G protein and is widely expressed in the brain and spinal cord. 5-HT$_{2C}$ receptor deficient mice are normal except they are overweight and experience sporadic seizures (Tecott et al., 1995). A small group of receptor deficient animals display seizures that are often preceded by repetitive grooming. This motor activity appears to generalize and progresses to seizures characterized by tonic–clonic movements. Mutant mice show a significant reduction in seizure threshold when pentylenetetrazole (PTZ) is injected intravenously. Occasionally, seizures progress to a tonic extension phase leading to respiratory arrest and death. The epileptic phenotype of 5-HT$_{2C}$ receptor deficient mice implies that this receptor subtype is involved in the maintenance of neuronal network excitability, consistent with previous observations that changes in the serotonergic system can alter seizure threshold. Within CNS neurons, the highest levels of 5-HT$_{2C}$ receptor transcripts are found in the hippocampus, a temporal lobe structure that is often involved in seizure and seizure initiation.

Synapsin I and II mutant mice

Synapsins I and II are phosphoproteins and found in synaptic vesicles. Mice lacking synapsins experience seizures that are precipitated by sensory stimuli such as vestibular stimulation (Rosahl *et al.*, 1995). The seizures develop only after two months of age. Mice carrying two or more mutant alleles (synapsin I and II double knock-out animals) exhibit an incidence of seizures proportional to the number of mutant alleles. Inactivation of synapsin genes leads to depletion of synaptic vesicles in nerve terminals without major changes in their distribution or in general synaptic structure. Pieribone *et al.* (1995) demonstrated that clusters of vesicles at synaptic release sites are composed of two pools, a distal pool containing synapsin and a proximal pool devoid of synapsin and located adjacent to the presynaptic membrane. The availability of the synapsin-associated pool of vesicles is required to sustain release of neurotransmitter in response to high-frequency bursts of impulses. Indeed, synapsin II and double knockouts, but not synapsin-I knockouts, exhibit decreased post-tetanic potentiation and severe synaptic depression upon repetitive stimulation that may form the basis of seizure predisposition in synapsin deficient animals.

Calcium calmodulin kinase IIa deficient mice

Multifunctional Ca^{++}/calmodulin-dependent protein kinase II (CaMK) phosphorylates proteins involved in diverse neuronal processes, and thereby coordinates cellular responses to external stimuli that regulate intracellular Ca^{++}. Mice deficient of CaMK exhibit profound hyperexcitability. For instance, administration of a single, normally subconvulsive stimulation of the amygdala evokes prolonged, often repeated and sometimes fatal seizures (Butler *et al.*, 1995). Morphologic studies disclosed extensive sprouting of mossy fibres in the supragranular region of the dentate gyrus in mutant mice. Mossy fibre sprouting is frequently found in animal seizure models and also in human epilepsies. For example, a consistent increase in mossy fibre projection has been identified following seizures induced by the glutamate receptor agonist kainate and in kindling (Tauck & Nadler, 1985). A hypothesis was formulated that hyperexcitability of the dentate granule cells is a consequence of a pathologic rearrangement of neuronal circuitry in which the excitatory granule cells innervate themselves, resulting in a recurrent excitatory circuit (Nadler *et al.*, 1980; Tauck & Nadler, 1985).

Jerky mice

A line of transgenic mice has been identified that shows neuronal hyperexcitability, handling induced behavioural seizure, and epileptic EEG, resembling human complex partial seizures with secondary generalization (Toth *et al.*, 1995). Similar to human epilepsies, the onset of seizures in the transgenic mice is age dependent, the seizure threshold is remarkably lowered, and the phenotype is variable in penetrance. Molecular and genetic studies demonstrated that the epileptic phenotype in the transgenic mice is caused by the disruption of a novel brain specific gene, mapped to mouse chromosome 15. Based on the phenotype, the gene was named '*jerky*'. *Jerky* encodes a putative 60 kD protein displaying homology to a number of chromatin proteins, including the centromere binding protein-B (CENP-B) and yeast autonomously replicating sequence-binding protein 1 (Abp1) (Donovan *et al.*, 1997).

Interestingly, deletion of only one *jerky* allele is sufficient to induce seizures, indicating that jerky has a dosage sensitive function in the brain. However, jerky has a non-dosage sensitive function as well, since the total absence of jerky in homozygotes results in abnormalities of somatic and sexual development (Donovan *et al.*, 1997). Some idiopathic epilepsies are dominantly inherited, and the pathomechanism of these epilepsies may be based on haploinsufficiency in the brain.

Mice deficient in glutamate receptor B subunit editing

Glutamate receptors sensitive to AMPA are ligand-activated cation channels that mediate the fast component of excitatory postsynaptic currents in CNS. These channels are assembled from four subunits and the GluR-B subunit renders the channel almost impermeable to Ca^{++}. An arginine residue at position 586 that is introduced into the molecule by pos-transcriptional editing is responsible for this property. Brusa et al. (1995) genetically modified the subunit that prevented editing, and the resulting mutation led to a rapidly developing neurologic syndrome that includes hyperexcitability and seizures. As a result of the mutation, the glutamate-activated Ca^{++} permeability and the Ca^{++} influx through these channels were increased, which can explain the seizure predisposition of editing deficient mice.

Inositol triphosphate receptor deficient mice

The inositol 1,4,5-triphosphate receptor ($InsP_3R$) acts as an $InsP_3$-gated Ca^{++} release channel in a variety of cell types. Type I $InsP_3R$ is neuronal, and is present predominantly in cerebellar Purkinje cells but also in the hippocampal CA1-region and cortex. Most of $InsP_3R$ deficient mice die prenatally, and animals that survive birth have severe ataxia and tonic–clonic seizures (Matsumoto et al., 1996). Continuous electroencephalographic recordings of these mice revealed paroxysmal polyspike activities, whereas only stable background activities were observed in wild type mice, indicating that $InsP_3R$, presumably by modulating Ca^{++} release, is essential for proper brain function.

Neuropeptide Y

Neuropeptide Y (NPY), a 36-amino acid neurotransmitter, is distributed throughout the nervous system. A subset of mice deficient of NPY display seizures characterized by jerking, tail erection and vocalization. NPY-deficient mice are hyperexcitable, as revealed by challenging them with a convulsive dose of pentylenetetrazole (Erickson et al., 1996). Seizures in NPY deficient mice are consistent with studies demonstrating that NPY selectively suppresses excitatory neurotransmission and blocks epileptiform activity when applied to isolated brain slices and neuronal cultures (Klapstein & Colmers, 1993). This action is thought to be due to presynaptic inhibition of glutamate release mediated by NPY2 receptors on the terminals of excitatory neurons.

Seizure phenotype of transgenic animals is reminiscent of symptomatic epilepsy rather than idiopathic

Table 2. Number of genetically determined symptomatic epilepsies is higher than that of idiopathic

	Idiopathic	Symptomatic
Human	< 10 (e.g. BFNC, JME)	> 100 with mendelian traits
Mouse	Jerky, 5-HT_{2C} knock-out ?	Synapsin I and II
		Calcium calmodulin kinase IIα
		Glutamate RB receptor subunit
		Inositol triphosphate receptor
		Neuropeptide Y

In humans, many types of epileptic seizures and epileptic conditions are recognized, presumably reflecting a number of pathophysiological mechanisms. Patients with idiopathic epilepsies show normal intelligence and no neurological symptoms other than seizures, and the disease is unassociated with specific structural pathology. Symptomatic epilepsies, on the other hand, are probably the consequences of existing biochemical or anatomical abnormalities. It is now recognized that both symptomatic and idiopathic epilepsies may have a genetic basis. As Table 2 shows, over a hundred inherited diseases are known that are associated with seizures, but only a small fraction of these disorders is considered to be idiopathic epilepsy. Similarly, the majority of the transgenic strains has a phenotype characterized by multiple neurological symptoms such as ataxia, convulsions and tremor. The only transgenic strains whose phenotype is reminiscent of idiopathic epilepsy are the jerky and perhaps the 5-HT$_{2C}$ knock-out mouse strains. The high number of symptomatic epilepsies in human as well as in animals is not surprising, taking into account that many different brain abnormalities can lead to hyperexcitability and seizures, but very few of these abnormalities are limited to seizures.

Heterogeneity of the phenotype of genetically homogeneous transgenic animals

Although heterogeneity in phenotype suggests a polygenic nature, single gene mutations can result in conditions with a variable expression of the phenotype. Indeed, most seizure-displaying transgenics show partial penetrance and highly variable seizure severity. This is an important point, since human epilepsies show a wide variation of phenotype between affected individuals even within the same families, which is presumably due to the unique combination of genetic and environmental factors. By using inbred strains, genetic factors as a source of heterogeneity can be excluded. Still, heterogeneity of the seizure phenotype is a consistent feature in transgenic mutants. For example, a relatively small group of 5-HT$_{2C}$ receptor deficient animals display seizures (Tecott *et al.*, 1995). Also, some InsP$_3$R deficient mice die prenatally, while others survive and show seizures (Matsumoto *et al.*, 1996). Similarly, jerky mice show a considerable variability in behavioural seizures and seizure susceptibility to pentylenetetrazole (Donovan *et al.*, 1997). Variation in susceptibility to pentylenetetrazole-induced seizures clearly correlated with the animal's tendency to display handling-induced seizures. Animals experiencing more clonus in the pentylenetetrazole test tended to show behavioural seizures as well, while animals responding to pentylenetetrazole with less clonus generally did not show seizures. However, phenotypic variability in susceptibility was probably not due to the differential expression of the non-deleted *jerky* allele, because there is an equal reduction of jerky mRNA levels in brains of seizure and non-seizure jerky mice (Donovan *et al.*, 1997). It is more likely that the variability of the phenotype in the genetically homogeneous population of jerky mice was due to non-genetic factors, such as environmental and/or developmental effects acting independently of jerky. There is a large number of such effects, including maturation, gender, circadian rhythm, seasonal changes, and stress. By measuring the individual sensitivity of jerky mice to pentylenetetrazole and handling-induced seizures, it was found that while 1-month-old jerky mice have a susceptibility comparable to that of wild type, the 4-month-old jerky mice show more pentylenetetrazole induced seizures than wild type animals and eventually half of them display handling-induced seizures. These data demonstrate that jerky mice undergo an age dependent increase in susceptibility that is necessary to bring the susceptibility level above seizure threshold. The late onset of seizure phenotype in jerky mice is reminiscent of the juvenile or adult onset of myoclonic jerks and abnormal EEG in several familial epileptic syndromes (Malafosse *et al.*, 1994; Kuwano *et al.*, 1996). Another feature of the epilepsy phenotype in jerky mice is that seizures no longer exist in animals older then 8 months of age, which could be due to an age-related process such as the selective elimination of numerous collaterals and synapses or neuronal loss. It is also possible that seizures activate compensatory mechanisms that reduce seizure susceptibility. However this possibility is not very likely, since repeated seizures sensitize the animal and lower the seizure threshold, a process termed kindling (McNamara, 1994).

Future directions

The availability of transgenic mutants with epileptic phenotype provides an opportunity to use new approaches in epilepsy research that may not be possible with other animal models. A few areas are enlisted below that could rapidly develop in the near future.

1. Sequencing and analysing human genes whose counterparts in transgenic animals have been associated with seizures.
2. Creating novel transgenic animal models in order to better understand the pathogenesis of

epilepsies by inactivating genes that have been found mutated in human epilepsies, such as the cystatin B gene (Pennacchio et al., 1996).
3. Modeling polygenic epilepsies and gene interactions in mice with multiple knock-outs.
4. Studying environmental /developmental factors in the pathogenesis of epilepsies in transgenic animals.

References

Brusa, R., Zimmermann, F., Koh, D.S., Feldmeyer, D., Gass, P., Seeburg, P.H. & Sprengel, R. (1995): Early-onset epilepsy and postnatal lethality associated with an editing-deficient GluR-B allele in mice. *Science* **270**, 1677–1680.

Butler, L.S., Silva, A.J., Abeliovich, A., Watanabe, Y., Tonegawa, S. & McNamara, J.O. (1995): Limbic epilepsy in transgenic mice carrying a Ca^{2+}/calmodulin-dependent kinase II alpha-subunit mutation. *Proc. Natl. Acad. Sci. USA* **92**, 6852–6855.

Capecchi, M.R. (1989): Altering the genome by homologous recombination. *Science* **244**, 1288–1292.

Donovan, G.P., Harden, C., Gal, J., Ho, L., Sibille, E., Trifiletti, R., Gudas, L.J. & Toth, M. (1997): Sensitivity to jerky gene dosage underlies epileptic seizures in ice. *J. Neurosci.* **17**, 4562–4569.

Erickson, J.C., Clegg, K.E. & Palmiter, R.D. (1996): Sensitivity to leptin and susceptibility to seizures of mice lacking neuropeptide Y. *Nature* **381**, 415–421.

Evans, M.J. & Kaufman, M.H. (1981): Establishment in culture of pluripotential cells from mouse embryos. *Nature* **292**, 154–156.

Joyner, A.L., Skarnes, W.S. & Rossant, J. (1989): Production of a mutation in mouse En-2 gene by homologous recombination in embryonic stem cells. *Nature* **338**, 153–156.

Klapstein, G.J. & Colmers, W.F. (1993): On the sites of presynaptic inhibition by neuropeptide Y in rat hippocampus in vitro. *Hippocampus* **3**, 103–111.

Kuwano, A., Takakubo, F., Morimoto, Y., Uyama, E., Uchino, M., Ando, M., Yasuda, T., Terao, A., Hayayma, T., Kobayashi, R. & Kondo, I. (1996): Benign adult familial myoclonus epilepsy (BAFME): an autosomal dominant form not linked to the dentatorubral pallidoluysian atrophy (DRPLA) gene. *J. Med. Genet.* **33**, 80–81.

Malafosse, A., Genton, P., Hirsch, E., Marescaux, C., Broglin, D. & Bernasconi, R. (eds) (1994): *Idiopathic generalized epilepsies: clinical, experimental and genetic aspects*. London: John Libbey.

Matsumoto, M., Nakagawa, T., Inoue, T., Nagata, E., Tanaka, K., Takano, H., Minowa, O., Kuno, J., Sakakibara, S., Yamada, M., Yoneshima, H., Miyawaki, A., Fukuuchi, Y., Furuichi, T., Okano, H., Mikoshiba, K. & Noda, T. (1996): Ataxia and epileptic seizures in mice lacking type 1 inositol 1,4,5-trisphosphate receptor. *Nature* **379**, 168–171.

McNamara, J.O. (1994): Cellular and molecular basis of epilepsy. *J. Neurosci.* **14**, 3413–3425.

Nadler, J.V., Perry, B.W., Gentry, C. & Cotman, C.W. (1980): Degeneration of hippocampal CA3 pyramidal cells induced by intraventricular kainic acid. *J. Comp. Neurol.* **192**, 333–359.

Pennacchio, L.A., Lehesjoki, A.E., Stone, N.E., Willour, V.L., Virtaneva, K., Miao, J., D'Amato, E., Ramirez, L., Faham, M., Koskiniemi, M., Warrington, J.A., Norio, R., de la Chapelle, A., Cox, D.R. & Myers, R.M. (1996): Mutations in the gene encoding cystatin B in progressive myoclonus epilepsy (EPM1). *Science* **271**, 1731–1734.

Pieribone, V.A., Shupliakov, O., Brodin, L., Hilfiker-Rothenfluh, S., Czernik, A.J. & Greengard, P. (1995): Distinct pools of synaptic vesicles in neurotransmitter release. *Nature* **375**, 493–497.

Rosahl, T.W., Spillane, D., Missler, M., Herz, J., Selig, D.K., Wolff, J.R., Hammer, R.E., Malenka, R.C. & Sudhof, T.C. (1995): Essential functions of synapsins I and II in synaptic vesicle regulation. *Nature* **375**, 488–493.

Tauck, D.L. & Nadler, J.V. (1985): Evidence of functional mossy fiber sprouting in hippocampal formation of kainic acid-treated rats. *J. Neurosci.* **5**, 1016–1022.

Tecott, L.H., Sun, L.M., Akana, S.F., Strack, A.M., Lowenstein, D.H., Dallman, M.F. & Julius, D. (1995): Eating disorder and epilepsy in mice lacking 5-HT2c serotonin receptors. *Nature* **374**, 542–546.

Thomas, K.R. & Capecchi, M.R. (1987): Site-directed mutagenesis by gene targeting in mouse embryo-derived stem cells. *Cell* **51**, 503–512.

Toth, M., Grimsby, J., Buzsaki, Gy. & Donovan, G. (1995): Inactivation of a novel gene related to CENP-B is associated with neuronal hyperexcitability and seizure in transgenic mice. *Nat. Genet.* **11**, 71–75.

Zijlstra, M., Li, E., Sajjadi, F., Subramani, S. & Jaenisch, R. (1989): Germ-line transmission of a disrupted β_2-microglobulin gene produced by homologous recombination in embryonic stem cells. *Nature* **342**, 435–438.

Chapter 27

The epilepsy of the GABA$_A$ receptor β$_3$ subunit knockout mouse: comparison to the epilepsy of Angelman syndrome

Timothy M. DeLorey[1], Adrian Handforth[2], Gregg E. Homanics[3], Berge A. Minassian[4], Antonio Delgado-Escueta[2] and Richard W. Olsen[1]

[1]*Department of Molecular and Medical Pharmacology, University of California, Los Angeles, California 90095,* [2]*West Los Angeles VA Medical Center, Los Angeles, California, and* [3]*Department of Anesthesiology/CCM, University of Pittsburgh, Pennsylvania 15261 USA; and* [4]*Division of Neurology, Hospital for Sick Children, University of Toronto, Canada M5G 1X8*

GABA receptors and animal models of epilepsy

GABA (γ-aminobutyric acid) is the major inhibitory neurotransmitter in the mammalian central nervous system (CNS), with GABA$_A$ receptors mediating the majority of rapid inhibitory synapses in brain. GABA$_A$ receptors are ligand-gated ion channels each composed of related but different polypeptide subunits (α, β, γ, δ, ρ, ε) selected from a gene family of currently 16 members (DeLorey & Olsen, 1992; Davies *et al.*, 1997). In the rodent brain the subunit subtypes show variable regional and developmental expression (Laurie *et al.*, 1992; Wisden *et al.*, 1992). Considering the importance of GABA in nervous system function, mutations in genes encoding subunits of the GABA$_A$ receptor family could lead to multiple deleterious effects on the CNS, including epilepsy.

GABA receptors have long been associated with epilepsy, with the GABA$_A$ receptor complex being a key target for several anticonvulsants in current clinical use, such as clonazepam and phenobarbital (Olsen, 1991). Although alterations in GABA$_A$ receptor levels or function have been reported in animal models of epilepsy (reviewed in Olsen *et al.*, 1986; Olsen & Avoli, 1997), evidence directly linking the GABA receptor to epileptogenesis has been limited. For example, GABA$_A$ receptors are abnormally low in the substantia nigra and other midbrain and brainstem regions of genetically seizure-susceptible gerbils and mice (Olsen *et al.*, 1986). However, it has not been determined whether these GABA$_A$ receptor abnormalities are related to the pathophysiology of seizures, nor is there any understanding of why these neurotransmitter differences exist.

Several seizure-related loci have been linked to the same general vicinity as the GABA$_A$ receptor cluster found on murine chromosome 7, an area that is syntenic to the Angelman syndrome (AS) region on human chromosome 15. These include the neurological mouse mutation, quivering (*qv*) (Yoon & Les, 1957), the seizure susceptibility locus (*Szf1*) (Frankel *et al.*, 1994), and the audiogenic seizure susceptibility gene (*Asp3*) (Neumann & Collins, 1992). The *Asp 3* gene is of particular interest because, in contrast to other epilepsy related genes, it is influenced by genomic imprinting (Banko *et al.*, 1995). In other words, the effects of *Asp 3* on audiogenic seizure susceptibility depends on whether the gene is transmitted through the male or female parent. Yet another murine model, involving a mouse with a chromosome aberration in the form of a translocation occurring between chromosome 7 and 15 (designated T(7;15)9H, Jackson Laboratories, Bar Harbor, ME), also seems to involve an imprinting phenomenon on chromosome 7 (Cattanach *et al.*, 1996). This mouse model is uniquely interesting as it carries a paternal duplication of the majority of the chromosomal region that is syntenic to the chromosomal region deleted in the human Angelman syndrome. Thus this mouse carries only the paternal imprint in the absence of the maternal imprint for this specific portion of the genome. Therefore, this mouse is equivalent to a paternal uniparental disomy. These mice are reported not to have seizures but they do have striking electroencephalogram (EEG) abnormalities, exhibiting prolonged 2–3 Hz spike and wave discharges and giant slow waves. Whether any of the loci mentioned are identical or associated with one another, or if they influence epilepsy by completely independent mechanisms, is yet to be determined.

Angelman syndrome

Clinical features

The neurodevelopmental disorder Angelman syndrome is characterized by early arrest of mental and

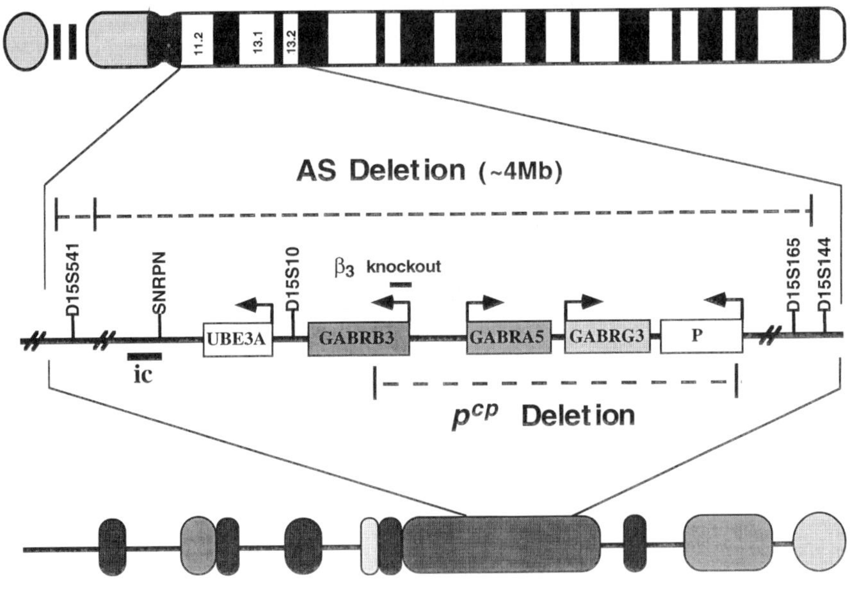

Fig. 1. *Arrangement of the GABA$_A$ receptor cluster (GABRB3, GABRA5, GABRG3), the P gene and the UBE3A gene on human chromosome 15 and mouse chromosome 7. The majority of Angelman syndrome (AS) probands have a large deletion on maternal 15q11–13 (indicated on the diagram with dashed line). The p^{cp} deletion (indicated) represents the extent of the deletion found in the p^{cp} mutant mice. The DNA region targeted for 'β_3 knockout' is shown above the GABRB3 gene. D15S541, SNRPN, D15S10, D15S165 and D15S144 are polymorphic (CA)n microsatellite markers used here for determining the extent of the chromosomal deletion. IC represents the region where the 'imprinting centre' is found.*

motor development, hyperactivity, absence of language, happy demeanor, inappropriate laughter, and epilepsy (Angelman, 1965; Williams & Frias, 1982; Clayton-Smith & Pembrey, 1992). This genetic disorder has a prevalence rate as high as 1:10,000 births (Petersen et al., 1995) and is associated with a deletion/mutation on maternal chromosome 15q (Fig. 1). While physical development progresses relatively normally, mental and motor development do not. Cognitive maturation seems to arrest at about a one-year-old level. The adult patient's behaviour and demeanor is that of a child not having reached age 2 years. The Angelman syndrome patient continuously smiles, has frequent easily elicited bursts of laughter, has no language beyond a few words, and is generally pleasant and happy. Another phenotypic feature is ataxia: the gait is wide-based with forward stooping at the pelvis, with the arms flexed at the elbows. Limb movements are jerky to the extent that the patients have been likened to 'puppets'. While the normal two-year-old child starts walking more 'normally' and acquires language, the Angelman syndrome child remains a one-year old in mental and motor function with relatively normal maturation of the body. Patients in their late 60s still walk and smile like toddlers. This conceptualization of Angelman syndrome should not mislead one to think that a sudden arrest occurs at one year of age: rather, there is a gradual slowing of postnatal development to a virtual standstill at the approximate equivalent of a one- to two-year old. Developmental delay can be noticed as early as 6 months of age and walking is usually acquired after 3 years of age. Feeding difficulties are commonly observed in early infancy. Decreased sleep, microcephaly, wide-spaced teeth and ophthalmological problems such as strabismus are other common features (Williams et al., 1995a).

Epilepsy

Seizure disorders are observed in over 90 per cent of Angelman syndrome probands. Multiple seizure types are reported, including myoclonic, atonic, generalized tonic–clonic, absence, partial motor and other. Most patients in the United States and Canada are treated with the antiepileptic drugs clonazepam or valproic acid with comparable degrees of improvement. The major features reported on EEG (Boyd et al., 1988; Sugimoto et al., 1992; Matsumoto et al., 1992) are spike-wave complexes, and an age-dependent evolution of seizure type with slow high-voltage bursts simulating hypsarrhythmia, in early childhood, changing to diffuse spike and waves in middle childhood, with atypical absences, and diminution of seizure discharges and clinical seizures after puberty. The EEG's of young (3–10 years old) Angelman syndrome patients are similar to those of the early childhood 'Lennox-Gastaut' syndrome. Atypical absence attacks in Angelman syndrome probands commonly appear in the second year of life, persist till mid-adolescence and tend to abate later in life. Although seizures improve with age, they are still present in adulthood, especially during sleep (Philippart et al., 1996; Delgado-Escueta et al., 1996; Guerrini et al. 1996). If untreated, the seizures are often continuous in the form of absence status epilepticus. Two recent papers (Viani et al., 1995; Guerrini et al., 1996) showed a pattern of high amplitude slow waves with some spike-waves (especially upon eye closure) associated with transient but quasicontinuous rhythmic myoclonus mainly involving hands and face; some patients showed atypical absences while others showed clonic or motor seizures.

With a prevalence rate of approximately 1:10,000, the epilepsies of Angelman syndrome represent ~1 per cent of all epilepsies. The association of severe mental retardation with a high incidence of epilepsy, as exhibited with Angelman syndrome, results in an overwhelming emotional burden to the Angelman syndrome family and a tremendous financial responsibility to both the family and society.

Neuropathology and neurochemistry

Reports of the neuropathology and neurochemistry of Angelman syndrome are limited. The most noteworthy features that have been reported, on one case, include cerebellar atrophy with loss of some Purkinje and granule cells, and extensive Bergmann gliosis (Jay et al., 1991). In addition, a mild reduction of dendritic arborization and dendritic spines of pyramidal neurons in the visual cortex was observed. Neurochemical studies by the same group reveal a marked reduction in GABA in the cerebellar cortex and elevated glutamate content in frontal and occipital cortices. The reduced GABA in the cerebellar cortex may be due to the loss of Purkinje cells and inhibitory GABAergic interneurons. The loss of inhibitory cerebellar influence could result in cortical myoclonus (Marsden et al., 1982). These observations need to be verified on further cases. Magnetic resonance imaging reveals most Angelman syndrome cases to be normal, with some individuals showing mild brain atrophy or mild ventricular asymmetry (Guerrini et al., 1996).

Genetics

Angelman syndrome is one of the best examples for the role of genetic imprinting in human disease (Williams et al., 1995b). Parental imprinting plays an important role in normal development; the disregulation of this process results in certain defined disease states (Lalande et al., 1997). Genomic imprinting can be defined as the epigenetic marking of chromosomal subregions of parental genomes in mammals that results in differential parent-of-origin specific expression of certain genes found within such subregions (Nicholls, 1993). To further demonstrate this point we can contrast Angelman syndrome with its 'sister' disorder, Prader-Willi syndrome. Both can result from a large deletion (~4 Mb) on chr. 15q11–13 with relatively consistent breakpoints at either end (Kuwano et al., 1992; Christian et al., 1995) (Fig. 1). The deletions are indistinguishable by cytogenetic or molecular analysis (Angelman, 1965; Knoll et al., 1989). The specific phenotype observed depends upon whether the deletion is on the maternal (Angelman syndrome) or paternal chromosome (Prader-Willi syndrome). These syndromes are clinically and genetically distinct neurobehavioural disorders. Prader-Willi syndrome is characterized by hypogonadism, mild mental retardation, and severe obesity resulting from hyperphagia (Butler, 1990). No seizure phenotype or EEG abnormality has been reported in association with Prader-Willi syndrome. Approximately 70 per cent of known Angelman syndrome cases result from large de novo deletions on the maternal chromosome 15q11-q13 (Fig. 1) (Knoll et al., 1989), resulting in the loss of many genes, one or more of which contribute to the full Angelman syndrome phenotype. Approximately 2 per cent of cases result from paternal uniparental disomy of chromosome 15 (Malcolm et al., 1991) in which the Angelman syndrome proband receives two copies of chromosome 15q11–13 from the father and no copy from the mother. Another 2–3 per cent are caused by what is referred to as a 'imprinting mutation' (Buiting et al., 1995). Instead of receiving the normal two alleles with their respective 'parent of origin' imprint, the Angelman syndrome individual receives an allele of chromosome 15q11–13 from each parent but with the paternal imprinting pattern on both alleles, the maternal imprint being absent. The remaining 25 per cent of Angelman syndrome cases are unexplained; they may result from microdeletions, point mutations or a yet undefined phenomenon, and can be familial. Recently, some examples of this last category were demonstrated (Kishino et al., 1997; Matsuura et al., 1997) to have mutations in the UBE3A gene, a ubiquitin-protein ligase gene (Fig. 1). How and if this particular genetic defect influences or causes Angelman syndrome is still to be elucidated.

In Angelman syndrome with large deletions, the deleted region contains several known genes including a cluster of $GABA_A$ receptor genes (GABRB3, GABRA5, and GABRG3) (Nakatsu et al., 1993; Greger et al., 1995). Importantly, two of the subunit genes in this cluster, the β_3 and the α_5 subunits, are widely expressed throughout the mammalian CNS. In addition, they are highly expressed during foetal and neonatal stages in rodents, with dramatic reductions occurring in some areas by adulthood (Laurie et al., 1992). This intense expression of these subunits in early life suggests that they play a critical role in early development, so that their absence could produce severe abnormalities in cognitive maturation.

Results and discussion

$GABA_A$ receptor $\beta3$ subunit knockout mouse

Recently we generated a mutant mouse line where the $GABA_A$ receptor β_3 subunit gene (gabrb3) was inactivated by gene targeting (Homanics et al., 1997a). Homologous recombination in embryonic stem cells was employed to disrupt the β_3 gene, which was subsequently passed through the germ line to generate mice without a functional β_3 gene, i.e. a null allele. The homozygous mutant animals ($\beta_3^{-/-}$) did not express β_3 mRNA. Approximately 90 per cent of $\beta_3^{-/-}$ mice died within 24 h of birth, and about 57 per cent had cleft palate. Thus far, we have been unable to determine the cause of death in the 30 per cent with apparently normal palates that die as neonates. The ~10 per cent that survived were runted, and required assistance in feeding for an additional two weeks after weaning, after which they grew normally to adulthood. These mice had a dramatically reduced life span and died at an average age of 18 weeks (normal age for wild type is ~119 weeks) although some have lived as long as 40 weeks. Adult knockout mice showed several behavioural and physiological abnormalities, including hyperactivity and seizures (Homanics et al., 1997a).

GABA$_A$ receptor density was remarkably reduced in the $\beta_3^{-/-}$ mice. Binding density of the GABA$_A$ agonist [^{3}H]muscimol and the benzodiazepine ligand [^{3}H]Ro15–4513 was approximately halved in brain homogenates of neonatal $\beta_3^{-/-}$ compared to $\beta_3^{+/+}$. There was no change in affinity (Homanics et al., 1997a). Similar reductions in GABA$_A$ receptor binding were observed in the pink-eyed dilution, cleft palate mutant (p^{cp}) mouse (Nakatsu et al., 1993). These mice had a large deletion on chromosome 7 eliminating the GABA$_A$ receptor subunit gene cluster (gabrb3, gabra5, and gabrg3) (Fig. 1). Neonatal homozygous p^{cp} mice were found to have a marked reduction (~60–80 per cent) in binding throughout the brain for the benzodiazepine antagonist [^{3}H]Ro15–1788, as compared to their normal control littermates (Nakatsu et al., 1993). The phenotypic characteristics of p^{cp} mice include cleft palate, early postnatal death, and neurological signs, including jerky gait, ataxia, and tremor (Lyons et al., 1992).

Both male and female $\beta_3^{-/-}$ mice were observed up to ~9 months of age. They displayed recurring hyperactive behaviour that was interrupted by periods of arrest lasting seconds to minutes. Myoclonic body jerks and epileptic seizures were observed in mice over 10 weeks of age, especially in older mice. Seizures varied in severity: the mildest seizures consisted of twitching of muscles of the mouth, face, whiskers, and ears. More severe seizures included head and bilateral forelimb jerks, with or without opisthotonos, arching of tail, and falls. In the most severe seizures, convulsions were succeeded by a wild running/bouncing phase. Seizures were noted clinically in 10 of 24 mice by chance observation. Closer observation during EEG analysis revealed seizures in three of three $b_3^{-/-}$ mice. Thus, seizures are likely present in all $\beta_3^{-/-}$ mice. It is interesting to note that the $\beta_3^{+/-}$ mice also displayed seizures although less frequently then the $\beta_3^{-/-}$ mice. The significance of the heterozygous mice displaying an abnormal phenotype should not be underappreciated. Although homozygous null mutants typically produce a more robust phenotype than heterozygous mice, genetic considerations suggest that the heterozygote may constitute a more accurate genetic model for Angelman syndrome.

EEG's of all $\beta_3^{-/-}$ mice examined ($n = 7$) had relatively normal background, especially during maximal alertness. The normal background was frequently interrupted by higher amplitude polymorphic bilateral slow and sharp waves (4–5 Hz) that corresponded to behavioural quiescence (Fig. 2A). This is possibly reflective of an absence-like state. This abnormal EEG pattern stopped on arousal. $\beta_3^{+/+}$ mice did not show these abnormal EEG patterns, whereas $\beta_3^{+/-}$ mice exhibited intermediate patterns between those of $\beta_3^{-/-}$ and $\beta_3^{+/+}$ mice (Fig. 2A). Seizures were associated with generalized spike-wave discharges. These were often initiated by an interictal spike and followed by electrographic depression (Fig. 2B).

Several features of the epilepsy in $\beta_3^{-/-}$ mice resemble the epilepsy associated with Angelman syndrome. The $\beta_3^{-/-}$ mice exhibit behavioural episodes of clonic seizure bursts that are accompanied by high amplitude symmetric spike-wave discharges. The nature of the seizures in the mice changes with age from three to seven months. Like the knockout mice, Angelman syndrome patients exhibit generalized high amplitude slow waves and spikes, myoclonias, a variety of convulsive seizure types, and changes in seizure type with age. In $\beta_3^{-/-}$ mice the anticonvulsant ethosuximide was found to suppress the epileptiform activity, whereas carbamazepine worsened EEG epileptiform activity. This

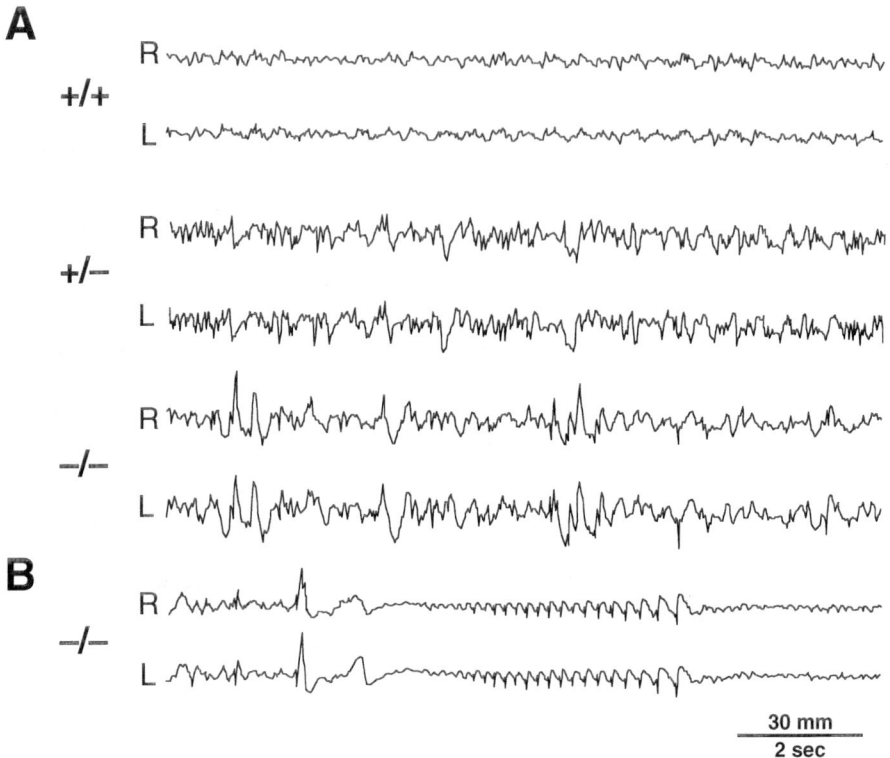

Fig. 1. Mouse electroencephalographic recordings. A. EEG from littermates of three different genotypes ($\beta_3^{+/+}$, $\beta_3^{+/-}$, $\beta_3^{-/-}$), recorded simultaneously at 2 months of age. The top recording of $\beta_3^{+/+}$ is an example of a normal pattern. The bottom recording of $\beta_3^{-/-}$ displays abundant paroxysmal slow and sharp wave activity. The middle recording is of a $\beta_3^{+/-}$ mouse which displays a pattern intermediate between the EEG recordings of $\beta_3^{+/+}$ and $\beta_3^{-/-}$ mice. B. An example of a seizure recording of a $\beta_3^{-/-}$ mouse at 5 months of age, followed by suppression of electrocortical activity (figure modified from Homanics et al., 1997a).

may be similar in Angelman syndrome patients where we have heard anecdotally that carbamazepine and phenytoin make seizures worse, and that ethosuximide may be effective.

No previous study has established that alterations in $GABA_A$ receptors underlie any type of animal or human epilepsy. This work represents the first direct evidence that impaired GABAergic inhibitory neurotransmission via reduction in a specific $GABA_A$ receptor protein, in this case the $GABA_A$ receptor β_3 subunit, can produce epilepsy. It is important to point out that another two $GABA_A$ receptor subunit genes have been knocked out in mice, the subunits γ_2 (Gunther et al., 1995) and α_6 (Homanics et al., 1997b). Neither of these appear to have a seizure phenotype, although this has not been thoroughly investigated. Further study of the behavioural phenotype of these β_3 knockout mice will reveal whether these mice are a model for some other aspects of Angelman syndrome.

Acknowledgements: Supported by NIH grants NS 28772 to R.W. Olsen, Angelman Syndrome Foundation research grant to R.W. Olsen, T.M. DeLorey and B.A. Minassian, NS 21908 to A.V. Delgado-Escueta, and AA10422 to G.E. Homanics. We thank C. Ferguson and A. Asatourian for expert technical assistance. We are especially appreciative of the continued support and encouragement of L. Firestone.

References

Angelman H. (1965): 'Puppet' children: a report of three cases. *Develop. Med. Child. Neurol.* **7**, 681–688.

Banko, M.L., Allen, K., Dolina, S., Neumann, P.E. & Seyfried, T.N. (1995): Genomic imprinting and audiogenic seizures in mice. Abst. *Soc. Neurosci.* **21**, 2109.

Boyd, S.G., Harden, A. & Patton, M.A. (1988): The EEG in early diagnosis of the Angelman (Happy Puppet) syndrome. *Eur. J. Pediatr.* **147**, 508–513.

Buiting, K., Saitoh, S., Gross, S., Dittrich, B., Schwartz, S., Nicholls, R.D. & Horsthemke, B. (1995): Inherited microdeletions in the Angelman and Prader-Willi syndromes define an imprinting centre on human chromosome 15. *Nat. Genet.* **9**, 395–400.

Butler, M.G. (1990): Prader-Willi syndrome: current understanding of cure and diagnosis. *Am. J. Med. Genet.* **35**, 319–332.

Cattanach, B.M., Barr, J., Beechey, C.V., Bressler, J., Sutcliffe, J.S., Beaudet, A.L., Martin, J., Noebels, J.L. & Jones, J. (1996): A mouse model for Angelman syndrome. Abstr. 307 *Am. Soc. Hum. Genet.* **59** supp., A59.

Christian S.L., Robinson, W.P., Huang, B., Mutirangura, A., Line, M.R., Nakao, M., Surti, U., Chakravarti, A. & Ledbetter, D.H. (1995): Molecular characterization of two proximal deletion breakpoint regions in both Prader-Willi and Angelman syndrome patients. *Am. J. Hum. Genet.* **57**, 40–48.

Clayton-Smith, J. & Pembrey, M.E. (1992): Angelman syndrome *J. Med. Genet.* **29**, 412–415.

Davies, P.A., Hanna, M.C., Hales, T.G. & Kirkness, E.F. (1997): Insensitivity to anaesthetic agents conferred by a class of $GABA_A$ receptor subunit. *Nature* (in press).

Delgado-Escueta, A.V., Minassian, B., Philippart, M., Van Ness, P., DeLorey, T.M. & Olsen, R.W. (1996): Epileptic seizures in Angelman syndrome (AS). Abstr. Amer. Epilepsy Soc., *Epilepsia* **37** supp.5, #3.014.

DeLorey, T.M. & Olsen, R.W. (1992): γ-Aminobutyric acid$_A$ receptor structure and function. *J. Biol. Chem.* **267**, 16747–16750.

Frankel, W.N., Taylor, B.A., Noebels, J.L. & Lutz, C.M., (1994): Genetic epilepsy model derived from common inbred mouse strains. *Genetics* **138**, 481–489.

Greger, V., Knoll, J.H.M., Woolf, E., Glatt, K., Tyndale, R.F., DeLorey, T.M., Olsen, R.W., Tobin, A.J., Sikela, J.M., Nakatsu, Y., Brilliant, M.H., Whiting, P.J. & Lalande, M. (1995): The γ-aminobutyric acid receptor $\gamma 3$ subunit gene (GABRG3) is tightly linked to the $\alpha 5$ subunit gene (GABRA5) on human chromosome 15q11-q13 and is transcribed in the same orientation. *Genomics* **26**, 258–264.

Guerrini, R., DeLorey, T.M., Bonanni, P., Moncla, A., Dravet, C., Suisse, G., Livet, M.O., Bureau, M., Malzac, P., Genton, P., Thomas, P., Sartucci, F., Simi, P. & Serratosa, J.M. (1996): Cortical myoclonus of Angelman syndrome. *Ann. Neurol.* **40**, 39–48.

Gunther U., Benson, J., Benke, D., Fritschy, J.M., Reyes, G., Knoflach, F., Crestani, F., Aguzzi, A., Arigoni, M., Lang, Y., Bluethmann, H., Mohler, H. & Luscher, B. (1995): Benzodiazepine-insensitive mice generated by targeted disruption of the $\gamma 2$ subunit gene of $GABA_A$ receptors. *Proc. Natl. Acad. Sci.USA* **92**, 7749–7753.

Homanics, G.E., DeLorey, T.M., Firestone, L.L., Quinlan, J.J., Handforth, A., Harrison, N.L., Krasowski, M.D., Rick, C.E.M., Korpi, E.R., Makela, R., Brilliant, M., Hagiwara, N., Ferguson, C., Snyder, K. & Olsen, R.W. (1997a): Mice devoid of γ-aminobutyrate type A receptor $\beta 3$-subunit have epilepsy, cleft palate, and hypersensitive behavior. *Proc. Natl. Acad. Sci.USA* (in press).

Homanics, G.E., Ferguson, C., Quinlan, J.J., Daggett, J., Snyder, K., Lagenaur, C., Mi, X.-P., Grayson, D., Wang, X.-J. & Firestone, L.L. (1997b): Gene knockout of the alpha 6 subunit of the GABA type A receptor: Anatomical, biochemical and behavioral studies. *Mol. Pharmacol.* (in press).

Jay, V., Becker, L.E., Chan, F.W. & Perry, T.L. (1991): Puppet-like syndrome of Angelman: a pathologic and neurochemical study. *Neurology* **41**, 416–422.

Kishino, T., Lalande, M. & Wagstaff, J. (1997): UBE3A/E6-AP mutations cause Angelman syndrome. *Nat. Genet.* **15**, 70–73.

Knoll, J.H., Nicholls, R.D., Magenis, R.E., Graham, J.M., Lalande, M. & Latt, S.A. (1989): Angelman and Prader-Willi syndromes share a common chromosome 15 deletion but differ in parental origin of the deletion. *Am. J. Med..Genet.* **32**, 285–290.

Kuwano, A., Mutirangura, A., Dittrich, B., Buiting, K., Horsthemke, B., Saitoh, S., Niikawa, N., Ledbetter, SA., Greenberg, F., Chinault, A.C. & Ledbetter, D.H. (1992): Molecular dissection of the Prader-Willi/Angelman syndrome region (15q11-13) by YAC cloning and FISH analysis. *Hum. Mol. Genet.* **1**, 417–25.

Lalande, M., Minassian, B.A., DeLorey, T.M. & Olsen, R.W. (1997): Parental imprinting and Angelman syndrome. In: *Basic mechanisms of the epilepsies*, Delgado-Escueta, A.V., Wilson, W., Olsen, R.W. & Porter, R.J. (eds), (in press). New York: Lippincott-Raven Publishers.

Laurie, E.J., Wisden, W. & Seeburg, P.H. (1992): The distribution of thirteen $GABA_A$ receptor subunit mRNAs in the rat brain. III. Embryonic and postnatal development. *J. Neurosci.* **12**, 4151–4172.

Lyons, M.F., King, T.R., Yoichi, G., Gardner, J.M., Nakatsu, Y., Eicher, E.M. & Brilliant, M.H. (1992): Genetic and molecular analysis of recessive alleles at the pink-eyed dilution (*p*) locus of the mouse. *Proc. Natl. Acad. Sci.USA.* **89**, 6968–6972.

Malcolm, S., Clayton-Smith, J., Nichols M., Robb, S., Webb, T., Armour, J.A., Jeffreys, A.J. & Pembrey, M.E. (1991): Uniparental paternal disomy in Angelman's syndrome. *Lancet* **337**, 694–697.

Marsden, C.D., Hallett, M. & Fahan, S. (1982): The nosology and pathophysiology of myoclonus. In: *Movement disorders*, Marsden, C.D., Hallett, M. & Fahan S. (eds), pp. 196–249. London: Butterworths Scientific.

Matsumoto, A., Kumagai, T., Miura, K., Miyazaki, S., Hayakawa, C. & Yamanaka, T. (1992): Epilepsy in Angelman syndrome associated with chromosome 15q deletion. *Epilepsia* **33**, 1083–1090.

Matsuura, T., Sutcliffe, J.S., Fang, P., Galjaard, R.-J., Jiang, Y., Benton, C.S., Rommens, J.M. & Beaudet, A.L. (1997): *De novo* truncation mutations in E6-AP ubiquitin-protein ligase gene (UBE3A) in Angelman syndrome. *Nat. Genet.* **15**, 74–77.

Nakatsu, Y., Tyndale, R.F., DeLorey, T.M., Durham-Pierre, D., Gardner, J.M., McDanel, H.J., Nguyen, Q., Wagstaff, J., Lalande, M., Sikela, J.M., Olsen, R.W., Tobin, A.J. & Brilliant, M.H. (1993): A cluster of three $GABA_A$ receptor subunit genes is deleted in a neurological mutant of the mouse *p* locus. *Nature* **364**, 448–450.

Neumann, P.E. & Collins, R.L. (1992): Confirmation of the influence of a chromosome 7 locus on susceptibility to audiogenic seizures. *Mamm.Genome* **3**, 250–253.

Nicholls, R.D. (1993): Genomic imprinting and candidate genes in Prader-Willi and Angelman syndromes. *Curr. Opin. Genet. Dev.* **3**, 445–456.

Olsen, R.W., Wamsley, J.K., Lee, R. & Lomax, P. (1986): Benzodiazepine/barbiturate/GABA receptor-chloride ionophore complex in a genetic model for generalized epilepsy, In: *Basic mechanisms of the epilepsies*, Delgado-Escueta, A.V., Ward, A.A. & Woodbury, D.M. (eds), pp. 365–378. New York: Raven Press.

Olsen, R.W. (1991): Antiepileptic action of benzodiazepines, In: *Drugs for control of epilepsy: Actions on neuronal networks involved in seizures disorders,* Faingold, C.L. & Fromm, G.H., pp. 463–476. Boca Raton: CRC Press.

Olsen, R.W. & Avoli, M. (1997): GABA and epileptogenesis. *Epilepsia* (in press).

Olsen, R.W., DeLorey, T.M., Gordey, M, & Kang, M.H. (1997): Regulation of GABA receptor function and epilepsy. In: *Basic mechanisms of the epilepsies*, Delgado-Escueta, A.V., Wilson, W., Olsen, R.W. & Porter, R.J. (eds) (in press). New York: Lippincott-Raven Publishers.

Petersen, M.B., Brondum-Neilsen, K., Hansen, L.K. & Wulff, K. (1995): Clinical, cytogenetic, and molecular diagnosis of Angelman syndrome: estimated prevalence rate in a Danish county. *Am. J. Med. Genet.* **60**, 261–262.

Philippart, M., Minassian, B.A., Zhang, Q.W., DeLorey , T.M., Olsen R.W. & Delgado-Escueta, A.V. (1996): The diagnosis of older patients with Angelman syndrome. *Neurology* **46**, A447.

Sugimoto, T., Yasuhara, A., Ohta, T., Nishida, N., Saitoh, S., Hamabe, J. & Niikawa, N. (1992): Angelman syndrome in three siblings: characteristic epileptic seizures and EEG abnormalities. *Epilepsia* **33**, 1078–1082.

Viani, F., Romeo, A., Viri, M., Mastrangelo, M., Lalatta, F., Selicorni, A., Gobbi, G., Lanzi, G., Bettio, D., Briscioli, V., Di Segni, M., Parini, R. & Terzoli, G. (1995): Seizure and EEG pattern in Angelman's syndrome. *J. Child. Neurol.* **10**, 467–471.

Williams, C.A. & Frias, J.L. (1982): The Angelman ('Happy Puppet') syndrome. *Am. J. Med. Genet.* **11**, 453–460.

Williams, C.A., Angelman, H., Clayton-Smith, J., Driscoll, D.J., Hendrickson, J.E., Knoll, J.H.M., Magenis, R.E., Schinzel, A., Wagstaff, J., Whidden, E.M. & Zori, R.T. (1995a): Angelman syndrome: Consensus for diagnostic criteria. *Am. J. Med. Genet.* **56**, 237–238.

Williams, C.A., Zori, R.T., Hendrickson, J., Stalker, H., Marum, T., Whidden, E. & Driscoll, D.J. (1995b): Angelman syndrome. *Curr. Probl. Pediatr.* **25**, 216–231.

Wisden, W., Laurie, D.J., Monyer, H. & Seeburg, P.H. (1992): The distribution of 13 $GABA_A$ receptor subunit mRNAs in the rat brain. I. Telencephalon, diencephalon, mesencephalon. *J. Neurosci.* **12**, 1040–1062.

Yoon, C.H. & Les, E.P. (1957): Quivering, a new first chromosome mutation in mice. *J. Hered.* **48**, 176–180.

Afterword

Samuel F. Berkovic

This volume documents the remarkable recent progress achieved in the genetics of focal epilepsies. This chapter will briefly summarize some of the novel concepts and provide an update of new material available just before publication.

Chapters 1 and 2 provide a background to the evolution of the concept of inherited focal epilepsies. Many new clinical syndromes have been described and doubtless more will be elucidated in the next few years. The clinical advances in this field have coincided with remarkable advances in the technology and promise of molecular genetics to unravel the basic biology of epilepsies (Chapter 3).

Benign childhood epilepsy with centro-temporal spikes

Although the most common form of idiopathic partial epilepsy, and the longest recognized, the genetics of this syndrome remain very difficult to disentangle. As described in Chapters 4, 5 & 6 it now appears that the clinical syndrome, and its associated electro-encephalographic trait, are multifactorial in origin. Attempts to find linkage and the basic underlying genetic defect in this disorder have been frustrated by the clinical and genetic complexities of the condition. More work needs to be done on carefully characterized families with this disorder in order to clarify its relationship to the idiopathic generalized epilepsies and to elucidate the relationship of the characteristic centro-temporal (Rolandic) spike to this disorder and other related conditions including Landau-Kleffner syndrome, epilepsy with continuous spike wave in sleep, rolandic epilepsy with speech dyspraxia (Chapter 13) and acquired dysphasias of childhood. The problems in molecular genetic progress in such multifactorial diseases are beautifully illustrated by the difficulties of identifying loci in the El mouse, a model of multifactorial epilepsy (Chapter 23). A variety of internal and external environmental factors appear to confound the genetic analysis in addition to interactions between putative loci. The difficulty that these investigators are experiencing in mapping and identifying mouse genes, where many generations can be studied, and the animals easily manipulated, must surely be greatly amplified in attempts to study human epilepsies with complex inheritance.

Benign familial infantile convulsions (BFIC)

An entrenched concept in epileptology was that afebrile seizures in the first year of life almost invariably indicated a severe neurological condition. The identification of numerous individuals with benign forms of infantile epilepsy by Watanabe and other Japanese workers (Chapter 8) and the subsequent identification of the familial nature of many of these cases was a major milestone.

Linkage studies of these conditions have entered an extremely interesting phase. The clear cut identification of a gene on 19q (Chapter 7) was followed by finding of a second locus in the peri-centromeric region of chromosome 16 in some French families (Szeptowski et al 1997) and the same locus has recently been confirmed in a large Chinese family (Lee et al 1998). In BFIC families with the chromosome 16 locus, there may also be paroxysmal dyskinesias in addition to rare afebrile seizures in later life. The association of infantile convulsions and paroxysmal movement disorders is tantalising as the biological basis of both groups of disorders involves ion channels. It seems extremely likely that the combination of BFIC and paroxysmal movement disorders will be due to a specific ion channel defect. The age dependence of human idiopathic epilepsies has always been a puzzling phenomenon and may relate to age dependent expression of specific channel molecules. In this new syndrome we presume that the same channel shows dysfunction at different ages but in different cerebral structures causing two forms of paroxysmal movement disorder.

Autosomal dominant nocturnal frontal lobe epilepsy (ADNFLE)

The discovery of ADNFLE in 1994 set the scene for recognition of the other inherited partial epilepsies (Chapter 9). Numerous families with this disorder have now been recognized and the original limits of the syndrome are now under going reconsideration. Two large series from Italy have suggested that there maybe an increased frequency of parasomnias in such families (Oldani et al 1998; Plazzi et al 1998). These parasomnias are rather brief events that are presumed to be non-epileptic, but the nature of these attacks remains uncertain. In the initial description of ADNFLE there was a relatively homogenous pattern of seizures within families (although the severity varied) but the full extent of the clinical pattern of this disorder requires further study. Furthermore, the relationship of the numerous sporadic cases of non-lesional nocturnal frontal lobe epilepsy to ADNFLE also needs clarification.

Other dominant partial epilepsies

Familial temporal lobe epilepsy (Chapter 10) is now very well established and numerous families are known from around the world with the usual pattern of relatively mild TLE with mesial temporal symptomatology. In its typical form the condition is mild and there is no discernible change on the MRI scan. A current challenge is to clarify the relationship of these common families to the rarer families, seen in surgical centres where there maybe unequivocal hippocampal atrophy. This may simply reflect the manifestation of a more severe case with secondary damage but could also reflect an entirely different pathological process. Regrettably, there has not yet been progress in identifying linkage in the typical mesial form of familial temporal lobe epilepsy.

The important syndrome of partial epilepsy with auditory features (Chapter 11) appears to be distinct from the more common mesial form. Linkage to chromosome 10 has been established and hopefully further families will be identified together with identification of the mutant gene causing this particular syndrome. The limits of the syndrome of partial epilepsy with variable foci (Chapter 12) remain enigmatic. By its very nature of having variable clinical patterns the limits of this disorder are very difficult to define and it is also difficult to proscribe diagnostic criteria. However, a number of families with similarities to the original pedigree have been described in France (Chapter 14) and Canada and it is likely that it will be shown to be a relatively important disorder.

The status of autosomal dominant rolandic epilepsy with speech dyspraxia remains uncertain. We have yet to identify a second family and thus the one described (Chapter 13) may be an "private syndrome". The relationship of this disorder to the more common forms of rolandic epilepsy remains an enigma as it does to the genetic forms of speech dyspraxia which are now being increasingly recognized in speech disorder clinics. A particularly interesting group is families with occipital seizures. The benign occipital epilepsies probably show multifactorial inheritance but detailed studies have not yet been done. Occipital foci can certainly be seen in some members of families showing apparently dominant inheritance and the relationship to epileptic photosensitivity would also need to be further explored.

Genetics of other focal epilepsies

A large number of established and emerging genetic syndromes provide special insights into the overall problem of the inheritance of focal epilepsies. As described in Chapter 15, a number of symptomatic epilepsies can have focal seizures. In some cases recent technological advances have allowed identification of these disorders which otherwise might have been regarded as "idiopathic" or cryptogenic. A good example is of the familial migration disorders such as periventricular heterotopia and subcortical band heterotopia, which have only been properly studied since the advent of magnetic resonance imaging. The gene products of many of these disorders are known and future laboratory studies on the pathogenesis of these disorders may provide insights into the understanding of the commoner idiopathic familial focal epilepsies. The idea that some of them may be due to quite subtle migration defects clearly needs to be considered.

The best studied form of focal epilepsy, temporal lobe epilepsy with hippocampal sclerosis is not directly inherited but the particular relationship to febrile seizures is carefully dissected in Chapter 16. Uncovering the nature of the genes causing febrile seizures and of the factors that may lead to more prolonged convulsions ultimately causing focal temporal lobe epilepsy is clearly a major priority in the next few years.

The remarkable syndromes of reading epilepsy and hot water epilepsy (Chapters 17 and 18) provide a great deal of food for thought in consideration of focal activation of seizures. These syndromes with their apparent relationship to idiopathic generalized epilepsy and febrile seizures challenge the conventional boundaries between generalized and focal epilepsy. Understanding the molecular basis of these conditions, although relatively rare, should provide considerable neuro-biological insights into the epilepsies as a whole.

Molecular defects in idiopathic focal epilepsies

The partnership of molecular biology with clinical epileptology is a particularly powerful one. Molecular genetic studies cannot be successful without carefully characterized families containing well defined phenotypes and this requires clinical epileptology of the highest level. On the other hand the molecular biologist can provide truly remarkable insights into the mechanism of diseases and at a more simple level, validate the clinical concepts of the nature of a clinical disorder by showing the underlying biological defect.

This was spectacularly shown by the discovery of the first molecular defect in an idiopathic epilepsy in ADNFLE. The molecular discovery came within twelve months of the clinical elucidation of the syndrome and provided confirmation of its clinical and biological validity. The discovery of a nicotinic receptor defect was, to say the least, a surprise. Most would have predicted that epilepsies might be due to mutations resulting in increased glutamatergic or decreased GABAergic activity. However, the importance of the cholinergic system to sleep and sleep/wake cycles perhaps is the explanation why this system is involved in this particular form of focal epilepsy. The mechanism by which the widely expressed cholinergic defect causes focal epilepsy remains unclear and further laboratory studies should be directed at this important question.

It now appears that mutations in the a-4 subunit of the nictotinic acetylcholine receptor are an uncommon cause of ADNFLE. A second locus has recently been described on chromosome 15 where there is a cluster of three cholinergic subunits and it may well be that one of these will be a more common cause of this syndrome (Phillips et al 1988).

The prediction (Chapter 21) that the idiopathic epilepsies may well be part of the enlarging channelopathy family appears to be confirmed. As discussed in Chapter 21 genes for both ligand-gated and voltage-gated channels are excellent candidate epilepsy genes. In addition to the first defect described in ADNFLE of a ligand gated cholinergic channel, benign familial neonatal convulsions were shown to be due to potassium channel defects resulting in channel hypofunction in 1998 (Biervert et al 1998; Charlier et al 1998; Singh et al 1998). This syndrome has been classified as a generalized epilepsy although in some children focal seizures have been recorded. This raises the challenging question of the distinction between focal and generalized epilepsies at a physiological level. A fourth ion channel, the b1 subunit of the sodium channel, has recently been identified as the cause of generalized epilepsy with febrile seizures plus in a large Australian family (Wallace et al 1998).

Clearly, channels are the principle candidates for epilepsy genes. However, other potential genes should not be forgotten. The elegant studies described in Chapter 22 of homeobox genes resulting in developmental abnormalities, often with epilepsy are of great importance whilst mutations in the EMX2 gene caused the very severe syndrome of schizencephally it is possible that more subtle defects could lead to subtle dysplastic abnormalities causing an apparently "idiopathic" focal epilepsy.

Animal models

Advances in understanding animal models of epilepsy will surely have a major impact on the direction of research in human epilepsies. We are fortunate in having a number of single gene and multifactorial epilepsy models in animals that allow for genetic dissection as well as neurochemical and neuropharmacological study of these models. The El mouse and the epileptic mongolian gerbil are excellent models of multifactorial focal epilepsy traits (Chapters 23-24). The ability to study these from both the mapping point of view and directly from neurochemical studies is extremely powerful and hopefully there will be a coming together of these techniques together with electrophysiology to gain a deeper insight into the biology of these important models. Similar considerations apply to the genetically epilepsy-prone rats (GEPR; Chapter 25). Finally, transgenic models provide a method to study the effects of specific genetic abnormalities in targeted genes. The number of knock-out models that have seizures as an associated phenomenon is rising quickly (Chapter 26). Many of these are "symptomatic" as the mice have numerous other neurological defects and these models may well be more relevant to the symptomatic focal epilepsies of humans described in Chapter 16.

The tools are now available to rapidly advance knowledge in this area with a combination of clinical, molecular genetic and basic neuroscience studies in man and experimental animals. The fact that the concept of familial focal epilepsies has only been with us for about five years is remarkable given the amount of progress that has already occurred. It is hoped that the pace of discovery will accelerate further, leading ultimately to better methods for treatment and possibly prevention of this important class of epilepsies.

References

Biervert, C., Schroeder, B.C., Kubisch, C., Berkovic, S.F., Propping, P., Jentsch, T.J. & Steinlein, O.K. (1998): A potassium channel mutation in neonatal human epilepsy. *Science* **279**, 403–406.

Charlier, C., Singh, N.A., Ryan, S.G. *et al.* (1998): A pore mutation in a novel KQT-like potassium channel gene in an idiopathic epilepsy family. *Nat. Genet.* **18**, 53–55.

Lee, W.-L., Tay, A.H., Ong, H.-T., Goh, D.L., Monaco, A.P. & Szeptowski, P. (1998): Chinese family with infantile convulsions and paroxysmal dyskinesias (ICCA syndrome): linkage to chromosome 16p12-q12. *Am. J. Hum. Genet.* **63** (suppl), A296.

Oldani, A., Zucconi, M., Asselta, Modugno, M., Bonati, M.T., Dalpra, L. *et al.* (1998): Autosomal dominant nocturnal frontal lobe epilepsy: a video-polysomnographic and genetic apraiasal of 40 patients and delineation of the epileptic syndrome. *Brain* **121**, 205–223.

Phillips, H.A., Scheffer, I.E., Crossland, K.M., Bhatia, K.P., Fish, D.R., Marsden, C.D., Howell, S.J.L., Stephenson, J.B.P., Tolmie, J., Plazzi, G., Eeg Olofsson, O., Singh, R., Lopes-Cendes, I., Andermann, E., Andermannn, F., Berkovic, S.F. & Mulley, J.C. (1998): Autosomal dominant nocturnal frontal lobe epilepsy: genetic heterogeneity and evidence for a second locus at 15q24. *Am. J. Hum. Genet.* **63**, 1108–1116.

Plazzi, G., Provini, F., Tinuper, P. *et al.* (1998): Nocturnal frontal lobe epilepsy (NFLE): clinical videopolysomnographic and genetic data in 100 cases. *Neurology* **50** (suppl 4), A67.

Singh, N.A., Charlier, C., Stauffer, D. *et al.* (1998): A novel potassium channel gene, KCNQ2, is mutated in an inherited epilepsy of newborns. *Nat. Genet.* **18**, 25–29.

Szeptowski, P., Rochette, J., Berquin, P., Piussan, C., Lathrop, G.M. & Monaco, A.P. (1997): Familial infantile convulsions and paroxysmal choreoathetosis: a new neurological syndrome linked to the pericentromeric region of human chromosome 16. *Am. J. Hum. Genet.* **61**, 889–898.

Wallace, R.H., Wang, D.W., Singh, R., Scheffer, I.E., George, A.L., Phillips, H.A., Saar, K., Reis, A., Johnson, E.W., Sutherland, G.R., Berkovic, S.F. & Mulley, J.C. (1998): Febrile seizures and generalised epilepsy is associated with a mutation in the sodium channel subunit *SCN1B*. *Nat. Genet.* **19**, 366–370.

Author index

An, I.	115
Andermann, Eva	125
Arzimanoglou, Alexis	125
Barker-Cummings, Christie	95
Baulac, S.	115
Beaussart, Marc	3
Berkovic, Samuel F.	7, 85
Bertrand, D.	187
Boncinelli, Edoardo	215
Brice, A.	115
Brunelli, Silvia	215
Buisson, B.	187
Bulman, Dennis E.	149
Carrozzo, Romeo	125
Choy, Y.S.	43
Curtis, L.	187
Dailey, J.W.	251
Delgado-Escueta, Antonio	267
DeLorey, Timothy M.	267
Dobyns, William B.	125
Doose, Hermann	57
Dulac, Olivier	125
Echenne, Bernard	69
Eeg-Olofsson, Orvar	35
Faiella, Antonio	215
Gavaret, M.	115
Genton, P.	115
Gericke, C.A.	115
Guerrini, Renzo	115, 125, 215
Guipponi, Michel	69
Handforth, Adrian	267
Hirsch, E.	115
Homanics, Gregg E.	267
Jobe, P.C.	251
Ko, K.H.	251
Lee, Joseph H.	95
LeGuern, E.	115
Loiseau, Pierre	3
Lopez de Munain, A.	115
Malafosse, Alain	69
Marescaux, C.	115
Mayer, Thomas	159
McLachlan, Richard S.	149
Minassian, Berge A.	267
Mishra, P.K.	251
Neubauer, Bernd A.	57
Olsen, Richard W.	267
Omar, Asma	43
Ottman, Ruth	95
Pandolfo, Massimo	15
Peterson, Gary M.	239
Picard, F.	115
Poderyck, Michael J. i	229
Poza, J.J.	115
Ptáček, Louis J.	203
Ranta, Susanna	95
Reith, M.E.A.	251
Ribak, Charles E.	239
Roger, Joseph	3
Rudolf, G.	115
Satishchandra, P.	169
Scheffer, Ingrid E	7, 81, 103, 109
Sebastianelli, R.	115
Seyfried, Thomas N.	229
Shankar, S.K.	169
Sinha, Anindya	169
Steinlein, Ortrud K.	179
Stephani, Ulrich	57
Tan, C.T.	43
Thomas, P.	115
Todorova, Mariana	229
Toth, Miklos	261
Ulla, Gautam R.	169
Vigevano, Federico	69, 115
Watanabe, Kazuyoshi	73
Wolf, Peter	159
Wolff, M.	115

Subject index

A
a4-subunit gene (CHRNA4) 182–3
AD *see* autosomal dominance
ADNFLE *see* autosomal dominant nocturnal frontal lobe epilepsy
ADPEAF *see* autosomal dominant partial epilepsy with auditory features
ADRESD *see* autosomal dominant rolandic epilepsy with speech dyspraxia
Agyria-pachygyria 131, 223
Aicardi syndrome 125–7
Algeria 115
Alzheimer disease 192
Ammon's horn sclerosis 231, 244
Andersen's syndrome 206
Angelman syndrome 133, 267–72
AR *see* autosomal recessive
ataxia, episodic 203, 206, 210
auditory features *see* autosomal dominant partial epilepsy with auditory features
auditory hallucinations 115
Australia 27, 103, 169, 173, 179, 182
autosomal dominance 49, 50, 52, 54, 60–1
autosomal dominant familial temporal lobe epilepsy 155
autosomal dominant frontal lobe epilepsy 116
autosomal dominant nocturnal frontal lobe epilepsy 81–3, 179–85
    a4-subunit gene (CHRNA4) 182–3
    with auditory features 95–6
    benign familial infantile convulsions 70, 71
    benign familial neonatal convulsions 180
    channelopathies 207, 209, 210
    clinical features 81–2
    dominant partial epilepsy 115, 117, 119, 120
    EEG studies 82, 180–1, 183

    familial partial epilepsy 25, 27
    familial partial epilepsy with variable foci 103, 106
    future directions 83
    genetic studies 83, 181
    misdiagnosis and differential diagnosis 82–3
    neuroimaging 82
    neuronal nicotinic acetylcholine receptor 181–2, 192, 193, 194, 196
    Ser248Phe mutation 183–5
autosomal dominant occipital lobe epilepsy 116
autosomal dominant partial epilepsy 120
autosomal dominant partial epilepsy with auditory features 95–101
    clinical description 97–8
    linkage analysis 95–9
    mutation identification 100–1
    statistical power estimation to replicate linkage 100
autosomal dominant partial epilepsy with auditory hallucinations 115
autosomal dominant partial epilepsy with variable foci 115, 116, 117, 120
autosomal dominant rolandic epilepsy with speech dyspraxia 109–13
    cognitive function 110–11
    epileptology 109–10
    genetic analysis 111
    hallmark 113
    molecular genetic studies 112
    relationship to familial speech disorders 112
    relationship to other epilepsy-speech disorders 111–12
    speech and language 111
autosomal recessive 50, 52, 54

B
bathing epilepsy *see* hot-water epilepsy

BCECTS *see* benign childhood epilepsy with centro-temporal spikes
Becker's myotonia congenita   208
benign childhood epilepsy with centro-temporal spikes   3, 24, 35–9, 43–55
    association with other epilepsies   54
    clinical symptoms   36
    data analysis   45–6
    EEG   36, 47–8
    exclusion criteria   44–5
    family history   46–7
    genetic studies   35–8
    inclusion criteria   44
    other clinical data   38
    pedigree analysis   49–53
    statistical analysis   53–4
    see also benign rolandic epilepsy
benign childhood epilepsy with rolandic spikes   35
benign childhood focal epilepsy   35
benign familial infantile convulsions   69–71
benign familial neonatal convulsions   69, 70, 71, 180, 181, 183
benign focal neonatal convulsions   25, 26
benign infantile myoclonic epilepsy   69
benign neonatal convulsions   69
benign partial epilepsy with centro-temporal spikes   35
benign partial epilepsy in infancy and early childhood   73–8
    with complex partial seizures   73–5, 76, 77, 78
    genetic background   77
    related syndromes and nosological problems   77–8
    with secondarily generalized seizures   73, 75–6, 77, 78
    study based on clinical criteria   76–7
benign rolandic epilepsy   3–5, 35, 109, 110, 111, 138, 154
bilateral periventricular nodular heterotopia   131–3
brainstem   252–5

C

CAG expansion   17, 18
calcium calmodulin kinase IIa deficient mice   263
calcium channel disorders   208
Canada   169, 269
cardiac muscle disease   206
cell lines collection   22
centro-temporal spikes   35
    see also benign childhood epilepsy
Chamarro Indians   152
channelopathies: ion channels and paroxysmal disorders   203–10
    cardiac muscle disease   206
    epilepsy   206
    episodic ataxia   206
    genetics of paroxysmal dyskinesias   209–10
    ion channels as molecular basis of paroxysmal disorders   208–9
    migraine headaches   206
    paroxysmal dyskinesias   204–5
    pathophysiology   208
    periodic paralyses/non-dystrophic myotonias   205–6
    similarities among paroxysmal disorders   207–8
    startle disease   206
childhood epilepsy *see* benign
chloride channel disorders   208
classical idiopathic focal epilepsy   120
cloning and analysis of candidate genes   25–6
Commission on Classification and Terminology of International League Against Epilepsy   109, 111
computed tomography   82
    autosomal dominant rolandic epilepsy with speech dyspraxia   110
    dominant partial epilepsy   118
    familial partial epilepsy with variable foci   105
    hot-water epilepsy   171
    reading epilepsy   163
continuous spike and wave during slow wave sleep   109, 112
convulsions   25, 26, 69–71, 180, 181, 183
cortical dysgenesis   223–4
cryptogenic focal epilepsy   120
cryptogenic partial epilepsy   120
CSWS *see* continuous spike and wave during slow wave sleep

D

dentate gyrus   242–6
DNA samples   22
dominant extra-frontal partial epilepsy   118
dominant frontal lobe epilepsy   119
dominant partial epilepsy   115–20
    clinical homogeneity   118–19
    general features   117–18
    genetics   119–20
    nosological position   120
    seizure localization classification   119
dynamic mutations   18–19
dyskinesias   206–10
dysplasia, focal cortical   223, 224

E

early infantile epileptic encephalopathy	126
Emx gene	220–2
episodic ataxia	203, 206, 210
Europe	5, 115
EXCLUDE analysis	105–6

F

familial epilepsy *see* autosomal dominant	
familial frontal lobe epilepsy	118
familial neonatal convulsions, benign	69, 70, 180
familial paroxysmal dyskinesia	206–7, 208
familial partial epilepsy	15–28
cloning and analysis of candidate genes	25–6
genetic research strategies	19–24
DNA samples and cell lines collection	22
families identification, clinical and EEG studies	20–1
genotyping strategies	22
linkage analysis for mendelian traits	22–3
linkage analysis when polygenic inheritance suspected	24
selection criteria for linkage studies	21
mendelian traits, complexity of	16–19
dynamic mutations	18–19
genetic heterogeneity	17
variable expressivity, pleiotropy and reduced penetrance	18
variable phenotypic effect of different mutations in same gene	17–18
mendelian versus polygenic inheritance	16
molecular genetic research in idiopathic epilepsy	26–7
multifactoriality	16
familial partial epilepsy with variable foci	103–7
differentiation from other familial partial epilepsies	106
EEG features	104–5
epileptology	103–4
genetic analysis	105–7
familial photosensitive occipital lobe epilepsy	117
familial temporal lobe epilepsy	85–92, 103, 115, 116, 117, 119, 120
clinical epileptology	86–90
EEG and neuroimaging	90
evolution and severity	90
genetic analysis	91
families identification	20–1
febrile convulsions genetics	149–54
focal cortical dysplasia	223, 224
focal epilepsy	120
idiopathic	3, 5
focal spikes and sharp waves	57, 58–9, 63, 64
genetics	59–63
occipital and frontal	59
forebrain	252–5
FPEVF *see* familial partial epilepsy with variable foci	
fragile X syndrome	138–9
France	4, 5, 69, 70, 81, 115, 254
frontal lobe epilepsy	115, 207
autosomal dominant	116
dominant	119
familial	118
idiopathic	120
see also autosomal dominant nocturnal	
FTLE *see* familial temporal lobe epilepsy	

G

GABA	134–6
GABAa receptor b3 subunit knockout mouse	267–72
Gaucher disease type III	140
gene mapping for benign infantile familial convulsions	69–71
generalized epilepsy, idopathic	15, 16, 20, 25, 26, 161, 164
generalized tonic/clonic seizures	251–8
genetic heterogeneity	17
genotyping strategies	22
GEPRs	253, 255–7
Germany	59, 64, 69, 81, 115
glutamate receptor B subunit editing deficiency	264
gray matter heterotopia	223, 224
Guam	152

H

hemimegalencephaly	223
hereditary hyperekplexia (startle disease)	206, 209
heterotopia	127–33
hippocampal gliosis	231
hippocampal sclerosis	231
homeobox genes in developing brain	215–24
areas and boundaries in forebrain	219–20
clues from analysis of mutants	222–3
cortical dysgenesis and epilepsies	223–4
Emx genes in developing cerebral cortex	220–2
expression of four genes in E10 mouse embryos	217–18
expression of Otx2	218–19, 220–2
regulatory genes in developing CNS	216
HOMOG program	23
hot-water epilepsy	169–75

clinical features	169–71	LINKAGE computer package	98, 154
genetics	172–5	lissencephaly and subcortical band heterotopia	127–31
pathophysiology	171–2	localization-related epilepsy, idiopathic	166
human idiopathic epilepsy	229	long-QT syndrome	203, 206, 210
human partial epilepsy	230		

M

Huntington's disease	112	magnetic resonance imaging	222, 224, 270
'hyperthermic kindling'	171–2	autosomal dominant nocturnal frontal lobe epilepsy	82

I

ICEES see International Classification of Epilepsies and Epileptic Syndromes		autosomal dominant rolandic epilepsy with speech dyspraxia	110
idiopathic epilepsy	179, 187, 210, 229, 235	dominant partial epilepsy	118
molecular genetic research	26–7	familial partial epilepsy	20
idiopathic focal epilepsy	3, 5	familial partial epilepsy with variable foci	105
idiopathic frontal lobe epilepsy	120	familial temporal lobe epilepsy	90
idiopathic generalized epilepsy	15, 16, 20, 25, 26, 161, 164	hot-water epilepsy	171
		partial symptomatic epilepsy	126, 129, 131, 137
idiopathic localization-related epilepsy	166	reading epilepsy	162, 163
idiopathic partial epilepsy	70	temporal lobe epilepsy and febrile convulsions	150
IGE see idiopathic generalized epilepsy		Malaysia	43–4
ILAE see International League Against Epilepsy		malformation syndromes with lissencephaly and subcortical band heterotopia	130–1
India	169, 171, 172, 173, 174	mendelian traits	16–19, 22–3
infantile convulsions	69–71	MERRF see myoclonus epilepsy with ragged red fibre syndrome	
infantile epilepsy see benign partial epilepsy in infancy and early childhood		migraine	203, 206, 207, 210
inositol triphosphate receptor deficient mice	264	Miller-Dieker syndrome with isolated lissencephaly sequence	130–1
Institutional Review Board	22	MLINK computer program	154
insulin-dependent diabetes mellitus	24	molecular genetic research in idiopathic epilepsy	26–7
International Classification of Epilepsies and Epileptic Syndromes	15, 16, 20, 35, 69, 73	mouse epilepsy models	229
International League Against Epilepsy	12, 15, 20, 57, 58, 98, 164	multifactorial epilepsy model	16, 229–35
		genetic studies	233–5
Italy	59, 69, 70, 81, 115	mapping epilepsy genes in man and mouse	235

J

Japan	59, 69, 77, 152, 169, 172, 232	neurochemical studies	232–3
jerky mice	263	neuropathology	231–2
juvenile myoclonic epilepsy	26, 70, 159, 162, 164, 165, 166	seizure phenotype and developmental expression	229–31
		mutation S248F: loss of function	192–3

K

'kindling'	171–2	myoclonic epilepsy, benign infantile	69
		myoclonus epilepsy with ragged red fibre syndrome	12

L

Lafora disease	140	myotonias	203, 205–6, 208
Landau-Kleffner syndrome	109, 111–12	myotonic dystrophy	112

N

Lennox-Gastaut syndrome	62, 129, 137, 269		
ligand-gated channel disorders	209	National Tuberous Sclerosis Association	136
linkage analysis	21	neonatal convulsions	
autosomal dominant partial epilepsy with auditory features	95–7, 98–9, 100	benign familial	69, 70, 71, 180, 181, 183
		benign focal	25, 26
for mendelian traits	22–3	Netherlands	129
when polygenic inheritance suspected	24	neurofibromatosis type 1	139–40

neuronal nicotinic acetylcholine receptor 181–2, 187–96
    human brain 191–2
    mutation S248F: loss of function 192–3
    structure and function 189–90
neuropeptide Y 264
New Zealand 169
nocturnal epilepsy see autosomal dominant
nocturnal paroxysmal dystonia 83
non-dystrophic myotonias 203, 205–6
non-kinesigenic dyskinesia 209
non-kinesigenic paroxysmal dyskinesia 210
North America 4, 81
    see also Canada; United States
Norway 27, 81, 185

N

occipital lobe epilepsy
    autosomal dominant 116
    familial photosensitive 117
Otx gene 218–22

P

paramyotonia congenita 205, 208, 210
paroxysmal choreoathetosis 209–10
paroxysmal dyskinesia 204–5, 208
    familial 206–7, 208
    non-kinesigenic 210
paroxysmal dystonia 83
paroxysmal hypnogenic dyskinesias 207
paroxysmal kinesigenic dyskinesias 207
paroxysmal non-kinesigenic dyskinesia 207, 209
partial epilepsy 7–12, 27, 155, 230
    autosomal dominant 120
    cryptogenic 120
    dominant extra-frontal 118
    genetic epilepsy syndromes 11–12
    genetic heterogeneity 10
    idiopathic 70
    mechanisms of familial partial epilepsy 7–9
    see also benign; dominant; familial
partial (focal) seizures and generalized tonic/clonic
    seizures 251–8
    brainstem and forebrain seizure circuitry 252–3
    brainstem seizure cicuitry ignition by forebrain
    seizures 254
    brainstem seizure predisposition in GEPRs 253
    forebrain seizure circuitry ignition by brainstem
    seizures 254
    forebrain seizure predisposition and brainste
    seizures 253–4
    forebrain seizure predisposition in GEPRs 253
    forebrain to brainstem seizure thresholds in
    GEPRs, relationship of 253
    GEPR–9s as model for secondary generalization
    of human partial seizures 255–7
    seizure mechanisms initiating interactions
    between forebrain and brainstem circuitry 254–5
partial symptomatic epilepsy 125–40
    Aicardi syndrome 125–7
    Angelman syndrome 133
    bilateral periventricular nodular heterotopia 131–3
    classical lissencephaly and subcortical band
    heterotopia (agyria-pachygyria-band spectrum) 127–30
    epilepsy 133–6
    fragile X syndrome 138–9
    neurofibromatosis type 1 139–40
    other genetic disorders 140
    tuberous sclerosis 136–8
periodic paralyses 203, 205–6, 208, 210
photosensitive occipital lobe epilepsy, familial 117
pleiotropy 18
polygenic inheritance 24
polymicrogyria 223
positron emission tomography 20, 82
    familial temporal lobe epilepsy 90
    neuronal nicotinic acetylcholine receptor 191
    reading epilepsy 164
potassium channel disorders 208–9
Prader-Willi syndrome 270
pseudo Lennox syndrome 62

R

Ramer-Lin syndrome 130
reading epilepsy 159–66
    case reports 162–3
    clinical features 160
    EEG 160–1
reduced penetrance 18
reflex or sensory epilepsy 169, 207
rolandic epilepsy 57–64, 166
    focal spikes and sharp waves 58–9
    genetics of focal spikes and sharp waves 59–61
    molecular genetic findings 63–4
    non-hereditary 61
    prevalence and EEG trait 59
    symptomatology in children with focal spikes and sharp
    waves of genetic origin 62–3
    see also autosomal dominant rolandic epilepsy
    with speech dyspraxia; benign

S

schizencephaly 223, 224

Scotland	81	transgenic animal models of epilepsy	261–72
Ser248Phe mutation	183–5	heterogeneity of phenotype	265–6
serotonin2C (5-HT2c) receptor deficient mice	262	single gene mutations leading to seizures in mice	261–5
Sherman's paradox	19	calcium calmodulin kinase IIa deficient mice	263
Singapore	69, 77	glutamate receptor B subunit editing deficiency	264
single gene mutations leading to seizures in mice	261–5	inositol triphosphate receptor deficient mice	264
single photon emission computed tomography	82, 105, 164	jerky mice	263
SLINK computer program	21, 100	neuropeptide Y	264
sodium channel disorders	208	serotonin2C (5-HT2c) receptor deficient mice	262
Spain	115	synapsin I and II mutant mice	263
SPECT *see* single photon emission computed tomography		symptomatic epilepsy	264–5
speech dyspraxia *see* autosomal dominant rolandic epilepsy with speech dyspraxia		tuberous sclerosis	17, 18, 136–8
		twin studies	
spontaneous non-reflex epilepsy	170	dizygotic	19, 36, 173
startle disease	203, 206, 210	familial temporal lobe epilepsy	85, 86
subcortical band heterotopia	127–9	monozygotic	19, 36, 60, 173
subcortical epilepsy	207	reading epilepsy	161
supernumeray GABAergic neurons and hippocampus disinhibition	239–48	temporal lobe epilepsy and febrile convulsions	152
		U	
Ammon's horn	244	United Kingdom	112, 169
animals	240–1	United States	69, 169, 171, 232, 269
cell counting	242	Unverricht-Lundborg disease	70
dentate gyrus	242–6	**V**	
hippocampal disinhibition hypothesis	247–8	variable expressivity	18
histology	241	variable foci	115, 116, 117, 120
statistics	242	*see also* familial partial epilepsy with variable foci	
synaptic interactions	242	variable phenotypic effect of different mutations in same gene	17–18
Sweden	38, 59, 69, 81	**W**	
symptomatic epilepsy	187, 235, 264–5	water-immersion epilepsy *see* hot-water epilepsy	
generalized	137	West syndrome	137
see also partial		Worster-Drought syndrome	112
synapsin I and II mutant mice	263	**X**	
T		X-linked lissencephaly with subcortical band heterotopia	131
temporal lobe epilepsy	27, 149–51, 154–6		
autosomal dominant familial	155		
see also familial			
Thomsen's myotonia congenita	208		